ADVANCE PRAISE FOR

Fire Burning in My Head

This extraordinary book, written by an extraordinary person, transforms the reader into a new and more dignified person. It shows how the forces of madness may be harnessed to serve creative purposes. Ho is a brilliant storyteller who entertains the reader with adventurous tales of his life as a spiritual journey. He is also a dialectical thinker who has succeeded in linking insights derived from his personal self-study with the science of mental illness versus health in diverse cultures.
—Evelin G. Lindner, Founding President, Human Dignity and Humiliation Studies

This book is the author's remarkable journey into the borderlands of madness and ordinary life. The reader is deeply enlightened by his power of integrating Oriental and Occidental perspectives within one inquisitive mind.
—Jaan Valsiner, Niels Bohr Professor of Cultural Psychology, Aalborg University

Ho is a relentless bridge-builder: His Chinese and Western selves are literal bridges between East and West, psychiatry and spirituality, poetry and prose, and internal struggle and cultural evolution.
—Rev. Dr. Tom Owen-Towle, Unitarian Universalist Minister

David Ho shows me that hypomania and hypercreativity form a happy couple that is powerful enough to open the gateway to East-West understanding. The account of his unusual mood elevations prompts us to realize that creativity and abnormality are rather mutually inclusive. Moreover, the over application of psychiatric diagnoses has the undesirable effect of viewing deviant experiences as dysfunctional and counterproductive.
—Hubert Hermans, Emeritus Professor, Creator of Dialogical Self Theory

Fire Burning in My Head

This book is part of Peter Lang Regional Studies list.
Every volume is peer reviewed and meets
the highest quality standards for content and production.

PETER LANG
New York • Berlin • Brussels • Lausanne • Oxford

David Y. F. Ho

Fire Burning in My Head

A Psychologist's Self-Study Reveals
How Madness May Enrich Your Life
in Diverse Cultures

PETER LANG
New York • Berlin • Brussels • Lausanne • Oxford

Library of Congress Cataloging-in-Publication Control Number: 2022052294

Bibliographic information published by **Die Deutsche Nationalbibliothek**.
Die Deutsche Nationalbibliothek lists this publication in the "Deutsche
Nationalbibliografie"; detailed bibliographic data are available
on the Internet at http://dnb.d-nb.de/.

ISBN 978-1-4331-9996-7 (paperback)
ISBN 978-1-63667-046-1 (ebook pdf)
ISBN 978-1-63667-047-8 (epub)
DOI 10.3726/b20464

© 2023 Peter Lang Publishing, Inc., New York
80 Broad Street, 5th floor, New York, NY 10004
www.peterlang.com

All rights reserved.
Reprint or reproduction, even partially, in all forms such as microfilm,
xerography, microfiche, microcard, and offset strictly prohibited.

To my daughters, Simin and Gigi, who have inspired me to be a better parent and brought forth the joys of fatherhood in my life.

If abnormality is so rich in its manifestations, surely normality should be no less colorful.

Contents

	Foreword	xv
	Preface	xix
Part I.	**Discoveries from a Self-Study of Madness**	
1.	Tales from My Two Worlds	3
	Psychohistory: Personal Experiences Reflect Historical Social Reality	4
	Family Background: Continuities and Departures from Tradition	7
	From Childhood to Grandparenthood	11
	The Age of Turbulence: Adolescence and Early Adulthood	17
	Reverse Culture Shock in an Anachronistic University	30
	The Golden Age of My Life	33
	From Marginality to World Citizenship: The Will to Master	38
	My Spiritual Journey Is Incomplete	44
2.	Episodes of Madness: All of Exuberance, None of Depression	47
	Glimpses into the Mystical-Transcendental	49
	Loneliness and Anguish amid Exuberance	56

	Aesthetic Sensibilities: Music, Art, Creative Writing	63
	Extraordinary Experiences: Audacity or the Courage-to-Be?	66
	The Empty Mind: Gone with Repression and Overcontrol	69
	Caught between the Challenges and Rewards of Hypomania	71
	A Hypomanic Episode in China	76
	A Living Buddha in a Schizophrenic City	84
	Later Hypomanic Episodes in America	86
	A Summation: Unanswered Questions	87

3. Madness Has Enriched My Life — 91
   A Self-Study of Unipolar Mania and Hypomania — 92
   On Being Strange in Normality as in Madness — 95
   Sequential Learning and Coping: Practical Suggestions — 97
   Body-Mind-Spirit Interconnectedness — 102
   Dialogic Action Therapy — 105
   Dynamic Relaxation and Meditation — 107
   Coping with Depression — 113
   Life as a Playful Journey: Intercultural Encounters — 120

4. From Psychiatry to Spirituality — 129
   An Early Case Study of and by My Own Self — 130
   Observing the Workings of the Mind — 137
   Spiritual Fulfillment Versus Spiritual Emptiness: A Dynamic Process — 140
   Relational and Ecumenical Spirituality — 147
   Witnessing My Ineptitude and Decline: Acceptance — 150

5. Glimpses of Enlightenment in the Midst of Madness — 155
   Fleeting Experiences of Enlightenment — 155
   Dialectics between Spirituality and Madness — 159
   In Love with Madness — 163
   Poetry and Spirituality Drive Each Other — 167

6. In Search of Transcultural Spirituality-in-Communion — 171
   Insights from the East: Psychological Decentering — 172
   Selflessness in Philosophical Daoism and Buddhism — 174
   Ambivalence Toward Christianity — 180
   Spirituality-in-Communion or Spirituality-in-Isolation? — 184

	Quakers and Unitarian Universalists	185
	A Religious Experience	188
7.	Epilogue: I'm Getting There	191
	Back to the Original Question	192
	Sharing My Karma with Fellow Travelers	193
	The Art of Loving for All Seasons	194

Part II.	Transcending the Clash of Opposites	
	Thematic Grouping of Chapters	197
	Rejecting the Pseudodichotomy Between Nomothetic and Ideographic Studies	198

Thematic Group 1. Normality Versus Abnormality   201

8	Madness as Creative Energy: Self-Observations	203
	A Self-Diagnosis	204
	Diagnostic Issues	208
	The Place of Madness in Creativity	210
	The High Costs of Cognitive Superefficiency	211
	Conclusion	213
9.	Psychiatric Diagnosis and Its Pitfalls	219
	Liberation from the *Diagnostic and Statistical Manual of Mental Disorders*	219
	Cultural Relativism and the Definition of Abnormality	220
	Dialectical Tension between the Particular and the Universal	222
	Is Your Child Suffering from ADHD?	226
	Concluding Remarks	229
10.	Psychopathology of Religious Luminaries	231
	Religiosity and Madness	232
	George Fox and Quakerism: The Tortuous Road of a Religious Movement	234
	Duality of Good and Evil	236
	Concluding Thoughts	238

Thematic Group 2. Individual Versus Collective Madness

11.	Societal Mental Health Crises in America and China	241
	The Mental Health Crisis in America	242
	Psychology and Psychiatry in China	247
	Concluding Thoughts	250
12.	Values Underlying Mental Health Practice	253
	The Limitations of Psychologism	254
	Self-Reliance Rooted in Individualism	255
	Crisis in Values	256
	Loneliness Is Lethal	258
	Reallocate Resources: Put Prevention First	259
	Concluding Thoughts	261
13.	The Trump Phenomenon and the Politics of an Unholy Alliance	263
	Trump and the Trump Phenomenon	263
	The Unholy Alliance	266
	Reportage: Personal Encounters with Evangelicals	269
	Absolutism and the Closing of the Mind	271
	The Price to Be Paid: A Surrender of Self-Ownership	272
	Will America Become a Theocracy?	273
	Concluding Thoughts	274

Thematic Group 3. Eastern Versus Western Culture — 275

14.	Two Ways of Life: Chinese and American	277
	Individualism and Collectivism: A Dialectical Approach	278
	Empirical Evidence: Dubious Comparisons between Americans and Chinese	284
	Two Ways of Life	287
	Concluding Thoughts	287
15.	Growing Up in the People's Republic of China: Culture, Ideology, and Policy	291
	Continuities and Departures from Tradition	292
	Socioeconomic and Psychological Costs of the One-Child Policy	295
	Conclusion	298

16.	The Oedipal Myth and Family Pathology in Literature	299
	Reinterpreting the Oedipal Myth	300
	Patricide Versus Filicide and Violence Toward Children	301
	Pathogenic Demands of Culture	309
	The Perils of Challenging Authority	310
	Concluding Thoughts	312

Thematic Group 4. Spirituality Versus Spiritual Emptiness — 313

17.	Transforming Madness for Dignified Existence	315
	Construct Explication	317
	Are Madness and Violence Necessarily Connected?	319
	Madness-in-Dignity and Dignity-in-Madness	320
	Summary and Conclusions	322
18.	Spirituality and Spiritual Emptiness: Toward Transcultural Applicability	325
	The Multidimensional Evaluations of Spirituality (MES)	326
	Dialectics of Fulfillment and Emptiness	328
	Strategies for Transcultural Applicability	328
	Dimensions of the MES	331
	Discussion	340

Appendix A. Multidimensional Evaluation of Spirituality (MES) — 343
- Reflectiveness-Decentering Versus Dogmatism-Egocentricity — 344
- Heightened Sensibilities Versus Psychic Numbing/Turmoil — 347
- Acceptance Versus Denial — 351
- Humility Versus Arrogance — 353
- Existential Quest Versus Hedonistic-Materialistic Pursuits — 357
- Transcendence Versus Self-Encapsulation — 357
- Self-Actualization Versus Alienation — 358

Appendix B. Strategies of Coping — 361
- Forbearance Versus Intolerance — 362
- Forgiveness Versus Vengefulness — 365
- Hope Versus Despair — 370
- Meaning Reconstruction Versus Entrenchment — 375

Appendix C. Highlights of 22 Episodes of Madness, Diaries, and a Free Association   379

Appendix D. Expressive Dance to Music: A Royal Road to Holistic Health (Explanatory Notes)   395

Appendix E. The Undiscovered Illness: The Opposite of Depression (Excerpts from Scientific American, March 2019, reproduced here with permission)   401

References   409

Index   415

Foreword

David Ho's latest offering is truly an extraordinary book. The author, himself a clinical psychologist, undertakes a self-study of his own "madness." He describes his episodes of mania and hypomania in great detail. His firsthand experiences lead to insights about spirituality and growth, both personal and professional.

Audacious assertions are made throughout the book. Suffice to select a few that stir up the mind as does an earthquake high on the Richter magnitude shake the ground. First, madness provides the creative energy that *may*, on balance, enrich rather than damage a person's life. Second, the psychiatric establishment, accustomed to the deficit model of thinking in terms of psychopathology, has largely failed to acknowledge the potentially positive or creative aspects of madness. Third, the *Diagnostic and Statistical Manual of Mental Disorders*, the "bible of psychiatric diagnosis," is largely responsible for the closing of minds in psychiatry. Fourth, the author has had only manic or hypomanic episodes and no depression of clinical severity; thus, to label such a person as a patient suffering from a bipolar mood disorder would lead to a "conceptual-linguistic conundrum."

The author has articulated his defense for these assertions logically and forcefully, backed by evidence derived from empirical research as well as his intensive self-study. He has also exercised caution against making excessive claims. He reminds himself, "Don't overgeneralize."

The book consists of two parts. Ho's encounters with madness described in Part I have enabled him to gain firsthand experiences of abnormality, a valuable resource for probing into the patient's mind. In his case, he is both doctor and patient. Taking advantage of his specialty, he can do a personal case study of abnormality.

Case studies may be invaluable for advancing knowledge. However, they have to be interpreted in the context of academic discourse and controversies. Accordingly, in Part II, Ho writes on the nature of abnormality, the current status of mental health in America and China, issues related to diagnosis and psychopathology, and research on the creative potentials of madness for spiritual development.

The reader will soon note that the style of writing differs largely between the two parts: writing more from the heart as a good storyteller in the first, and articulating arguments backed by reasoning and evidence in the second.

To integrate the two parts of the book has been a most demanding task, which requires an in-depth knowledge of diverse disciplines, psychiatry, comparative religion, and East-West learning. Being thoroughly bicultural, Ho has an immense advantage in bringing Buddhist, Daoist, and Christian values and beliefs to advance his own ideas about spiritual fulfillment. In the end, he points to novel avenues for answering profound questions about the place of madness in human life.

The book's major achievement is the integration of several central ideas, madness as creative energy, human dignity, self-transformation, and enlightenment into a coherent theme. Ho achieves this integration by weaving these ideas together to tell the story of his journey in quest of new directions to lead a dignified life—in short, spiritual fulfillment.

This book reminds me of Kay Jamison's *Touched with Fire*, a best-selling account of her own bipolar mood disorder. David Ho, also a professor of clinical psychology, writes about his own experiences of mood disturbances. But then the similarity ends there. Ho's mood disorder is unipolar. He says he has had "22 episodes of exuberance, none of depression"! This is truly an exceptionally psychiatric condition, replete with imbalances such as hyperactivity coexisting with mental or physical fatigue, tranquility punctuated by inner turmoil, and ecstasy intermingling with anguish. During episodes, Ho's mind alternated between bursts of creativity and cognitive disturbances such as extreme forgetfulness or confusion.

What I find most fascinating is Ho's rich description of his extraordinary experiences. During fleeting moments of enlightenment, he glimpses into mystical magnanimity. He feels connected with all of humanity, at home in society, nature, and the cosmos. Gone are the prejudices, obsessions, and fixations of his "normal" life. Now, life is sweet, meaningful, and fulfilling.

What are some of these extraordinary experiences that exemplify the author's mystical magnanimity? Visualizing himself being nailed on a cross and feeling intense pathos for the sufferings of humankind; experiencing androgyny, the yin and the yang, united in one body; a cosmic experience of visualizing himself lying in a coffin about to be interred, hearing nails being pounded as the cover of the coffin closes, followed by absolute darkness, silence, and nothingness—without any fear at all! These are just a few examples of many.

Ho is a brilliant storyteller. He entertains the reader with adventurous tales of his life as a spiritual journey. The one I find most fascinating is named A Living Buddha in a Schizophrenic City. The city in question is Macao because it is characterized by a schizophrenic split between its casino district and the rest. Once our storyteller ventured into a "casino nightclub." Typically, the manual staff, many of whom are Buddhists, come from the poorest countries in Southeast Asia. They are treated like enslaved workers. With a state of mind filled with compassion, our storyteller told a few of these Buddhist workers that he was a Living Buddha, there to make an appearance for their consolation. They seemed to have no trouble believing what he told them. Our storyteller says, "Looking back at my adventure now, I can still feel the same compassion I felt then."

Written in an accessible style, the book will appeal to readers from diverse backgrounds, especially those interested in the interface between psychology and spirituality, comparative religion, or bicultural development. It is particularly useful not only to mental health professionals but also to readers who have had experiences similar to those of the author. I have tremendously enjoyed the passion and the sparking prose with which the book is written.

Evelin Gerda Lindner
Founding President
Human Dignity and Humiliation Studies

Preface

This book results from the blessing of circumstance. In separation, being a psychologist steeped in a bilingual-bicultural background, experiencing glimpses of enlightenment, or having episodes of madness may not be that uncommon. But the confluence of all these is rare, if not unique.

The book comprises two main parts: Discoveries from a Self-Study of Madness and Transcending the Clash of Opposites. The first part consists of a detailed self-study of unipolar mood disorder, from which reflections and insights about madness are derived. It belongs to the long tradition of ideographic studies that attend to the uniqueness of each individual. The second part adheres to the nomothetic tradition of knowledge generation. Extensive coverage is given to various aspects of mental disorders from a scientific perspective. It provides the psychiatric as well as ethical, political, and sociocultural contexts for understanding mental disorders in general and my own case in particular.

The chapters in Part II are categorized into four thematic groups: Normality versus Abnormality, Individual versus Collective Madness, Eastern versus Western Culture, and Spirituality versus Spiritual Emptiness. The use of the word *clash* implies coexistence, for there would be no clash between opposites if they do not coexist. The application of dialectical thinking confronts the clash of opposites, leading to a resolution of contradictions.

Dialectical psychology rejects the pseudodichotomy between the idiographic method of investigation of an individual over a prolonged period of time (as in Part I) and the nomothetic designed to discover general laws or principles (as in Part II).

It takes a fundamental stand in rejecting any contention that the psychopathology of an individual may be adequately understood without reference to the whole society of which the individual is a part. That is, the microcosm of an individual's disorder reflects the macrocosm of societal disorder within which it is embedded. In particular, intrapsychic conflicts reflect contradictions found in external reality; and the condition of each individual reflects societal health and pathologies.

Why is the main title of my book named *Fire Burning in My Head*? Because it is an apt and accurate description of exactly what I have experienced during episodes of abnormal mood elevation, physically and psychologically. Physically, I can feel the "fire burning" when I put my hands on my head, as if there were an active volcano erupting inside my brain. Psychologically, I experience creative ideas raining down on me faster than I can absorb. These extraordinary experiences, described in detail in the book, come when I enter into a state of selfless-oblivion.

The subtitle sharpens the focus on the thesis that madness may enrich a person's life. In this book, I reveal my own experiences of madness to the reader; explain how madness may be conceived as creative energy; and specify the conditions under which madness may enrich one's life. Such a sharing of personal experiences would provide hope for countless others who have had their own encounters with madness or, to use a more technical but disparaging term, mental disorders.

I had no history of psychiatric disturbance prior to age 58. Then something happened that profoundly changed my life. For about two weeks, I listened to music in a way I had never listened before. Music came to life, evoking emotions that brought me to the lofty realm of spirituality. As I listened, I began to move—first my arms, then my whole body. I was on my way toward a rediscovery of my artistic and literary bent. People around me said I had become strange—stranger than my usual self. Then, this brief episode of exuberance ended as unpredictably as it came.

What happened? Even as a clinical psychologist, I was and I am still perplexed. I knew I showed hypomanic symptoms during the episode, such as abnormally elevated mood. But I didn't think I suffered from a psychiatric disturbance. Why should I? I enjoyed the episode immensely; it caused me or others no harm.

Since then, more episodes have occurred, two of which approached the severity of mania. Symptoms like inflated self-esteem, racing thoughts, and excessive talkativeness appeared. I acted in ways that went beyond the bounds of social acceptability. People around me were bewildered and became very concerned about my mental condition. Yet, my mind retained its logicality and self-reflectiveness with undiminished prowess. At no point was there any threat of losing contact with reality or of acting in destructive or violent ways.

Altogether, I have had 22 episodes—all of exuberance, none of depression. That is to say, the episodes are all unipolar, not bipolar, mood disorders, defying the typical pattern seen among patients who have had hypomania or mania. This intriguing fact alone would occasion a rewriting of psychiatric textbooks. Further, the deeper I delve into my case, the more I become aware of how limited psychiatric approaches to understanding and coping with abnormality are. Fundamentally, psychiatry has failed to address the creative forces of madness.

These episodes of exuberance afford me precious opportunities to gain unhindered access to the unconscious, experience the extraordinary, and glimpse into the mystical. All the good things are present, in enhanced magnitudes. Gone are fixations, prejudices, and obsessions. Life is sweet, meaningful, and fulfilling. The enlargement of love dominates my being, leading me to act in selfless ways for the betterment of humankind. I became a colorful person, more sensitive, generous, and loving *during* episodes of madness. What's more, I had glimpses of enlightenment, a mystical state of magnanimity.

I was forced to ask myself, "Am I enlightened or mad?" The response to this question is a self-study of my life. I dig deep into my past to better understand the present and future. I struggle to harness the creative forces of madness without incurring unnecessary social costs, which is quite a feat even if it is only partially successful. But what does madness have to do with either enlightenment or spirituality? Everything. This audacious assertion I will defend.

Writing this book affords me the opportunity to fulfill one of my lifelong aspirations: to be an agent of East-West understanding. I take advantage of my bilingual-bicultural background to tell select tales of intercultural encounters along the way of my spiritual journey. I draw upon the religious-philosophical traditions of the East, Confucianism, Daoism, and Buddhism, to enlarge our understanding of spirituality.

So this book is not meant to be just a report on my bouts of madness, extraordinary experiences, and glimpses of enlightenment. It is about my personal journey in quest of an integrated identity, sense of self-mastery, and new directions to lead a good life—in short, spiritual fulfillment. The journey is at once arduous and rewarding. Often I see no end in sight; I may come close to facing despair. Along the way, however, hope invites me to go on, and I also experience tranquility, interspersed with intense feelings of exhilaration and ecstasy.

Confronting episodes of madness one after another is a process of consecutive learning. Gradually I learn to view these episodes as high points in my journey of spiritual discoveries, where the dynamics of spirituality and spiritual emptiness play out. The benefits, both professional and personal, I have derived from my encounters with madness are immense. This realization propels me to share my spiritual discoveries with fellow travelers in search of a good life.

Spirituality then provides the unifying theme and context to interpret all my experiences, normal and abnormal, in China and the United States. What have I learned? Madness has the potential to energize spiritual journeys. Spirituality derives creative energy from madness to reach new heights; madness receives the healing, calming effects of spirituality to become benign. Wedded to ecumenicity, spirituality dissolves ethnic or cultural boundaries, fosters universal love, and promotes world citizenship.

In closing, I wish to express my gratitude to *Scientific American* and to the article's author Simon Makin for approaching me to serve as an informant. This book includes portions of the article "The Undiscovered Illness: The Opposite of Depression" in the March 2019 issue of *Scientific American*.

Writing this book is the closest experience to conception, and getting it published is the closest to giving birth to a baby I will ever have. This new life is my karma. Fortunately, I have help from a competent and encouraging "obstetrician": Evelin Gerda Lindner, a holder of doctorates in psychology and medicine, who has kindly consented to write a foreword for this book. To her I owe the trust that the fruit of my labor is a book worthy of my readers—a baby that will live its life to the fullest.

David Y. F. Ho

Part I

Discoveries from a Self-Study of Madness

Helping others is the royal road to help oneself.

How would my experience enrich your Life? This question entails generalization from my case to yours. Some readers may react with the question, "I have not been mad. So how relevant is your experience to my life?" My counterquestion is: "How can you be sure?" As I have made clear in various chapters in Part II, the demarcation between madness and normality is far from being clear cut (see Thematic Group 1 in particular).

Others may ask, "You have unipolar disorder, which is unusual. I have a different mental disorder. To what extent is your case applicable to mine?" My answer is that it has taken me decades to learn and benefit from encounters with my disorder. Each person has to go through a process of learning to cope with whatever disorder he might have. The reflections and discoveries from my self-study may energize your learning process.

And it is important to recognize that madness does not necessarily benefit your life; in fact, it is more likely that madness has damaged your life. It is unsound to overgeneralize from a case study of a single individual. This is why I have used the words *may enrich your life* in the subtitle of this book. In Chapter 17, I have spelled that several preconditions for enrichment have to be met; moreover, sustained effort is required to transform madness in the service of life enrichment.

Regardless of your own condition, you are free to extract whatever you find useful in this book to enrich your life, in addition to gaining knowledge about madness in diverse sociopolitical, religious, and cultural backgrounds.

A major thesis of this book is that the best way to help oneself is to help others. In various chapters, illustrations are provided to clarify and expand on its implications. Yet, there are times I feel that I can't even help myself, let alone others. Experience has taught me, however, that I may elevate my mental health most effectively through a synergistic engagement with others. This, above all, is what I wish to share with my readers.

1

Tales from My Two Worlds

Faith begins where, and only where, reason ends.

The will to master marginality leads only to world citizenship.

My aim in life is to be shameless—but not to lose the sense of shame.

This chapter is a self-study of my life. It serves as the background case history found in standard psychological "clinical reports." But there is more. It may be viewed as oral history: My life overlaps with a period of turmoil in Chinese history. In many ways, my psychological development mirrors that turmoil. It is no less a case study of intercultural fertilization, which my bicultural-bilingual background facilitates.

I belong to two worlds, one Eastern and the other Western. It is quite natural, therefore, that much of the narrative takes the form of an imaginary interview, in actuality an internal dialogue between my two selves, David and YF (initials for Yau Fai, my given name), different but complementary.

The interview is dialogic action at work. David is my Western-educated self, analytic, informed, and thoughtful. He sees things from different perspectives, Eastern and Western. He puts things in context and spells out their implications. He also functions as a detached observer, summarizing periodically and giving feedback to YF. He tempers YF's extremist proclivities and keeps him on track. Occasionally, he functions as a therapist for YF. He acts as a catalyst, challenging YF to go deeper or to clarify issues, thus pushing the interview forward.

YF is my Chinese self, born and raised in Hong Kong. He derives knowledge from firsthand experiences, including those of "madness." His mind is complexity itself, critical, incisive, and self-reflective. Characteristically direct, he minces no words. He is intense in both action and thought, single-minded in the pursuit of his goals. He has a low threshold for enthusiasm and is almost incapable of doing things halfway.

Psychohistory: Personal Experiences Reflect Historical Social Reality

I tend to be an iconoclast. My frankness may cause embarrassment. I dare to speak the unspeakable—in public. It is a truism that things unsaid may be more meaningful than things verbalized, and things stated openly in public may not be as revealing as things whispered in private. Yet things unstated in public often require frank and open discussion. So the dialogue between YF and David begins.

> YF   I don't want to pontificate about the shortcomings of Western psychology and how they may be remedied. What may interest the reader is *how my personal transformation mirrors the turmoil of modern Chinese history*, particularly with regard to the pains and rewards of intercultural fertilization.
>
> David   You may be a daunting person to interview. The Yau Fai I know is an atypical psychologist and an eccentric, in normality as in madness. You have an unusual social and educational background. You get into all sorts of intellectual pursuits, many of which do not fall within academic psychology proper. You are steeped in revamping psychology, drawing from, as you say, the treasure trove of Chinese culture; yet you don't behave like a typical Chinese. You conduct research on filial piety, toward which I can detect you harbor great antipathy. You study face, like a person saving his own or giving face to another, yet you yourself pay little attention to face in social interactions. Paradox incarnate?
>
> YF   Chinese society has undergone radical, often convulsive, changes during the last hundred years and more. This compels me to engage in soul searching, in response to relentless onslaught from the West—military, political, cultural.
>
> David   Intense debate has focused on the road that China should take to rid itself of foreign domination externally and feudalistic backwardness internally; reassert itself as a strong, modernized nation; and assimilate Western culture, while preserving China's cultural identity. This is no armchair debate, for

YF China was embroiled in a life-or-death struggle for national survival; wars were fought and revolutions broke out that were to determine its destiny. Personal experiences reflect social reality: Struggles within my psyche mirror external conflicts in society. I have felt the pain of domination and humiliation by foreign powers. I have wrestled with the question of who I am: Chinese or American. This is a question of paramount importance. Ultimately, it concerns my identity and being. An integrated identity, enriched by bicultural-bilingual competence, is a happy ending; a fragmented identity, with divergent aspects of itself in uneasy coexistence, is not.

David Your experiences constitute data on intercultural fertilization. You are a psychohistory resource, witness to an ongoing historical process pregnant with paradoxes and ironies. But, in a larger sense, the issues you have struggled with are universal: to preserve, protect, and defend human dignity in the face of humiliation.

This interview is then an exploration of a psychologist who has witnessed the tumultuous events of Chinese history, of epic proportions, in the 20th century. It is Chinese history seen, felt, and interpreted through the eyes of a psychologist, and his psychological transformation in response to historical changes.

It is also a personal story of endeavoring to lead a life of dignity. What was the Chinese intellectual and social climate in which you found yourself during childhood? What internal psychological conflicts have you experienced? How are they resolved? What self-transformation has taken place? Can you relate the historical process to your firsthand experiences?

Mother Worship and Infantilization

YF Take an example from everyday life. Chinese women are supposed to be modest with regard to their bodies. Yet, in my childhood, women in Hong Kong could be seen breast-feeding their infants in public places (e.g., inside a tram) without embarrassment. That came to an end when the likes of Marilyn Monroe and Jayne Mansfield introduced the worship of the big breast into local consciousness.

I have nothing against fascination with the workings of Mammalia, but I do lament the decline of breast-feeding in the name of progress. Asian ideas of physical beauty have changed, and a multibillion-dollar industry to exploit gullible consumers has developed. In Korea today, surgical operations to make female faces look more Western are big business.

David Aside from your fascination with. . . .

YF The worship of motherhood in Chinese culture is of great significance to psychohistory. It goes hand in hand with maternal mollycoddling, an extreme of which is what I call *infantilization*, especially of males well into their adulthood.

Psychologically speaking, the umbilical cord is never cut, thus blocking the road to autonomy and maturity. For males, never weaned psychologically, the chances of attaining manhood are dim. A Chinese popular saying states, "Tender hearted mothers produce mostly rotten sons." Of course, the mouth that utters it is typically a paternal mouth.

Tragic outcomes of infantilization are predictably more likely to occur in well-to-do families, where sons grow up with a sense of entitlement, without a corresponding sense of responsibility. In contemporary Western societies, I might add, entitlement without responsibility is an endemic problem, for children as well as grown-ups.

I've come across such tragic outcomes, actual or potential, in my professional practice. One case involves a boy from an upper-upper class family. By age 12, the boy has never been allowed to do much by himself, except to study; to go anywhere without accompaniment; to take a bus or a taxi; to cross a street by himself; to go to a supermarket, make a purchase, and learn money changing; and so forth. He goes to an international school and returns home in his family's Rolls-Royce driven by a chauffeur, as do many of his classmates from "filthy rich" families in Hong Kong.

> **David** You saw in this boy the dark shadow of what you could have become, even though your family came nowhere near his in terms of wealth and social standing.
>
> **YF** My mother felt the need to take care of my elder brother (e.g., preparing meals for him on a daily basis), even after he had reached the age of 30. Of course, I too did not escape overprotection.

At one time, my family was well-to-do, and this enabled my mother to carry infantilization to new heights. She assigned a servant to take care of me; her duties included accompanying me to school. The servant brought my lunch and stayed in school all day, everyday, even though I was already in the third year of primary school. This made me the laughing stock of my classmates. I felt humiliated. Protesting my mother did nothing to change my situation.

Maternal Guilt Induction

> **YF** Like many other Chinese children, I worshipped my mother, unshakable in my belief that she was, in her own words, "the greatest mother on earth"—until I began a serious study of psychology in early adulthood and came under the onslaught of new ideas that questioned overprotective, possessive parenting. Inculcated into my mind was my mother's subtle message (not directly

verbalized), "You need me, and you will continue to need me in the years to come. So do what I say."

I am no stranger to guilt, given that my mother was a past master of guilt induction. Her guilt-induction messages were pervasive. Made explicit, they read: "I have made sacrifices all my life for you. Now that you are grown up, you are the source for supporting me in my old age. How can you ever abandon me?"

I am convinced that all these originated from insecurity, originating in large measure from the discrimination against women that made my mother bitter all her life. In addition, she had no trust in her marital relationship. My mother was a very anxious, insecure person.

> **David** It's no wonder why Chinese men are hobbled by feelings of indebtedness to their mothers throughout their lives. The debt that they owe can never be repaid.

Awakened from Disillusionment

> **YF** Finally, I woke up from "the greatest illusion of my life." Disillusionment, however painful, is the mother of psychological growth. I came to realize that overprotection prolongs dependency, which serves to maintain maternal control over children.

Thus, antipathies to things Chinese that smacked of conformity, control, or inhibition came to me naturally. They sowed the seeds for rebelliousness. I was rebellious more in thought than in action, for I remained basically an obedient child.

Later, my exposure to Western education, psychology in particular, accentuated these antipathies. It has, moreover, awakened me to be freed from the yoke of backward Chinese values, to be myself. So I have engaged in thorough soul searching and embarked on the path to freedom and personal liberation—tortuous but never boring.

Family Background: Continuities and Departures from Tradition

I was born into an extended family in Hong Kong. My father had seven siblings; my mother had five. I have five siblings: one elder and one younger sister; two elder brothers, the older of whom died of illness when I was one year old.

My paternal grandfather, a classmate of the founder of the Republic of China Dr. Sun Yat Sen (Chinese surnames precede given names), was one of the earliest Christians in Hong Kong. His grandfather was an influential Christian in Southern China. So I was a fifth-generation Christian (according to the available genealogy of my family) and was baptized in a Methodist church when I was an infant.

According to my grandmother, my grandfather was also the first Chinese person in Hong Kong who dared to fly in an airplane. He had a will prepared before doing it, so the legend goes!

Close Relatives Have Become Strangers

The disintegration of the extended family reflects dramatically a fundamental change that has taken place in Chinese society in the past century and more. In my childhood, I had dozens of cousins, some of whom I played with on a frequent basis. Chinese New Year was a festive season. We paid visits to relatives for weeks. After my grandparents died, visits became infrequent. For years, the only time I saw my cousins was at funerals. Now that most members of the elder generation have gone, I seldom see them. Some have emigrated; some I have lost touch with. I wouldn't recognize most of my nephews and nieces if I were to meet them.

All these changes have taken place within the lifetime of a single generation! Forces brought about by changes in kinship overwhelm individual intentions. In mainland China, the one-child policy tolls the death knell for the extended family. It has altered fundamentally familial and more generally interpersonal relationships.

The fabric of Chinese society is based on kinship. Imagine then in the future a Chinese child growing up without a sibling, a cousin, an uncle or an aunt; but with two parents and four grandparents, six doting adults in all in his life, each competing for his attention and affection. Why wouldn't he mature into a superegotistic individual and consequently Chinese society be altered beyond recognition?

Never before in human history has the world seen a social "experiment" on such a massive scale, conducted at such a rapid pace, affecting such a large portion of humanity. The socioeconomic and psychological consequences are unprecedented and will remain so for generations to come. How can we be prepared for the onslaught of these megatsunamic forces?

Girls Will Become More Precious Than Boys in China

YF   Here is another fantastic story to tell about my extended family: Two girls for one boy. My number one paternal aunt had only one son who died in early adulthood, followed by eight daughters. When I was a baby, she made a proposal to my parents: to exchange two of her daughters for one son, me. Of course, my mother said, "No deal." I only learned about this story at the age of 68, when my elder sister told me out of the blue.

David   In the old days, adoption within the extended family was not all that unusual. A male child may be raised by a paternal uncle by blood (with the same surname) acting in the role of his adoptive parent, especially when the uncle has no male heir of his own. Still, two-girls-for-one-boy would take such adoption to a new level. If the exchange did materialize, undoubtedly you would have been surrounded by indulging females in your childhood. How enviable!

How do people console a mother who has given birth to a baby girl? They would say, "First the flower, then the fruit": A boy will follow the girl as surely as the fruit will come after the flower. In the case of my aunt, the fruit never came even after eight flowers. I can imagine how desperate she might have been.

However, a consoling thought is that girls will become more precious than boys in future! That would be revolutionary in altering man-woman relations in China. But where have all the flower babies gone? The answer to this question is just about too horrible to contemplate. Human life by the millions has vanished, mostly by design (e.g., induced abortion), not by natural causes.

The measure of a civilization lies largely in how it positions and treats the better half of humanity. As Mao Zedong says, women can hold up half the sky.

YF   Now I know what male-centeredness really means. But I don't know what my life would be like if my parents had agreed to my aunt's proposal. How different would the book I am now writing be?

David   Years later, in the middle of your second manic episode, you wrote: "Life does not need a reason for its existence. It must, however, be welcomed." What is the reason for one's existence? How many of you, dear readers, are here in this world because of an accident? Or of negligence, because your parents forgot or failed to take prophylactic measures? You are lucky, YF. You were welcomed. Overall, your childhood was a happy one. You were loved, perhaps even favored, by the adults around you—parents, relatives, and teachers.

YF   Right, except that obsessive-compulsive traits were manifest as early as age six. I recall I used to throw temper tantrums when I couldn't fit everything perfectly into my school bag. The negative experiences I had were not so much about me personally as the domination of the old over the young, subjugation of women under men, and exploitation of the poor by the rich and powerful. In response to these conditions, I felt moral indignation. So my sympathies have always been with the underdogs since early childhood.

My First Heavenly Experimentation

One incident, involving my very first sexual contact with the opposite sex, stands out in terms of provoking my moral indignation. At age 14, I went to stay with my maternal grandparents for the summer. My grandmother put me and a maid, some three years older, in the same room with a bunk bed. I slept in the lower bunk; she slept in the upper.

Days passed without mishap, until one day my brother, four years older, came for a visit. Somehow, the three of us ended up in the upper deck in physical intimacy and exploration. My brother and I caressed the maid's shapely body. Her willing participation took me by surprise: Until then, women had been put on a pedestal, sacred and inviolable.

In the midst of our heavenly experimentation, my grandmother burst in. From her mouth came language as foul as anything I had ever heard, untranslatable and unfit for print. It could have been uttered only by one woman directed at another much below her status. But my brother and I were not scolded or punished. What injustice, I thought to myself.

> **David** It was your grandmother who set you up for a natural occurrence. What on earth did she expect? Apparently, she had no conception of adolescent sexuality—strange as it may sound to American parents. And, of course, the incident was but one of countless others like it in traditional Chinese society.
>
> **YF** I now look back at the incident with more compassion for my grandmother. She had bound feet (also known as "lotus feet"). It's hard to imagine how crippling a woman's being that can be. I have faint memories of my grandmother unwinding her foot binding cloth at night, revealing her feet no more than a few inches long.
>
> **David** Renowned for his use of lifelike metaphors, Mao Zedong spoke of the foot binding cloth, "as smelly as it is long," to characterize long-winded, empty articles that ideologues in the Chinese Communist Party loved—and still love—to write.

Classic Antagonism Between Mothers-in-Law and Daughters-in-Law

Strife within the extended Chinese family is much more common than orthodox Confucians would like us to believe. A case in point is the classic antagonism between mothers-in-law and their daughters-in-law.

YF   One day my mother gathered all her children for instruction. The occasion: My paternal grandmother was about to move into our household, despite my mother's protest to my father. My mother instructed us not to be nice to our grandmother, under whose dominance she had suffered. She even taught us to sing a vengeful song she had composed just for her nemesis, "I don't want to be a parasite in the world. . . .." Years later, during psychotherapy workshops I conduct in Confucian-heritage communities, when I mention marital strife caused by antagonism between the wife and her mother-in-law, women participants immediately recognize the phenomenon and describe their own experiences with it.

David   Control and ownership of the most important man in their lives underlie perennial battles between mothers-in-law and daughters-in-law. What can men caught between two women do? Poor menfolk! By the ethic of filial piety, a man is supposed to side with his mother and persuade his wife to accede. But not all wives are docile or open to persuasion. Some may be fearsome and prone to strike back, as did your mother against her mother-in-law. Psychological illiteracy appears to be more pronounced in men than in women. In the final analysis, psychotherapy for Chinese families is basically limited in what it can hope to achieve. We need to redefine the role of women and of male-female relationships in Chinese societies. Again, I see individual struggles in a larger context; they must be linked to collective struggles involving society as a whole.

YF   In my own family, quarrels between my parents seemed endless. Eventually they were separated when my mother left Hong Kong to live in the United States. I was then ten years of age. So I grew up in a broken family, pained but unbroken.

From Childhood to Grandparenthood

Dramatic changes in my roles as a son, a father, and a grandfather reflect not only my personal transformation but also changes in Chinese cultural values concerning socialization that have taken place over the past hundred years and more.

Socialization: What Is Filial Piety?

Overall, traditionally Chinese children are socialized to be obedient, timid, controlled, inhibited, and dependent. Like their counterparts in the West, they love to play and make noise. But their childhood impulses are increasingly subdued as they grow older. While children in the West climb up trees, Chinese children tend to sit still to avoid physical risks because they have been reminded constantly of the filial injunction, "The body, hair and skin, have all been received from one's parents. One does not dare to do them harm. That's the beginning of *xiao* [filial piety]." Right, sit still they do, at home and in school—too much, especially in the presence of authority figures. It's quite a sight to see an entire class of kindergarten or primary schoolchildren sitting still, with both hands held firmly behind their back. Meanwhile, the teacher looks over them like an owl.

YF Like other children of my generation, I was expected to be respectful and obedient toward my elders and stay out of trouble. Misbehavior that reflected poorly on the family invited shaming. Generally, I was well behaved. But I didn't sit still.

One of my childhood memories, of age 11, stands out. Once I ran down a hilly path at "lightning" speed, to the horror of my onlooking uncles and aunts, who showed great disapproval of my unruly behavior. Inwardly, I harbored delight in having horrified them with my physical agility.

David Understandably, hyperactive children cause formidable difficulties to their parents and teachers. Of special interest here is a cross-cultural comparison between Western and Chinese standards of hyperactivity. Many a child considered normal in the West would be regarded as a hyperactive trouble-maker in a Chinese context.

YF And so it is painful to witness the deadening developmental path of Chinese children: lively in nurseries and kindergartens, overcontrolled in primary schools, half-dead in secondary schools, and brain-dead by the time they enter universities.

David The reader will surely forgive you, driven by moral indignation, for making such hyperbole. Let's touch on another cross-cultural comparison. The difference in reaction to animals between Western and Chinese children is dramatic. While Western children delight in seeing small animals, dogs in particular, Chinese children are prone to retreat in fear to hide behind their mothers.

YF Why? Because the mothers, afraid of dogs themselves, frequently frighten their children with the remark, "Watch out! The dog will bite you." Another scare tactic that adults use to control children is to say to them, "If you continue to misbehave, I will take you to the police station." This reinforces the generalized fear of authority figures typical of Chinese children. In addition, young girls are frequently reminded by elderly women, "Men are not to be trusted."

David Women might rebut that the reminder to young girls is based on reality. Still, it is an overgeneralization, not helpful to maidens in courtship for developing skills to discriminate between suitors who can or cannot be trusted. Can you be trusted?

YF Being trusted by a woman imposes on the trusted man heavy responsibilities not to betray her trust. Wouldn't you rather be released from all bondage, on occasion, and plunge with abandon into the "pleasures of cloud and rain" (Chinese euphemism for sexual union)?

David I retreat back to psychohistory. Unwittingly, the adults create an unsafe world full of dangers in the minds of the young. How can trust and security be established? The unsafe world extends into the home when mothers deal with their misbehaving children with the threat, "Wait till your father comes home."

In translation, this threat implies three messages. One, I have failed to discipline and control you by myself. Two, the real authority resides in your father. Three, in our home your father is the fearsome person you should be afraid of. The first two messages undermine the mother as a disciplinarian.

The last one is pernicious, for it drives a wedge into the father–child relationship emotionally and predisposes the child toward a generalized fear of authority figures. The child has reasons to be fearful of the father, who is more likely than the mother to administer harsh discipline. A popular Chinese saying sums it up: "Stern fathers, softhearted mothers." No wonder Chinese children tend to be emotionally attached to their mothers, but detached from their fathers.

Battling Against Psychological Illiteracy

All these I have seen and heard, all too frequently, in my professional practice as well as daily life. Even as a child, I thought to myself: With such emphasis on impulse control, obedience, and fear inducement, our traditional upbringing produces enslaved nations!

After becoming a psychologist, I was determined to bring about changes in upbringing children for the better through parental education. It was an uphill battle—to put it bluntly, against centuries of psychological illiteracy.

To begin with, being a psychologist invited people to look upon me with circumspection. I had to earn their trust, before I could begin to educate. It is pleasing to witness how generally Chinese parents have become more democratic and sensitive to the child's psychological needs, with far-reaching consequences for Chinese society as a whole.

After becoming a father, I went to an extreme to give my daughters what I was deprived of in my childhood. I engaged them in dialogues. I encouraged them to express their own opinions, even to argue with me. A dialogue with my elder daughter at age seven ran like this:

Father   "Is there a God?"
Daughter "Yes. If there is no God, who made you? Grandma?"
Father   "Who made God?"
Daughter "Chemical liquids."

At age 17, after a day of job hunting, she said, "I discovered something today. Everybody wants to know if I can type, take shorthand, and so forth. Nobody asked me about philosophy. I don't see anything like 'Philosopher Urgently Needed' in the newspaper ads. I am angry."

At age four, my younger daughter gave me a lecture: "You taught us to do.... Why haven't you done so yourself?" I didn't interrupt her. The lecture lasted some 20 minutes, as recorded by my stopwatch, after which she resumed her usual sweetness. In her first year of primary school, I went to receive her report card. Her teacher complained, "She talks too much." Intimidated, I dared not reveal I was a psychologist. Back home, I asked her, "Why do you like to talk so much?" She replied, "The mouth is not just for eating, but also for talking."

David	Like daughter, like father!
YF	Apprehensive, I let my paternal protectiveness take over: "You are right, of course. Fortunately, you have only one mouth. What matters the most is not so much what you say, but where. You can say what you want at home. But you need to be more careful at school. I don't want you to get into trouble with your teacher."

She didn't argue with me. Now she is a teacher herself. I asked once, "How do you keep the kids under control?" She replied, "I have learned from all your mistakes." Suddenly, I was at a loss for words. As a mother of two children, she makes me a grandfather. Noah is the first born, followed by Harper. In this case, the fruit arrives before the flower. My troubles fly away when these kids smile in response to my stimulation.

On Being a Grandfather

No less than fatherhood, grandfatherhood requires new learning. In the traditional pattern, there is a dark side to grandparenting, in the form of extreme indulgence. In particular, grandmothers tend to mollycoddle, pamper their grandsons beyond belief, to the point of smothering them with excessive care that leaves little room for independence. Enforcement of discipline by male adults would be sabotaged, rendered virtually impossible. The Chinese term, "drowning love," captures aptly the essence of such extreme indulgence—even plants may wither from too much watering. Drowning love reinforces infantilization. Thus, women have the awesome power to turn the very boys they love into good-for-nothing men.

My guiding principle for grandparenthood: "Just enjoy it. Be helpful, without interfering. Avoid giving advice or expressing too many opinions." Surprisingly, I find it quite easy to do, for a professor who has been expounding a lot of opinions on parenting. Grandparents and their grandchildren form a natural alliance, against their common "enemies." Why not indulge Noah and Harper a little? That's my grandparental privilege.

I can't help comparing the superb quality of parenting and material abundance (baby strollers, books, toys, etc.) that my grandchildren enjoy with what most children of my generation received. Family life has been turned upside down, from traditional elder-centeredness to modern child-centeredness. Everything revolves around my grandchildren's needs; their sleeping and feeding schedules dictate adult schedules. In the words of my daughter, they are "the center of the universe for us."

David So, in place of filial sons and daughters, nowadays you find plenty of filial parents. One child commanding the attention of two parents and four grandparents: This is the modern reality. We belong to a sandwiched generation, expected to be filial sons and daughters to our elder generations and filial parents to our children. What's more, we can't expect the same filiality from our children that our parents expect from us.

YF Some years ago, my younger daughter asked, "Dad, what research are you doing?" I replied, "Filial piety." She shot back, "What's that?" The times have surely changed. Changes I have witnessed in my own family are just a few examples of changes in the Chinese family as an institution, which are symptomatic of changes in the wider society.

Confucianism, Shame, and Thought Liberation

David Your account strengthens the impression that you are not a typical Chinese. Why are you so atypical? Not by choice, I suppose, for atypicality typically makes life more difficult. You simply accept it as a fact of your existence. Perhaps you can even exploit it to your advantage.

YF Not typical of anything, anywhere. I have always been a minority among minorities, being different, wherever I find myself. The typical Chinese is one oversocialized, subdued in Confucian culture. For as long as I can remember, I have had instinctive antipathies to Confucianism. It strangles the Dionysian spirit. I discern no dialectical thinking in the *Confucian Analects*. Confucius says—end of dialogue. In contrast, the Daoist philosophers Laozi and Zhuangzi come across as dialectical thinkers. They have inspired me in my journey of spiritual discoveries. Zhuangzi speaks of the equality of all things: "The great Dao is all-embracing without making distinctions."

David	Equality ascends when no categorical distinctions among people are made. This strikes at the heart of Confucian societal order founded on well-defined status hierarchies, which you regard as a barrier to bidirectional communication and the formation of egalitarian relationships.
YF	I recall the apprehensive thought I had when I obtained my doctoral degree: "The degree transforms my social identity. It can place a distance between me and other people. Beware." Does "PhD" stand for "permanent head damage," in a manner of speaking?
David	An important point you make is that Confucianism has inculcated in the Chinese mind not just a sense of shame, but also feelings of shamefulness. As Mencius declared, "Those who do not have a sense of shame and dislike are not human," that is, no different from beasts. That's why you say one of your goals in life is to become "shameless"—getting rid of not the sense of shame (i.e., the capacity to feel repugnance toward things evil), but feelings of shamefulness about oneself. Your thoughts about shame are captured in one of your epigrams (3 Jan 2009): "The sense of shame has been a shackle on the Chinese soul. Ridding ourselves of it would open the door to creativity."

Alas, the sense of shame is now eclipsed by avarice in mainland China in its blind quest for economic development. On the other hand, strengthening the sense of shame would restore time-honored standards for conduct in American society, especially for celebrities and politicians. The horrors of shame I have experienced are portrayed in a poem I wrote (March 2004):

Shamefaced

I dreamt I was on stage, naked,
In front of a thousand piercing eyes, staring
At me. My face is a face that does not dare
To show itself. Nowhere to hide—
Not even from myself.
But what have I done wrong?

YF	Being Chinese, I have an entrenched sense of shame. To become shameless is a most formidable goal, which I have yet to reach after a lifetime of self-therapy. Only in episodes of madness do I find total relief.
David	That said, I wish to add that in many ways what America lacks China has in abundance, and vice versa. Strengthening the sense of shame would be good for American society, just as loosening thought control would be for Chinese society.
YF	Central to the Confucian tradition is to have no depraved thoughts—think not what is contrary to propriety. Underlying propriety is the basic virtue of sincerity. Because sincerity means purity of thought, "impure" thoughts must be purged. Not only impulse, but also thought control! No wonder we had the campaign against "spiritual pollution" in China not long ago.

David Confucian thinking on morality has always assumed that there is a fundamental distinction between right and wrong, that the human mind is able to grasp this distinction and to act accordingly. The distinction cannot be disputed, because it is an extension of the cosmic principle into the social realm. Of course, Confucian scholars are anointed to decide what constitutes right versus wrong. You have traced some of your negative personal experiences to Confucian origination.

YF I draw on my multicultural experiences that span decades in North America, Hawaii, and Asia (mainland China, Taiwan, Hong Kong, Singapore, the Philippines). At every turn, I see pernicious traces of Confucianism in Chinese family life: paternalism, prejudice, and discrimination against women; overprotection, overindulgence, infantilization of children, especially of males, by mothers and grandmothers.

In the midst of my mother's funeral in New York, a Chinese funeral director proclaimed, "Chinese people do not include the names of female descendants in elegiac couplets." My sisters and I protested. The funeral director, who saw himself as a defender of tradition, became nasty and began using foul language. It was one of the most painful experiences I have had in my life. The legacy of Confucius lingers in the land of the free.

Yes, I openly declare, in the spirit of Thomas Jefferson, eternal hostility to all forms of oppression over freedom of thought and speech. This is a celebration of my way to personal liberation. Unfortunately, however, I am also all too aware that the battle for freedom in China is far from over.

The Age of Turbulence: Adolescence and Early Adulthood

This was the period when I was most susceptible to the impact of changes, biological, sociocultural, and educational, on the development of my personality. It was also the most turbulent years of my life.

The "Dark Ages" of My Education

Reflecting on my educational history now helps me to understand more deeply how education shapes the destiny of nations and is, therefore, a critical component of psychohistory. I have two educational parents, Chinese and American, a comparison of which demands attention across the Pacific.

My childhood education can only be described as the "Dark Ages" of my intellectual development. It was mostly uneventful and uninspiring. It did not prepare me well for anything. First, it was imbued with British colonialism. Hong Kong, where I was born and raised, was under British colonial rule. In my school days, students spent endless hours on arithmetic problems involving guineas, pounds, crowns, half-crowns, shillings, and pence—sterling units, now antiquated, they had never seen or touched. Do you know 1 half-crown = 2 shillings 6 pence = 1/8.4 guinea? That was surely an infamous chapter in the history of mathematics education.

In contrast, modern Chinese history was given truncated coverage by design. What was not in the syllabus was not examined and, therefore, would not be taught. Most young people, even if educated, had no or only fuzzy knowledge of Chinese history after 1911. Even today, you can find university students confusing the founding of the Republic of China in 1912 with that of the People's Republic of China in 1949.

David   Depriving a people of knowledge of its history is a powerful instrument of colonialism: It multiplies the effects of individual memory loss, even if reversible; it warps the normal development of selfhood and identity, at both individual and collective levels. Colonialism and missionary schools often go together. To what extent were you exposed to Christian education?

YF   I attended a Jesuit school for boys for six years. Its approach to religious education was dogmatic and impoverished through and through. I can still recite parts of the Catechism of the Catholic Church that provided me with the main diet of religious education in those years. So, such religious education did nothing to awaken my spirituality.

As a schoolboy, I was rather mischievous. The youngest and the smallest in my class, I horsed around and cracked jokes that caused the entire class to burst into laughter. This brought punishment upon me by humorless or, worse, sadistic teachers. Chinese schoolchildren commonly have tales of horror to tell about their teachers and principals, don't they?

Many years later, in one therapy case I worked on, the school principal made a schoolboy stand in the hallway, wearing a humiliating placard for all to see. On the placard was written: "I received a zero-egg [literally, a zero mark]." The schoolboy became utterly resentful of all authority figures.

Many Chinese schoolchildren react to their teachers typically with fear, docility, silence, negativism, resentment, and outward compliance (but inward defiance) in front of their teachers; disrespect, noncompliance, and passive-aggression behind their backs. When they grow up, they react to authority figures likewise. Is the Chinese nation condemned to be made up mostly of people without guts? Under ordinary circumstances, resentment and aggression are held in check or expressed indirectly. Students would ventilate anger in the form of passive or displaced aggression. They would "dare to be angry but not to voice a protest" and "forbear and swallow one's voice."

Under extraordinary circumstances, however, control mechanisms break down and aggression might erupt into the open. During the Great Cultural Revolution, aggression did erupt, this time in the form of unprecedented collective violence. Prompted by Mao Zedong, students revolted against institutional authority. Many got out of control, humiliated and acted with physical violence toward their teachers and professors.

David In terms of psychohistory, your personal experiences both as a student and as a therapist make it easier to understand the phenomenon of student violence during the Great Cultural Revolution. But there must have been some exceptional teachers whose good words or deeds made enough of a difference to your life to be remembered.

YF Yes, a Jesuit teacher who taught us the true meaning of manhood comes to mind. In a self-study class, many students, including myself, were reading books outside of the curriculum (e.g., novels) we weren't supposed to read. We did it surreptitiously, hiding the books under desk covers. The teacher stood up and said to the class: "Bring your books out, into the open. It's all right. Don't act like you have something to hide, as if you were a scoundrel. I'd rather see you act with openness and courage."

Unfortunately, most of the teachers were uninspired and uninspiring, morally or intellectually. Yet, they had great talent for reducing joyous learning to painful drudgery. They habitually repeated the same boring lessons time and again. Incredibly, the thought of boredom reduction seemed to have never once occurred in their minds. They have forgotten the days when they themselves were students. So, to bring some life into the classroom, I made fun of teachers, targeting those and only those I held in low regard. What else was there to do?

Intellectually speaking, those years were the "Dark Ages" of my life. Never once, however, was I destructive or openly defiant. Years later, I became a teacher yourself. Having gone through the "Dark Ages" of my intellectual life, I've learned that there is a connection between cowardice and being boring. So, as a teacher I shall summon all the courage to be true to myself—inspired and inspiring, never to bore.

Across the Pacific on My Way to Discover a New World

In 1955, at age 16, I took a step to leap out of my intellectual "Dark Ages." Together with my elder brother, we went overseas to study in Canada. Before that, I had never traveled away from home for a distance of more than 20 miles or so. I was academically and emotionally unprepared. Living in a foreign culture added complications, especially to heterosexual relations. All these propelled me to enter into adulthood prematurely; my life as an adolescent was foreclosed and shortened. My brother and I traveled by ship and train, as it was rather expensive to travel by plane in those days. I still remember *President Cleveland*, the ocean liner that took us to continental America, with nostalgia. The voyage took 18 days across the Pacific to reach its destination, San Francisco, from where we continued to travel to Canada.

David You are the reincarnate of Columbus—from the East. I bet you were highly conscious of being among the lucky minority who had the privilege of studying overseas. Full of hope, you looked forward to getting the most out of not only a university education but also Western culture.

YF That's right. The voyage marked a turning point in my life. It was not until 12 years later that I would set foot on Chinese soil again. There were more than a hundred students on board *President Cleveland*, enough to create much excitement. Playing around and mingling with these fellow passengers for the entire voyage, I put to the back of mind my intention to study. I wrote in my diary (circa Aug 1955): A huge fish jumping out of the surface of the sea, swimming faster than the ship; watching sunrise at four a.m., together with some female passengers; a risqué burlesque in Japan; watching the hula dance and using the surfboard in Hawaii: These are all my first experiences, which I enjoy. I remember how exhilarating it was to watch a snowfall and other natural wonders of a Canadian winter for the first time.

David Don't you now envy the youthful you who had such capacity for delight in the simple, wondrous things of the world? I also sense that the original emotions you had are being reawakened in the present as you describe the past. It is in your being to preserve youthfulness for as long as you can. It is part and parcel of spiritual striving. What was your first exposure to university education in a foreign land like?

YF I found myself among giants, physically speaking, something I experienced initially as rather bewildering. I was the youngest student at Carleton College (now Carleton University). On one occasion, a bus driver issued me a ticket for a primary schoolchild. It was amusing. I was awfully unprepared academically. My major was physics. I learned more in the first physics lecture than in the previous three years combined.

English was my major headache. I still remember the textbook I had for freshmen English. It was bulky, many more times thicker than the texts I had in Hong Kong. In it, close to half of the words on every page were words I had never before seen. Naturally, I failed freshman English and had to take a supplementary exam. My self-esteem suffered little loss. I simply construed the failure as a discovery of ignorance. Then, I had the audacity to go to the dean and asked for permission to take a survey course in English literature in place of the required course in geology in my sophomore year. I argued with him until permission was granted. In hindsight, I feel that I made the right choice. I took to the survey course in English with a level of keenness that would have well-nigh impossible to attain for geology.

Being academically unprepared was not the main reason why my grades were bad: Unlike other Chinese students, I was not a "good" student. Attending university was like a child entering a playroom full of intriguing toys. Finally, I thought to myself, I was out of the dark age of my secondary school days in Hong Kong. Homework was no longer doing repetitive exercises; composition was no longer drudgery; and learning was no longer unrelated to life, but joyous and meaningful.

Mingling with Canadian students in extracurricular and social activities was an eye-opening experience. They worked together, they practiced democracy, and they knew how to have fun. In sharp contrast, my fellow Chinese students, all of whom were from Hong Kong, did not know how to work together. Most of them were reluctant to assume leadership positions but treated those who did as targets of animosity. During meetings, they bickered endlessly among themselves, with nothing much accomplished in the end. I felt ashamed of being Chinese. They were not just "a pile of loose sand," as Dr. Sun Yat Sen, the founder of the Chinese republic, used to say, but an assembly of warring cliques. Defying stereotypes (unwittingly reinforced by cross-cultural psychologists), the Canadians were behaving like "collectivists" and the Chinese like "individualists."

Naive and Fearless: The Seeds of Spiritual Adventure

My life as an adolescent was shortened. But the life of my adolescent playfulness and sentiments was not. So a belated adolescence would pop up now and then in my later years—as my friends trying to make fun of me might say. My youthful naiveté combined with fearlessness served me well. I welcomed the opportunity to explore new frontiers. An intrepid traveler, that's what I was. On the front page of my 1958 diary were these words:

> In this little book, I will give my most honest account of passion, lamentations, and joy; laziness and industry; shame and pride; hatred and love; action and thought; endless intellectual explorations. Let this be an adventurous tragic song, and pages of glory, for these are the years of foundation. Holding my present fast, upon the past shall I build my future, in the service of mankind.

David	These diaries and correspondence with friends and relatives are revealing of your state of mind.
YF	Reading these materials again today refreshes my memory of some forgotten aspects of my youth, most notably my inclination toward spirituality and my desire to write poetry. Writing was one way of satisfying the yearnings for expression of my "lonely soul." I felt the sentiments of a "poet in love, in ecstasy." Writing to a friend, I wrote, "If I were a poet, I would . . . immortalize our friendship" (18 Dec 1962).

But my proficiency in the English language was simply no match for the demands of expressing my thoughts and sentiments. In those days, the difference between words like *circumcision* and *castration* were fine distinctions I was ignorant of. Once I asked a Jewish friend of mine, "Is it true that Jewish infant boys are castrated?" Fortunately, my friend distinguished between linguistic goof and social ineptitude. Much of what I wrote now strikes me as rather uncouth or melodramatic. It has taken me decades of hard work to approach meeting the demands of poetic expression.

David	Nonetheless, the dynamism, passion, and resolute determination of a young man in search of himself leap out of the diaries and correspondence. So do the idealism and extremism characteristic of youthful minds.
YF	"I am a person of extremes," I wrote in my diary (31 Jan 1959). This terse statement summed it up well. There were fluctuations between supreme self-confidence and self-doubt, and between elation and sorrow. Ideas of striving toward "spiritual beauty" and "a finer inner being" may be found in abundance. Often, however, the emotional tone was very negative: "[I suffered from] spiritual disease" (1 Jan 1960); "My soul drowns in anguish. . . . My spiritual emptiness is very acute" (28 Aug 1960).
David	I can't help but notice the theme of spirituality in your writings. It is significant that you expressed your inner turmoil in the language of spirituality rather than of psychology. Thus your articulation of a dynamic conception of spiritual fulfillment versus spiritual emptiness years later should come as no surprise. You have acquired the requisite firsthand experience of struggle and emotional foundation for articulating the dynamic conception. The highly charged negative tone reflected your feelings of frustrated spiritual striving. What saved you from collapse?
YF	My love of life remained unshakable: "My passionate love of life never dies" (20 Feb 1958). I maintained an intense sense of purpose. My writing was replete with expressions like "meaning," "destiny," "transcendence," "self-discovery," and "quest for the ultimate truth."
David	Your fighting spirit would not allow you to surrender; you were ready to "plunge into battle." But I must also say that you were neurotically driven, overwhelmed by ambition. You were a tormented soul. There was a pressing

	sense of urgency: Expressions like "make haste to live, to love" dotted your diaries everywhere. Constantly reproaching yourself for "wasting time," you pushed yourself to the limit. To excel was the only way you knew how to deal with your self-doubt and feelings of inferiority. Psychologists call it compensation. So you exploited your intellectual endowment to the fullest—at a terrible psychological cost to yourself.
YF	Yes, I wanted to know, to learn everything, to be schooled in scholarly pursuits as well as martial arts. To equip myself, I took violin, singing, dancing, and fencing lessons. I wrote a short story, "On the Other Side of Hate" (19 April 1959), for submission to a literary contest. My notebooks were filled with all kinds of ideas for writing projects, such as an autobiography (9 June 1960) and "The Future of Mankind" (25 Aug 1960).

One was to write "The Outline of Philosophy" (27 Dec 1959), even though I had taken only an introductory course in philosophy. I had the audacity to make assertions like God is "the origin of evil." Another project was "The Great Dialogue between Reason and Faith" (28 Dec 1959). In it, I find this statement: "Faith has its beginning where reason ends" (which may be taken as a paraphrase of Voltaire's famous dictum "Faith consists in believing when it is beyond the power of reason to believe," of which I had not heard then). This provides proof that many of my present thoughts have their origins in my early adulthood.

The fact that I was uninformed of the topics I wrote about was of no concern to me. I wanted to give my imagination free rein. I protested against "the creative writer [being] forced to write as a scholar." This was a presage of my career as an academic author in the decades to come. Amazing!

Occasionally, however, I was unsettled by reality checks. I would write, "Damn it. There is not much of value in what I have written." Poor me, as I look back: I had the makings of a Renaissance man, but without the requisite genius to generate momentous knowledge or objects of beauty. Was my maker playing a trick on me? It is a good thing that I know, and accept, my limitations. Otherwise, my ambition would have consumed me in the awful predicament of endless frustrations.

David	Years later, you say to your students not to dwell on the final outcome or achievement, but to enjoy of the process of creating. Revisiting your turbulent age has deepened our understanding of subsequent periods of your life, particularly the golden age, to which we shall turn shortly. In all, literary-artistic-spiritual aspirations during your energetic student days in North America match those of your golden age, but they were also intertwined with neurotic entanglements. Or, to put it differently, your golden age may be viewed as a distillate of your former aspirations, more mellowed and less turbulent than before.

Did Psychology Turn Me into an Unfilial Son?

Back in the 1950s, studying psychology was virtually unheard of among overseas Chinese students. How did you become a psychologist? Although my major was physics, I could not resist the temptation of exploring other subjects. I roamed the library and read books unrelated to physics. I sat in courses in which I had not registered and made diagnostic assessments of professors on the inspiring-boring spectrum.

One psychology professor, Harold Breen, was particularly fascinating. He had deep-set blue eyes and a mustache, looking rather like the philosopher Friedrich Nietzsche. I followed him around, looking for opportunities to talk with him. Sensing that I had an interest in psychology, he invited me to audit his Personality Dynamics course. That was my very first exposure to psychology; it took place during my freshman year. There were no lectures, only discussions. No syllabus, no lecture notes, and no formal examination. Textbook learning was not emphasized. To a Chinese student, this must have been strange indeed!

The students did not appear knowledgeable, even to one as ignorant as I was. Yet the remarkable thing was that most of them seemed genuinely interested in the subject matter and participated actively in discussions. They struggled to apply psychological principles to understand life better. They expressed their opinions freely, arguing with one another and even with the professor.

At first, I was hesitant to speak. One day, I mustered enough courage to open my mouth. No one laughed at me. Professor Breen encouraged me to speak up more. Since then, I have found it difficult to keep my mouth shut. This got me into lots of trouble after I returned to Chinese societies many years later. I was not sure what I had learned, probably not much that could be measured in a traditional examination. Nonetheless, I began to ponder questions I had never before thought of. The seeds for a lifelong quest had been sown.

Professor Breen was also instrumental in arousing my interest in psychiatry because he brought me relief from my conflicts over sexual impulses. I had more than the usual adolescent angst concerning sexuality.

When I was around 14, my father told me that masturbation was damaging to the body, like "cutting your artery open and letting the blood flow out"; worse, it would lead to intellectual deterioration. Naturally, I was terrified. Conflicts between sexual impulses and control over them reached intensities that brought me great distress and turmoil. I had fallen victim to a culturally induced psychoneurosis. With trepidation, I sought advice from Professor Breen, who set me straight about the normality of masturbation. I felt much relieved after talking with him.

At age 20, I left Canada and moved to the United States. After obtaining a degree in physics, I decided to enter graduate school to study psychology—to the dismay of my parents and the bewilderment of other Chinese students. That is why I am a psychologist today. Had I been deprived of these opportunities in North America, I would have suffocated under the Hong Kong educational system or have been eliminated altogether by it. That's why I remain grateful to Canada and the United States to this day.

I took to psychology as a fish to water. My specialization was clinical psychology. Studying psychology was like eating the forbidden fruit of knowledge. Eyes opened, I read the psychopathology within my own family. I became critical of the repressive, conservative, and authoritarian aspects of Chinese culture.

My mother complained that I had become a bad, unfilial son after I began studying psychology. "It's largely on account of you that I have decided to study psychology. I want to know how to deal with my mother," I informed her.

Engineering a Social Revolution in a Mental Hospital

David So knowledge can lead to, or accentuate, conflicts. Psychological knowledge, in particular, can be outright dangerous. But for you the pursuit of knowledge is a cardinal drive that has seen no diminished intensity for more than half a century. I bet you were eager to apply the knowledge you had acquired.

YF I engineered a revolution in a mental hospital (Elgin State Hospital in Illinois), where I did my internship and later worked as a staff psychologist in the 1960s. The hospital was a monstrosity, with over 5,000 mental patients. It was like a small town unto itself, with its own electric generator, canteens, laundries, and staff quarters.

David Like other total institutions, such as prisons and concentration camps, it encompassed the inmate's whole being, subjected him to regimentation and undermined his individuality and dignity. Institutionalization rendered patients increasingly dependent on the hospital, and turned them into chronic patients with nowhere else to go. It was a place of hopelessness, much like the setting of the film *One Flew over the Cuckoo's Nest*.

YF Soon after completing my internship, I conducted milieu therapy in the hospital. I declared that the first target of treatment was none other than the hospital itself, not the patients. I challenged the hierarchical authority structure of the institution. I wrote one of the earliest articles I ever published, entitled "Staff Too Can Be Institutionalized" (Ho, 1965), which ruffled feathers.

I introduced democracy to a ward of chronic patients, some of whom had been hospitalized for more than thirty years: I empowered the patients to organize themselves, elect their own leaders, and insofar as possible make their own decisions. I organized the staff, and won them over to participate in the process of democratization.

> David You also stepped on people's toes, when you challenged their habitual ways of operation or threatened their vested interests.
>
> YF My supervisor said I took on a job he wouldn't have for a million dollars. However, statistics spoke to the fruits of my labor: Within a few months, discharge rate went up three times. Not that the discharged were cured; it went up largely because the discharged patients were reconnected with their families, deinstitutionalized. The milieu therapy continued, even after I left the hospital; by that measure, I regard the therapy as having its greatest success.
>
> David Like a dreadnought battleship in World War I, you were a force to be reckoned with; and like a bull in a china shop, you were fearless.
>
> YF As a Chinese saying puts it, "A new born calf does not fear the tiger"—because it is too ignorant or stupid to fear. Acquiring knowledge was not enough; I wanted action. It is ironic that what I succeeded in doing in a mental hospital I couldn't even begin to try in an institution of higher learning, namely, the University of Hong Kong, where I spent most of my professional life after returning to Hong Kong.
>
> David Your experience at Elgin State Hospital speaks to an admirable feature of American society: its receptivity to new ideas. There is still more room than probably most other places for an individual, through heroic effort, to make a difference.

Locked Up in Jail

> YF More action: Back in 1964, I took part in a demonstration against the war in Vietnam. A group of protesters sat down in the middle of a street, right in the heart of downtown Chicago. I was the only Asian among them. Arrested, I was locked up in a crowded cage, together with other male protesters, for some 36 hours. I cherish that experience, for now I know what it means to lose one's freedom, if only for a short time.
>
> David Speaking about the Vietnam War, horrors come to mind: napalm that consumed human flesh and bones; "saturation bombing of suspected targets"—in translation, indiscriminate bombing in the absence of reliable intelligence; Buddhist monks who set themselves on fire, as a *nonfinal* act of protest.

Remember Agent Orange? A chemical agent dropped by the tons to defoliate forests, so the North Vietnamese and Vietcong (Vietnamese communists) had nowhere to hide. Now, by the third or later generation, deformed children continue to be born.

> YF I lived through those exciting years—of the civil rights movement, Martin Luther King, protest against the war in Vietnam—as a graduate student in the United

States. While other Chinese students were preoccupied with getting a PhD, a job, and a wife/husband, nearly always in that unchanging order, I became an activist.

Sad to say, America seems to have lost its sense of direction, its compassion for the needy or the oppressed, and its place in the world of nations as a beacon of hope, as it enters into the 21st century. Some say that the American Dream is dead or dying. I feel that one-half of my being is under threat. Trump as a person only sickens me, but I despair over Trump and his followers as a sociopolitical phenomenon (see Chapter 13).

Trumpery, Trumpery, and More Trumperies!

Trump plays his trump to deafen
Our ears. Out on the stump,
With nothing better to say,
Trump trumps up charges of foul play.
The stump speeches Trump makes
Make the Trumpers dull and dumb.
Oh, what great pleasure there will be
To trump and stump Donald Trump!

David So the actions you took on your path to personal liberation were linked to social conflicts in America, not China. In effect, you were saying: Personal liberation derives greater meaning and potency when it is enlarged to include liberation for all humanity. But actions for liberation typically invite suppression. Did you get into any trouble?

YF I suspected that the FBI opened a file on me. After I became naturalized, I exercised my right to request access to surveillance information gathered on citizens. The FBI sent me a copy of my file. How disappointing: There was nothing in it about myself that I didn't already know! Nonetheless, it was a concrete demonstration of how the United States is run by the rule of law, and how the individual may stand undiminished against the might of government.

Some years ago, I visited Vietnam. I fired an AK-47; none of the bullets hit their target. I crawled into a tunnel where the Vietnamese used to live for extended periods of time and fought the Americans with untold sacrifice; I felt extremely uncomfortable after only some 20 minutes.

I made it a point to go around asking how people felt about the war and Americans. This is what Chinese people call octogrammic (*bagua*, meaning nosy) investigation. I found no trace of hatred or animosity toward Americans! The people actively practice forgiveness. I suspect that being Buddhist has much to do with it.

Encounters with Prejudices and Discrimination

There was yet another challenge that I had to face in my age of turbulence. Prejudices and discrimination against Asians in North America during my student days were more pronounced and overt than they are today. Readers who would like to know how I faced them may see Chapter 2.1 "Ethnic Stereotypes, Prejudice, and Identity: An East-West Dialogue" in *Rewriting Cultural Psychology: Transcend Your Ethnic Roots and Redefine Your Identity* (Ho, 2019a).

I had my share of unpleasant experiences. One, in particular, threatened my personal safety. In 1956, a summer job landed me on a construction site in Canada, working as a laborer. Immediately I found myself met with unconditional rejection and hostility. The workers ganged up to bully the teenage Asian, alone in their midst, with menacing threats of physical violence. I stood my ground, although I knew I could have been hurt seriously. Fortunately, physical violence did not materialize; unfortunately, I was fired.

In my freshman year in Canada, a female student refused to sled down a slope on the same toboggan with me during a group outing in the snow. (Other students disapproved of her behavior.) I tasted the first rejection by the opposite sex. To a teenage boy, rejection by males is no comparison with rejection by females.

A few years later, upon learning that my elder brother had found a Canadian girl he intended to marry, I wrote him a letter (30 March 1959): "You know I have never been against interracial marriage. . . . It demands exceeding firmness and courage, especially when you may find yourselves alone against society. . . . We need pioneers to open the way toward . . . material progress, spiritual well-being, and universal brotherhood."

> **David** Significantly, you saw interracial marriage as a natural avenue for achieving all kinds of good things for humankind.
>
> **YF** At the same time, I sensed that the marriage would be opposed and run into difficulty. Sure enough, my apprehension was not groundless. Subsequently I received a letter from my brother (3 March 1960), informing me of "a tremendous change" in his life: "[My girlfriend] told me that we should part. The reasons: 1) She is not mentally strong enough to be insulated from violent family opposition and social pressure, 2) I am 'too good' for her in 'every way'; she is incapable of 'catching up' with me."

I also experienced racism in academic-professional circles. An example is the use of medical term "mongolism" or "Mongolian idiocy," a misnomer with pointed racist overtones. The term has been largely replaced by Down syndrome. One of my most memorable experiences speaks to this very point. In a clinic for children with cognitive impairment, where I had my first job as a psychologist, I examined hundreds of children with Down syndrome and counseled their parents. One day, during a consultation session, the head of the clinic suddenly asked me how I felt about the term "mongolism," which was still commonly used. Mentally unprepared, I lied and told her that I didn't care—to avoid further embarrassment. To this day, I still feel embarrassed that I resorted to lying.

As a budding psychologist, I formulated a relationship: As understanding approaches infinity, condemnation and bitterness drop to zero. The rationale: There are always reasons that account for why people act in foolish, destructive, or self-destructive ways; once the reasons are fully understood, it would be pointless to condemn (oneself or others) or to be embittered.

This formulation acknowledges that there are fools who do foolish things in the world. The important thing is to remind oneself not to be one of them: "I am the one who might become no less of a fool, when I dwell on the negativity of fools and suffer unnecessarily"; and equally, "I will become more of a fool than I am now, if I persist in dwelling how much of a fool I have been."

Although I did not think of it as such then, this formulation strikes me now as a workable way to approximate enlightenment. It has evolved into forgiveness as a coping strategy for those who have to face life's misfortunes I have articulated in my late professional life (see Appendix B). Needless to say, the formulation does not always work because our understanding is nowhere near infinity.

Nevertheless, I have benefited greatly when I do apply it. My unpleasant experiences from prejudices have not made me bitter, diminished my faith in universal brotherhood, or derailed me from my path to world citizenry.

I say to myself, "There are always bad or uninformed people in any ethnic or national group who need to be educated." I simply define prejudices against me as an educational problem, to be linked to the larger context of intercultural understanding. In a letter to a Canadian friend (1 Feb 1961), I wrote, "I see bridging the gulf of misunderstanding between the East and the West as a sacred mission. . . . We need people who are well acquainted with both sides."

Uprooting Myself from Chinese Culture

David "Gulf of misunderstanding" and "sacred mission" are expressions laden with emotion. I sense a deeper psychological meaning here. You came from a broken family; your parents had been separated since you were a child of ten years.

I have two cultural parents, Chinese and American. Certainly I don't want to relive the pain of separation, this time between my cultural parents. So I "transform pain into strength," as a Chinese saying puts it, to preserve their marriage, a marriage of cultures. In doing so, I deal with an internal psychological conflict through directing my energy outwards for a worthwhile cause.

My extracurricular activities, such as engineering a revolution in a mental hospital and being jailed for antiwar protest, are integral to my education in America. These activities have undoubtedly contributed to making me a new person.

> **YF** However, they pale in comparison with cultural uprooting. While working in the mental hospital, I made the drastic decision to uproot myself from Chinese culture! This was the most radical of my decisions in life. Why such a drastic measure? Because I thought that it was necessary if I wanted to be true to my chosen profession: Rid me of the cultural roots that breed psychological illiteracy. For several years, I had little or no contact with Chinese people. I spoke only English, even in my dreams. The psychology I absorbed into my being was devoid of Chinese content.

Uprooting oneself from one's culture is not something I would recommend to other people without great caution. It is probably irreversible. Moreover, it does not mean rooting oneself in another culture. Neither Eastern nor Western: That makes a marginal person.

For years, I walked on tightropes, continually trying to balance myself between conflicting demands. After much anguish, I acted to transform marginality into strength. I began to look at the East and the West alike with both attachment and detachment. I worked to absorb the best and discard the worst from both worlds, even to create an East-West synthesis. Since then, I stand in and out of the two worlds with greater ease. Values are no longer anchored in any one culture. To serve as an agent for intercultural understanding has become a cardinal motive that impels my lifework. Still rootless, I have become a world citizen.

Reverse Culture Shock in an Anachronistic University

After an unbroken absence of 12 years, I returned to Hong Kong as a liberated, transformed person, imbued with democratic, egalitarian values strengthened by my North American experiences. I cherished the opportunity to serve as an agent of East-West understanding. The stark reality, however, was that Hong Kong remained what it had always been: mercantile and colonial.

> YF   I sense trouble. Going overseas for higher education was no culture shock. My student days in North America were formative of my worldviews. In contrast, my reentry into Hong Kong was traumatic. The society where I was born and raised had become alien to me. Nothing had prepared me for the shock of reentry. My academic career was marked by contradictions and agonies.
>
> David   The University of Hong Kong, where you worked, was dense with anachronism. Hoity-toity Oxbridge pretensions and Mandarin scholasticism (some say academic warlordism) were marital partners made in heaven. External examiners, mostly from the UK, descended on the local scene, to be treated like overlords. American scholarship was treated with condescension, as second class ("The American doctorate is equivalent to the British master's degree" was uttered with predictable regularity—a defensive reaction to the threat of increasing American dominance and corresponding decreasing British status). Chinese language and learning were relegated to third-class status.
>
> YF   An English lecturer in philosophy once asked, "Is there such a thing as philosophy in Taiwan?" Status distinctions were nonnegotiable, as in the glorious days of Empire. Even washrooms were differentially marked for "gentlemen" (reserved for senior staff) and for "boys" (reserved for minor staff). Pomp and circumstance received more attention than intellectual pursuits. I saw precious little evidence of universities functioning as centers of East-West learning or intercultural exchange. Most expatriates led self-imposed ghetto-like lives, with little or no meaningful interaction with the local people, as if they had never left their home country. They had no need and were unable to converse in the local language (Cantonese), even after having lived in Hong Kong for decades.

All these factors make good material for a case study of how intelligent and knowledgeable people can be self-encapsulated. The University of Hong Kong was a place of racial separation and thinly disguised racial discrimination. Entering the Senior Common Room, into which minor staff were not admitted, you would find with few exceptions the expatriates in one quarter and the local Chinese in another. Expatriate (mostly British) staff had generous perks (e.g., heavily subsidized housing, paid long-term leave) that local (i.e., Chinese) staff did not have. Of course, such discrimination was rationalized on high principles that most people today would find blatantly hypocritical.

Thus, colonialism corrupted academic institutions, which corrupted the academic staff that in turn, acting as negative role models, corrupted the students.

Even by design, it would be difficult to achieve the efficiency with which these institutions produced students with a turtle-like syndrome: refusing to stick their necks out, speak up, or act like young adults with a vision or passion for living.

> **David** Inequality in political, military, and economic power between ethnic groups produces unhealthy intergroup relations and breeds prejudices. What were the relations like?
>
> **YF** Unhealthy intragroup relations as well. I had never encountered so much emotional masking, distancing, and frigid embitterment. On the face of a self-proclaimed "world-class" professor was written his untold story: Every maxillofacial muscle was twisted, betraying inner rage. I shuddered when I saw him, even though we never exchanged a word.

When I first arrived at the university, I had the habit of greeting colleagues spontaneously. Some responded with a mixture of hesitation, embarrassment, condescension; some with autistic-like avoidance of eye contact. Some people showed determination not to allow collegial relationships to move an iota closer, no matter how sincerely I tried. I experienced unconditional rejection, without being given any opportunity for interaction—possibly because I did not belong to their clique.

Academics at the University of Hong Kong excelled in games of one-upmanship. One such game was peculiarly popular: treating you as if you did not exist. On quite a few occasions, I interacted with some expatriate colleague at a party, only to find later that the same colleague behaved as if he had never seen me before. A scholar from Japan invited some expatriates to a banquet; on the next day, one of them did not "recognize" his Japanese host from the evening before. Chinese colleagues played the game as well, apparently having acquired the requisite mindset from their expatriate counterparts. To an educator, most disconcerting was to witness students emulating their teachers—pretending upon seeing their teachers that they did not exist, especially after graduation.

There were moments when I doubted my sanity. Social validation reassured me that I was not the one insane. Friends, both Chinese and non-Chinese, shared with me similar experiences they had. Painfully I learned to adjust my emotional temperature in the midst of a refrigerator. I learned to value the resilience of many of my colleagues and students; they were exemplars of being sane in "insane" places.

Before turning to a more pleasant topic, I must make clear my intent: to indict evil conditions that produce toxic relations in which human nature is warped. Nothing I have said implicates individuals, expatriate or local, as evil. As an interesting postscript, Hong Kong, unlike Singapore and India, shows little vestige of Anglophilia after the end of colonial rule.

Now times have changed. There are indications of exchange on a more egalitarian basis and an increasing flow of knowledge in the East-to-West direction. These indications reflect a changing global balance of economic prowess. If history is a guide, political and military might will eventually follow.

The Golden Age of My Life

Fast forward to the years from 2003 to 2007, which I say is the golden age of my life. The age is golden not because it came during the "golden years" of old age, but because of three developments. First, my work environment could not have been better; my relations with coworkers were warm and mutually satisfying. Second, I derived great joy from teaching and felt affirmed as an educator. Third, my literary-artistic impulses, long repressed, found expression. Of great significance is the fact that the golden age is also the period during which four of my episodes of madness occurred. This runs counter to the usual pattern wherein abnormal conditions occur during periods of stress, traumatization, or depression.

> YF   In the summer of 2003, I was invited to join the faculty in a teaching and research center at the University of Hong Kong. Thus began the golden age of my life, at least as far as work was concerned. I was freed from administrative duties and conflicts arising from vested personal interests that abound in academia. I was above the fray of backstabbing and petty power struggles that were all too common elsewhere in the university.
>
> David   For decades, your working environment could be described as an emotional refrigerator, with temperatures sometimes dropping to those of a freezer. There, one could observe self-contained individualism in a not-so-collectivist Chinese society: academics locked in their offices, caring little about their colleagues, passing each other by in the hallway often without greeting or acknowledging the other's existence.

Looking Forward to "Play" While Working

> YF   Here, in contrast, the atmosphere at work couldn't be better. So coming to the center was like diving into a hot spring from an icy cave. I have had many appointments in diverse locations: Canada, the continental United States, Hawaii, the Philippines, Taiwan, mainland China, and, of course, Hong Kong. The center surpassed them all. It was like a family, where people really cared for one another. At lunch, we would eat together, making jokes. I never

laughed so much, so heartily in all my life. If laughter be the measure, then it was surely the happiest time I have had. My relations with coworkers were excellent. I maintained no distinctions based on status or age.

David It appears that Daoist ideas of spontaneity and "the equality of all things" underlie the golden age of your life, particularly with regard to removing psychological barriers stemming from differences in status. Generally, you find putting on professorial airs, all too common by academics in Chinese societies, to be distasteful. . . ..

YF My spontaneous, mischievous ways were a source of collegial joviality. My coworkers viewed me as humorous, scholarly, and talented. I didn't mind being the object of laughter, most often because of my well-known gullibility. I was not easily offended. In short, my coworkers, most of whom were much younger than I was, viewed me as a jovial, harmless father figure they could trust. To many, I was their unofficial mentor. (By mutual consent, they refer to me privately as their Black Market Mentor.) Each day, I would look forward to going to work—actually to "play" while working.

David I can't resist saying the obvious. In some ways, you match the stereotype of a nerdy professor. For instance, you don't normally dress like a professor, do you? How did your coworkers react to your nerdiness?

YF I attach more importance to what's underneath the clothes I wear than to clothing. I hate shopping, especially for clothing. That's enough to prompt many a student to buy me articles of clothing as gifts. I feel rich, not impoverished, no matter what I wear. However, my work at the center involved meeting VIPs, local and overseas. So it was fitting for me to pay more attention to my attire. My coworkers were all too ready to help. A trendy research assistant volunteered to accompany me for a shopping excursion. The end result: Not a trace of nerdiness could be found anymore.

A Self-Liberated and Transformed Teacher

David I wish attaining enlightenment could be that easy. What about your role as a teacher?

YF As a teacher, I felt liberated and affirmed. In a message to several of my close relatives about workshops I conducted (22 May 2005), I wrote: "People were moved to tears, transformed. They gained self-respect. They learned to communicate more effectively, and less defensively. They dared to do things they had never done before (like speaking before a large audience, confronting their hidden selves). They began to face life with renewed conviction."

In no small measure, they were touched by my intellectual, moral, and spiritual presence. It gives me great comfort that I have brought greater happiness to the world through my actions.

David	It sounds as if you were self-liberated. In teaching, as in therapy, one cannot liberate others unless one is self-liberated first. Self-liberated from perfectionism, you encourage your students to accept and not to conceal their imperfection at the expense of authenticity. Having greater courage to be yourself, however imperfect, you insist on their being authentic.
YF	In a message I wrote to my students (27 Sept 2006), I stated: "You are what you are, always. Everything you say or do reveals what you are as a person, imperfect, with your strengths as well as foibles. In a sense, therefore, it is impossible not to "self-disclose." Better to be an imperfect, but real, therapeutic agent than to play the phony role of a counselor."
David	Acceptance of imperfection facilitates authenticity by reducing the need to conceal one's imperfection behind a facade. That's a central idea implied in your message. You abhor spurious role playing among helping professionals. Authenticity ranks no less in ordinary life as in therapy. But I must also ask: Do you know how much students may be scared of you?
YF	Of course. They come into my office like scared rabbits or mice seeing a cat, formal, stiff, uneasy. But I am no cat. I dislike status distinctions, and I don't humiliate students, ever. Those who are not afraid of me have no problem.

My standards are high. My logic is as sharp as a knife. And I speak my mind. That makes me enough of a cat to make a student feel like a little mouse. On top of that, one of my teaching assistants once said to me point-blank: "You look too solemn. You don't smile much. So students find it hard to approach you, even though you are actually approachable. Remember to smile!" I listened, and I was thankful. She was one of those who weren't afraid of me.

David	So you like those who aren't afraid of you. What about those who are? As a psychologist, you ought to know how strong an emotion jealousy can be.
YF	Oh, yes. Some years ago, I became aware of a strange "scale of favor" my clinical psychology students once invented. It was like the Hang Seng Index, except that instead of tracking the Hong Kong stock market it purported to track the favor I showed to specific students on a daily basis. This home-made scale came to me as a wake-up call. I do have a problem of being too transparent. When I like someone, I make no effort to hide my feelings. That can be a problem for a group I interact with intensively.

On one occasion, a student gave me this wise counsel: "In a group situation, it's best if members feel that your attention is evenly divided." It could have come only from a woman. After much reflection, I changed some of my ways. But it is liberation from guilt and self-doubt that has truly enabled me to seize the opportunity to educate, now that external circumstances have changed for the better.

David As a high-impact teacher, you have heavy responsibilities. You must remain sensitive to the fact that many students yearn for your recognition—just as your daughters need their father's approval. Finally, you have mellowed, much like a fully-flavored fruit asking to be plucked from a tree. This enables you to become far more effective, influential, and inspirational as a teacher. The courage to be your true self, in and out of the classroom, holds the key.

YF I maintain correspondence with my students after formal teaching has terminated. Here is one of the email messages I received: "It's always a pleasure to read your emails (and of course a bigger pleasure and honor to attend your class) … I am so impressed by your knowledge, wit, and heart." Another one says, "You already are our master-mentor-friend. I do not have any doubt about it." And another, "Indeed, your teaching has touched my life and I will always bear that in mind." These are messages that have sustained me, even in my darkest moments.

David You define a facilitative teacher-student relationship as *the relational context in which the student and the teacher discover, apply, and generate knowledge.* This relationship forms the source from which teaching and learning proceed. A facilitative relationship has to be created; it is not present at the beginning. Creating this relationship is a joint endeavor. The act of creation transforms its creators. In an important sense, then, learning is self-learning, and education is self-transformation.

YF My priorities are to be, in ascending order, a clinical psychologist, psychologist, social scientist, scientist, educator, thinker, writer, person of integrity. I want to be a member of the human family dedicated to ecumenical ideals, an educator committed to whole-person development, a social scientist with broad intellectual interests, a psychologist with research and clinical skills. Humility comes from knowing how far I have fallen short of realizing my ideals.

Liberation from the Repression of Artistic-Literary Impulses

David Your golden age is an age of generativity during which you direct your energy to guide and nurture younger generations, such as mentoring budding colleagues and touching the lives of students. There is still another side of you, long unrecognized. "Be the artist that you are": That's the inner voice you have been hearing, most loudly during your golden age.

YF Actually, I heard this inner voice no less loudly in my student days in North America. It subsided after I returned to Hong Kong and became absorbed in my academic career. For years, I did not think of myself as artistic in temperament.

A visit to my historical self, however, contradicts this assessment. As a Chinese student in the United States, I did many things that were singularly unusual. I went dancing on the south side of Chicago, where I found myself the only non-African-American present. I also took up folk dancing. The music of the Middle East got into my blood after a while.

Once I went to a folk dance camp and danced for three days and nights, with little rest. My body was dead tired, but the music drove me onwards. I love music and dancing, but I never thought I had much artistic talent. And I still don't think I have. Fortunately, talent is not necessary for reveling in the performing arts, as I have said to my students:

> I would rather be a third-rate musician or performing artist than a first-rate psychologist. But, without talent, what could I do? This is why I stand before you today as your psychology teacher. Please don't look at this negatively. For, to know and accept one's limitations is the beginning of wisdom.

The episodes of madness, in which heightened aesthetic sensibilities, self-expression, and ecstasy figure prominently, have reawakened my artistic impulses. On account of this alone, I would have reason to be grateful. But there is more: the artistic impulses have joined forces with my literary bent, which I discovered only several years before my first episode. It was as late as December 1995 that I attempted to wrote my very first poem.

Rewriting the Golden Rule

Pronominal reversals
Are symptomatic of infantile autism.
What audacity it is,
Therefore, to rewrite the Golden Rule,
"Do unto others as you would have others do unto you,"
By a humble pronominal reversal,
And end up with "Do unto others
As *others* would have *you* do unto them."

Yet, this humility brings forth
The karma of selflessness.
And self-consciousness, now wedded
To the Dao of empathy,
Has taken a quantum leap.

Untutored, I was groping in the dark. A few more years brewed before I took writing poetry seriously, and many more meandered before I began to take myself seriously as a writer. Actually, however, my literary bent had been present, though not cultivated, long before that. I have always loved Chinese poetry. But I never dreamed that I had the ability to write poetry, in Chinese or English.

My interest in literary pursuits, creative writing in particular, is negatively correlated with my interest in academia. Increasingly, I find writing for scholarly journals unbearably dreary. It drains me of the energy and time that I would rather spend on more meaningful activities, such as writing this book. During Mania 2, I did a free association in which I wrote about the escape from the compulsive perfectionism in writing I have long suffered from.

> **David** Ordinarily, you impose on yourself the task of making everything easier for the reader: to connect and organize ideas in ways that allow them to flow smoothly and logically; to anticipate the reader's reactions, queries, or doubts; to save the reader time by high-density writing, to pack as much as possible in the least number of words; to double check the factual accuracy of contents; and so forth.
>
> Readers of this book may have sensed this perfectionism by now. In all, the episodes have forced you to realize that temperamentally you are much closer to the artist than to the academic. To that extent, you have not been leading an authentic existence. Your desire to be an artist in living and relating has found expression in your golden age. Surely this is a milestone in your personal journey of spiritual discoveries.
>
> **YF** I did worry that the golden age would not last long. It was simply too good to last. I was determined to enjoy it as much as possible while it lasted. And in fact, by the summer of 2005, the environment at work began to decline. Some left the center under unhappy circumstances. By the summer of 2007, when I left the center, also under unhappy circumstances, the golden age had ended.

From Marginality to World Citizenship: The Will to Master

Now that I have given my life account from childhood to the golden age, it's time to reflect. To pursue a career in clinical psychology, to be politically active, to be immersed in American culture, for instance, were almost unheard of among overseas Chinese students in the 1960s.

Of the things I have said, cultural uprooting stands out because it is so drastic. Yet I don't reject myself as a Chinese, and I am not anti-Chinese. In fact, I am proud of the treasure trove of Chinese history and culture; I practice Chinese martial arts, and I love Chinese poetry.

David   This has to be pointed out, if only to rectify the misleading impression of being anti-Chinese you might have given on account of your critical comments about Confucianism. Please expand and clarify on this point.

YF   To be precise, I was uprooting myself from Confucianism, rather than Chinese culture per se. After my return to Hong Kong, I dug deep into my cultural roots. The result: I felt more holistic as a Chinese person. By then, however, being Chinese is only a part of my identity as a world citizen; being American figures prominently in that identity.

David   The will to master marginality leads only to world citizenship. World citizens live in appreciation of diversity.

YF   But I also tend to be more critical of the "ugly Chinese" when I live in China and of the "ugly Americans" when living in the United States. In the midst of Hypomania 8, I wrote: "I sometimes get the feeling that Americans treat dogs better than humans. In the past I have also heard remarks made by Chinese people that they would rather be a dog in America than a human in China" (9 April 2010).

The Joys and Pains of Being Bicultural

David   Such musing is indicative of the comfort you feel in being a Chinese American. So is this is a happy answer to the question of who you are, Chinese or American? Have you achieved an integrated identity?

YF   Not quite entirely happy. Being bicultural magnifies my being atypical and different from others. It is certainly an asset, but it also complicates my life, particularly in terms of interpersonal relationships.

I don't mean I have a fragmented identity, with divergent aspects of itself in uneasy coexistence. I do have one foot rooted comfortably in Chinese culture and the other in Euro-American culture. These two cultures are synthesized in my mind, such that the specter of a schism between them would not arise. I switch between the two with ease, functioning appropriately depending on the cultural background of the people I interact with. Rather, my unhappiness refers to complications in communicating and relating with other people that being bicultural can bring. I experience anguish when I wish others to fully understand me as a bicultural person.

David   You are expecting too much! Being so fully understood rarely happens, unless you are in the company of people who have been immersed in both cultures. Be prepared that, most of the time, you are going to be only half-understood. People from a Chinese background would have trouble comprehending your American side; likewise, people from a Euro-American background would have trouble comprehending your Chinese side. Moreover, you will find yourself often caught in reciprocal stereotypes and prejudices that people from one background have toward those from the other.

YF A highly educated Chinese woman decided to terminate her brief acquaintance with me after I sent her some materials I had written on intercultural interaction. The reason: She found American culture alien to her and was apprehensive about the cultural distance between us. This happens rarely; in fact, most people I know view my bicultural background favorably. Nonetheless, being bicultural can be a cursed predicament; and it is difficult to explain the anguish it may bring, especially to people without a bicultural background.

David This accounts for why you want so much "to serve as an agent for intercultural understanding." You envision the day will come when bicultural or even multicultural persons are no longer viewed as marginal individuals but as models for advancing world citizenship. In this connection, psychologists speak of multicultural competence. I don't think competence can be achieved without having a solid self-identity and self-esteem to begin with; at least, competence would be much more difficult to attain.

Self-esteem is as important as it is badly misunderstood. It's important because without it you would not dare to engage in dialogues (or play Ping-Pong) with your teachers or supervisors. Lacking in self-esteem, we would be misers in both giving and receiving: not knowing how to show or to respond to appreciation. Worse still, we might be lavish in belittling others. It's misunderstood because educators and therapists often confuse the promotion of self-esteem with that of self-deception (e.g., saying to a child, "You can do whatever you set out to do," irrespective of the child's aptitudes).

YF From this perspective, the self-esteem movement in America is largely misguided. There are cultural differences: People in the United States are more generous and direct in giving compliments than people in Chinese societies. In the United States, sometimes I take with a grain of salt compliments people give me. In Hong Kong, some former students tell me, rather unexpectedly, how they have been influenced by what I had done or said years before; that makes me very happy. Self-esteem has not been much of a problem for me. Trouble comes with episodes of madness, during which my self-esteem becomes inflated.

David More fundamental than self-esteem is the will to master. Self-esteem grows out of achieving a sense of mastery in life—not to be equated with the Confucian preoccupation over scholastic, occupational, or any other kind of achievement. It requires patience and hard work. Being appreciated by significant others for what one is and what one has done helps to foster its growth.

But self-esteem based on empty slogans, "positive reinforcements" given mechanically or unconditionally, and other artificial means rests on a pile of loose sand. Feelings of self-doubt and self-torment can no more be decreed out of consciousness than self-acceptance be decreed into existence. They do not necessarily imply an absence of self-esteem. They are an essential part of human experience; they may be restructured into a new, kinder concept of the self. If they activate the will to master and impel us to take constructive *actions*, then they too have a positive value.

> YF   I accept the generalization that Asians tend to lack self-esteem vis-à-vis Americans, just as Americans lack modesty vis-à-vis Asians. I therefore pray that there will be more promotion of self-mastery and modesty, less of self-deception in the United States; more of self-esteem, less of shaming and self-debasement, in Chinese societies.
>
> David   You have had plenty of unpleasant experiences, such as being rejected on account of prejudice or racism, on your path to world citizenry. In view of these experiences, how has the will to master developed in your personal journey?

There are experiences for which the word "unpleasant" would make a gross understatement. My encounters with discrimination, racism, and rejection during my student days in North America were hurtful, but they did not damage my self-esteem or self-identity. Observing self-rejection by members of my own group was harder to bear than rejection by an external group.

Witnessing self-rejection by my own mother was the hardest of all. Embedded in her utterances were subtle, infiltrating messages that Chinese were inferior to Americans and that Chinese-Americans would always be second-class citizens. This was ultimate self-rejection that shook my self-identity to its core. I got really angry, enough to write to her (25 Dec 1965):

> Maybe you like Americans better than we poor Chinese. . . . Why bother with the backward Chinese? The hell with self-respect, as long as we are in America. We Orientals are inferior; but that is all right, as long as we . . . have a degree to make money.

> David   In fairness to your mother, to be able to live in America by any means and to "have a degree to make money" were (and are still) common preoccupations among Chinese people.

YF	But self-rejection is something else. I knew that nothing would change my mother's attitude or put an end to her messages of racial self-degradation. This did not prevent me from trying. Predictably the result of trying to move an immovable object with an unstoppable force was more frustration and anger, sometimes reaching volcanic proportions. The unstoppable force for change inside me was simply no match for my mother's immovability. This was an engine that made my early adulthood more turbulent than it already was. I was almost driven mad. Ironically, around that time I was working as a psychologist in a mental hospital. The thought of my being locked up there, with a change of roles from staff to patient, did arise.
David	Readers may rest assured that it was just an entertaining thought.
YF	Besides, if I were to become "insane," I would still know enough about insanity to conceal it from detection by psychiatrists—just as easily as to feign insanity to get myself locked up in insane places.

Cut the Chain from Rejection to Self-Rejection

David	Admitting the need for change is a beginning, if not a battle half won. But as you have probably found after many costly lessons, changing yourself is difficult enough; changing another person may well be impossible when that person sees no need or doesn't want to be changed.
YF	At least changing myself is under my own control; changing another person is not. So eventually I abandoned my utterly futile, even counterproductive, attempts at changing my mother. Out of necessity, I redirected my "unstoppable force" to reconstruct my self-identity, onwards to self-mastery. Coming face-to-face with self-rejection strengthened my resolve to go through with cultural uprooting. This was the most formidable task I had ever undertaken. It entails undoing the past, ridding myself of unwanted familial and cultural viruses in my mind. In particular, I performed a kind of psychological surgery, to identify and extirpate the pernicious *influences* of my mother's messages one by one from my mind and cleanse my soul.
David	Note that this does not involve an erasure of memories: Unlike computers, the human mind cannot rid itself of specific memories. The messages themselves will remain in your mind until the day you die; all you can do is to neutralize their effects.
YF	This realization helps me to formulate my ideas on forgiveness as a therapeutic strategy: To forgive is not only possible but also desirable; to forget *at will* is not only impossible but also undesirable.

One therapeutic weapon I use is to "cut the chain from rejection to self-rejection." Too often, rejection by others activates self-rejection, thus amplifying the damage caused. The chain of progressive self-rejection goes something like this:

I am rejected by others. There must be something bad within me to cause people to reject me. I also reject myself because I am bad. I am a disgrace to my family, to my country, to humankind, and to myself. I am ashamed of myself. Moreover, there is nothing I can do about it. I am not only unloved but also unlovable, even to myself. I can't and I don't love myself. My shame comes with my birth, a mistake to begin with. It is intrinsic to my being and will accompany me until the day I die. Therefore, my self-rejection is total, unconditional, and unalterable.

Shame accompanies the rejected self; it aggravates self-rejection, resulting in yet more shame. It may penetrate into the core of one's being, and is much more difficult to deal with than guilt.

The possible conditions leading to shame are much broader than in the case of guilt: One can feel ashamed of not only one's thoughts and actions, but also one's body (e.g., lack of attractiveness), incompetence (despite having tried one's best), humble condition in life, heritage, and country. Shame may be experienced under conditions over which we have no control, and hence personal responsibility is not necessarily involved.

Note that the "progressive self-rejection" above mentions nothing about what the person involved has done wrong. The effects of shame can be pervasive and devastating. They may persist like a psychic scar, for which there is no easy prescription for healing. "Cutting the chain from rejection to self-rejection" would be a workable prescription, because putting an end to self-rejection destroys the underground factory in which shame is manufactured.

YF It is not enough just to remove the negatives; I need to be pulled forward by positive visions. I reaffirm my belief in the dignity of each and every person, without exceptions. This augments my "unstoppable force." So, positive visions are essential to the will to master.

David Going a step further, I would say that spirituality is based primarily on the pursuit of the most positive of goals, rather than on negating the negatives. It is the well-spring from which selfhood and identity grow into maturity; it guides the formation of worldviews; it confers meaning and adds color to life. For psychohistory, a more significant question concerns how collective experiences figure in your personal identity and esteem. Chinese people have suffered repeated insults to their national and ethnic pride in modern history.

YF "No dogs and Chinese allowed" was a sign erected in a park in one of the foreign concessions in Shanghai. It probably did more damage to the Chinese national psyche than anything else ever did. Similarly, recent media coverage of Chinese astronauts venturing into outer space shows clearly how they bear a heavy burden: Failure would result in a collective loss of face. As it turns out, their success, far from personal, brings pride to the Chinese people as a whole.

So, you see self-esteem is not entirely a personal matter. Individual identity is interwoven with collective identity. Each partakes in the pride of the collective and bears its humiliation. Even now, the collective Chinese identity still runs deep in my psyche. I am not totally a world citizen—at least not yet.

My Spiritual Journey Is Incomplete

I felt affirmed as a teacher-educator and that my literary-artistic impulses found expression sometime during my golden age. However, the more I dig into my past, the more I find that the germs of spirituality may be discerned much earlier. Going through my personal papers one day, I found a letter of recommendation (5 Oct 1959), written on my behalf by Professor Breen, the one who introduced me to psychology. In it he wrote, "It is nice to be able to add that his fine qualities are linked to an unusual sense of purpose in life. David genuinely wants to make a contribution to the spiritual well-being of his fellow man."

David To contribute to the spiritual well-being of others is a recurrent theme of your spiritual journey. This is your karma, a Buddhist idea that we will explore further in later chapters. It says that your journey is not an individual undertaking and must involve others. The main ideas that appear recurrently in this interview are personal liberation, will to master, creative synthesis, intercultural fertilization, and psychohistory. That's a lot to digest.

YF The strands of thought do weave into the overarching theme of self-transformation, by which I mean something more than growth. Transformation is quantum change. It is a dynamic process that entails not only quantitative, but also qualitative, change; and not only alterations of previously observed patterns, but also emergent patterns of thought and action that were previously dormant or unobserved. Self-transformation goes a step further: It is self-initiated, self-directed quantum change.

David You summarize and learn from firsthand experiences amassed from your family life, your education in Hong Kong and overseas, your career as a teacher-educator, and your intercultural encounters. Early on, you decided to embark on a course of personal liberation from the constraints of Chinese culture, particularly Confucianism.

The most drastic action I took was cultural uprooting. I then balanced this uprooting with the will to transform my marginal status into strength, and end up being a world citizen dedicated to the betterment of humankind. Creative synthesis of my two worlds, Eastern and Western, plays a crucial role in this process. This is self-transformation, self-initiated and self-directed. Moreover, I am quite conscious of the parallels between my personal transformation and the historical transformation of the Chinese nation as a whole.

YF It hasn't been a smooth process. A lot of fumbling along the way. What has helped *us* move forward is the dialogic action that you (David) and I (YF) have engaged in. Thus, our different selves can work together synergistically. This interview is, in itself, an illustration of how therapeutic dialogic action can be.

David I must draw your attention to a perplexing question. There is hardly anything in your childhood or early adulthood to foretell, or even to suggest, that you would turn "mad" episodically in your later life.

YF That's right. But I did mention obsessive-compulsive traits in passing. In actuality, I have been driven by the desire to resolve the contradiction between compulsivity and creativity virtually all my life. Creativity triumphs over compulsivity during episodes of madness, when artistic-literary impulses are unleashed, especially during my golden age. So the will to creativity is a cardinal force that drives self-transformation, and ultimately enlightenment.

David More and more, you have come to conceptualize self-transformation as part and parcel of your journey of spiritual discoveries. But your journey is obviously incomplete. What kind of self-transformation is it, if you continue to alternate between creativity when you are mad and compulsivity when you are normal?

Enlightenment is holistic: It can be reached when, and only when, creative self-transformation is continually sustained. In the following chapters, we shall see how you confront the contradiction between madness and normality. Particularly in Chapter 6, we shall see how being a world citizen dovetails and blossoms into the idea of spirituality-in-communion.

2

Episodes of Madness: All of Exuberance, None of Depression

A person in a manic state may be quite attractive in some ways, but he might also drive you crazy if he stays manic much longer.

This chapter presents a description of episodes of "madness" I have had. At first, I thought I had only a few. However, as I assembled my records, including diaries, it became clear that the number is significantly higher. I am sure there were no episodes prior to 1997, that is, before I turned 58 years of age.

Here, I should point out that I am using the term *madness* rather loosely. Madness is a nontechnical term that refers, in a broad sense, to mental disorders or abnormal conditions. It lacks specificity and does not refer to a specific disorder. Madness connotes insanity, frenzy, and severity: For instance, psychosis is madness, but we would not refer to a common anxiety disorder, which is mild in relative terms, as madness.

In my case, at no point was there any threat of my losing contact with reality or of acting in ways that endangered myself or others. I was never destructive or violent. I remained intensely aware of what was happening in my mind and surroundings. In referring to my case, madness is delimited to mean mania or hypomania.

A hypomanic episode is a period of persistently and unusually elevated, expansive, or irritable mood. Common symptoms include inflated self-esteem or grandiosity, more talkative than usual or pressure to keep talking, subjective experience that thoughts are racing, decreased need for sleep, and excessive engagement in pleasurable activities that have a high risk of adverse consequences (e.g., engaging in unrestrained buying sprees). Social functioning during the episode is clearly uncharacteristic of the person. The mood disturbance and changed social functioning are observable by others.

You may find a person in a hypomanic state quite attractive in some ways, but you might also be driven crazy if he stays hypomanic much longer. He feels unusually high, euphoric, and overly self-confident, coupled with a lack of self-doubt; he can be funny. Disinhibited, he can be too forward or audacious. He talks a lot, at a fast pace, jumping from one topic to another. He's got a lot of energy. You can't catch up with him. Under the influence of inflated self-confidence, his judgment is compromised. In short, he is feeling and acting in ways that are uncharacteristic of his usual self.

From 1997 to 2021, I have had altogether 22 episodes of abnormal mood elevation, occurring on average nearly once a year (see Appendix C for details). Two episodes were the most severe, in some respects reaching mania. By definition, manic episodes are basically similar to but more severe than hypomanic episodes. Psychotic features, like delusions, may be present; there may be marked impairment in social, interpersonal, or occupational functioning.

These features were absent in my case. Furthermore, it was during the most severe episodes that I gained the most dramatic of my extraordinary, mystical experiences: for instance, total access to the unconscious and what Dance Movement therapists speak of as authentic movements, so called because they come directly from the unconscious and are uncensored. In Mania 1, I experienced the empty, selfless self; self-healing of an injured knee; transforming myself into a woman; *willful* hallucination, in which I saw myself vividly on a cross and felt great pathos for the sufferings of humankind. In Mania 2, I performed a free association. Mania 2 was the most costly to me in occupational and social terms.

In the following, I record my struggles and lessons learned. Informed by these lessons, my personal journey continues in quest of spiritual discoveries. The episodes afford me opportunities to gain unhindered access to the unconscious, experience the extraordinary, and glimpse into the mystical-transcendental state of enlightenment. The data on the episodes are drawn, in whole or in part, from diverse sources: epigrams, correspondence, email messages, poems, a free association, internal dialogues, and diaries by myself, most of which were written during or around an episode (diaries and poems are dated whenever possible). Editorial changes are kept to a minimum.

Glimpses into the Mystical-Transcendental

Although they share commonalities, the episodes varied greatly in intensity, duration, and social costs to me. Each has its own individuality. Mania 1, however, stands out particularly in terms of access to the unconscious, extraordinary experiencing, and glimpses into the mystical-transcendental. It is also the episode on which I have the most comprehensive and revealing information, which is now shared with the reader below.

Though lasting no more than two weeks, Mania 1 was probably the most dramatic. Exceeding the hypomanic episodes, this one was serious in terms of social costs. My behavior exceeded what most other people regarded as the bounds of normality. During a staff retreat, I played tricks or antics that annoyed others; I shouted at the top of my voice to demonstrate my *qi* (literally air, breath, meaning energy), in locations where few people were around but where I could still be heard; I had a quarrel with a friend in the middle of night, loud enough to be heard by others.

My colleagues at work, with whom I had formed the most congenial of relationships, became very concerned about me. They knew I had difficulty sleeping during this episode. Afterward, they would become nervous whenever I mentioned sleep disturbances. They had become sensitized to the trigger of my manic-like behaviors. Here is an imaginary dialogue between two of my different selves, David and YF, I wrote around the end of the episode.

David You often refer to your personal experiences. The most private portion of these is a precious resource for gaining insight into the inner workings of the human psyche. What can you share with the reader?

YF I have had the good fortune of gaining the most extraordinary, mystical experiences, each time during a period of about several weeks. My inner-private and outer-social selves merged. The child inside came out. I became unusually playful, spontaneous, disinhibited—in a sense, more genuine.

David To be disinhibited is not valued in Confucian societies, given their emphasis on impulse control and social order. I sensed a willful disregard of social convention when you speak of "good fortune." Rather self-indulgent, you didn't want to bow down to how others viewed your behavior. Perhaps your "mania" represented a rebellion against Confucian control, under which you felt you had suffocated long enough.

Here is an excerpt of what one of my close friends wrote down (translated from Chinese, added comments or explanations in square brackets) about my condition during Mania 1.

> You couldn't sleep. You talked a lot, often with yourself.... From your words, I felt at times you were exceedingly mature; at times innocent, like a child. No matter, whether you were an adult or a child, your thinking was always so genuine; everything uttered came from your heart, expressing your true thoughts... self-confident, praising yourself.... Your blood pressure was high. Your face was radiant, flushed. [On special occasions] you were in a state of complete intoxication, as if you were not in this world, uttering a lot of words of enchantment, like in a nightmare.... Listening to music every day, you let your thoughts and emotions run unbridled, nonstop. You took a pen and wrote [Chinese characters] on paper without stopping, telling me that [different writing styles represented different emotional states]. Sometimes, when you got excited, you would close your eyes, move both hands beating to the music. Or, you might suddenly cry out aloud for a while.... When going out to eat, walk in the street, travel, you were invariably different from the crowd.

I was indeed talkative. I phoned my friends, old and new. Actually, the talkativeness, interspersed with periods of contemplation, was impelled by an intense desire to communicate, to be understood, and to share my newfound self.

David Your professional colleagues thought that your condition met the criteria for hypomania, if not mania: difficulty in falling asleep, emotional lability and intense reactivity, and so forth. They were simply following the psychiatric bible on diagnosis, the *Diagnostic and Statistical Manual of Mental Disorders*.

YF In retrospect, I did cross the boundary of social and cultural acceptability. But I retained the master switch: metacognitive awareness and control of my actions. Critical reflectiveness and scientific doubt were fully operative. I was aware that other people viewed my behavior as weird. However, I caused no harm, to myself or to others—only a great deal of worry to bewildered people close to my life. My impulse control was intact. At no point would I do anything that I considered morally wrong or reckless.

David What was your physical condition?

YF Imbalance: My body was near exhaustion, yet my mind remained active, running on fast time. I was mentally hyperactive. I was thirsty most of the time. I felt hot where others would feel cold. Aware that my energy reserve might be depleted, I moved around slowly. Sometimes, I would half-close my eyes, a conservation technique that I had learned from a yoga master.

David	Your brain's consumption of energy must have been extraordinarily high. Coupled with prolonged sleeplessness, this led to disturbances of cognitive functioning.
YF	At worst, I found it difficult to perform even simple arithmetic. I got confused easily. I could perform only one task at a time. I could be extremely forgetful, like forgetting what I had done or where I had put something just a few seconds ago. At times, I could focus on just one thought at a time. While I was staying focused, I would make myriad associations. The next moment, no trace of what I had just been thinking about could be found. The thought was gone.

I became obsessive about lost memories—lost in the cosmos forever. I tried to record some of my thoughts on paper or in a computer file before they got lost. At some point, I said to myself, "Let go of lost memories. They will come back. Let my mind rest." That helped to put an end to the obsession.

When my energy level improved, I was unusually focused and efficient. At home, I performed different household tasks very efficiently. Often my hands and legs maneuvered and performed complex tasks without conscious direction, as if the "wisdom of the body" had extended to the executive ego: They accomplished what my mind had intended, without deliberation or being aware of its own intention. Freed from obsessive-compulsive tendencies, I read rapidly, without worrying that I might have missed something; unencumbered by perfectionism, I wrote fluently.

David	Perhaps your retrospective account may throw fresh insights into brain functioning. With regard to memory, your forgetfulness probably reflected a disturbance of registration (encoding) and/or storage of information. At the same time, however, retrieval of information already stored in your long-term memory was amazingly efficient.
YF	I enjoyed doing even "tedious" tasks, such as throwing the garbage out. Every second of life was enjoyable. When I was a schoolboy, a Jesuit teacher once said, "You can pray twenty-four hours a day, even when you are brushing your teeth." Finally, I really know what he meant, for I have experienced it. Better still, I felt a sense of tranquility, at peace with myself, at home in the cosmos. I have had my share of self-torment, overattachment, compulsivity, embitterment, which I had tried to overcome for decades. All vanished.

I achieved shamelessness. I became more tolerant and compassionate. I cherished the simple joys of just being alive. Walking around in the streets, I would say to myself, "Life is wonderful. The world is so beautiful." I felt humbled by the commanding heights of human achievement, the vastness of the cosmos. I wrote, in the midst of this period, "Nothing in the cosmos is alien to humans. Therefore, speak not of what is alien." (In response to Terentius, Latin playwright, who wrote "I am human, therefore nothing human is alien to me.")

> **David**   Clearly, your manic period was marked by extraordinary creativity, heightened aesthetic sensitivity, depth of feelings, and deep humility. These positive, delightful features are significant: They define the nature of your mania.
>
> **YF**   The more I knew, the more I became aware of my profound ignorance. Knowledge and humility were like twins. I experienced the near-despair of trying to fathom the infinite with a finite mind.

This prompted me to write the following poem around 2003:

> **Sea of Learning**
>
> The sea of learning
> Knows no bounds.
> No shore in sight
> To return to land,
> I drift on, lost
> In her bosom—
> Only to lift
> From the depths of the deep,
> To receive the love that moves
> Upon the face of the waters.

The poem gives a new twist to the Chinese idiom:

> The sea of learning knows no bounds,
> No shore there is, save diligence.

It also invokes biblical imageries in the opening of Genesis. But love, rather than the Spirit of God? They should be identical. "Lost in her bosom" brings to mind the immortal lines of Tennyson:

> Now folds the lily all her sweetness up,
> And slips into the bosom of the lake:
> So fold thyself, my dearest, thou, and slip
> Into my bosom and be lost in me.

> **David**   The difference is that you long to be "lost in her bosom," rather than inviting her to slip into yours. The deeper meaning I read: Ultimately, salvation comes from love, not knowledge. Along with creativity, you probably experienced

	what psychiatry calls "flight of ideas," or rapid succession of ideas or verbalizations with abrupt shifting from one idea or topic to another.
YF	Definitely, racing thoughts, faster than usual, appeared. Sometimes I was obsessed with losing these thoughts, which I couldn't utter fast enough, let alone put down in writing. Speed was also manifest in an extraordinary sensitivity to cues in social interaction.

Watching films or TV shows provided delightful occasions for predicting the next scene, what the actors would say and do. My predictions showed uncanny accuracy, as if I had overtaken the role of the director. That was empathy: The director and I became one. Probably, I conducted some of my best psychotherapy sessions or workshops, during which my empathy joined forces with the courage to be myself.

Things of beauty appeared in plentiful ways. More precisely, I keenly perceived many things as never before—ordinary things, like people's faces; the sound of running water; tree leaves, through which the rays of the setting sun penetrated.

My friends once showed me a Japanese painting, which instantaneously absorbed my attention. In my early days as a graduate student in clinical psychology, I developed an interest in the clinical use of drawings. Now, that interest was elevated to aesthetic appreciation. I talked with my friends about the aesthetic features of the painting, and in so doing also about the artist endowed with the faculty to create it. I surprised myself, because I never thought I had much capacity for appreciating visual art.

Music evoked strong emotions. Reactions to J. S. Bach were total and could not be described as anything short of spirituality. Tears would flow profusely from my eyes whenever I listened to the *Largo* from his *Violin Concerto in G Minor*. This emotional response was specific to this piece of music and to none other. I was in touch with the deepest pathos—without despair. Real catharsis! Listening to music induced spontaneous movements, involving my head (inside and outside), my limbs, my whole body, and being. My artistic impulses, long subdued, demanded expression. I rebuked myself:

You coward, where is your courage-to-be?
The artist that you are,
To fulfill your potential
In working, living, and relating?

David	As a Chinese saying puts it: "There is no greater grief than the death of one's heart." The capacity for depth of feelings, both positive and negative, versus

	psychic numbing, is the watershed that separates emotional health from sickness. Dysphoric feelings do not necessarily incapacitate. I have long wondered if prolonged inhibition of artistic or creative impulses can lead to neurosis. Dance Movement therapists speak of authentic movements, so called because they come directly from the unconscious, uncensored. Did you experience anything like that?
YF	There were times when the body moved involuntarily. The movements differed from aimless automatism described in neuropsychiatry. They were clearly meaningful, albeit raw, expressions. I liberated myself. I danced. I entered into a state of dynamic meditation. In that state were incorporated elements of hypnotherapy, martial arts, music, dance, meditation, yoga, and qigong, which I had learned imperfectly in past years. I experimented with different forms and techniques. For instance, independently one arm might move slowly and softly, draw an imaginary circle of varying size, and so forth, while the other was doing something different.

I engaged a personal instructor to teach me expressive dance. She did not instruct, but taught through a classic master–disciple relationship, mostly nonverbally. I learned to express myself in ways I had not known before. My body was transformed.

David	My psychologist friend Bruce Bain says that the self-conscious mind is formed through acts of speaking with others and with oneself. This assertion resonates with your ideas about the dialogic self: The self engages in both internal and external dialogues, in the process of which it may participate in its own transformation. Thus, the self has immense potentiality for creative self-transformation, even self-creation. What do your experiences tell us about the dialogic self?
YF	During meditation, at times the self seemed to have vanished. I experienced the no-mind state of emptiness. I felt energy flowing within my body. So I thought of taking advantage of it. Several days before, I injured my left knee; the pain was so bad that I was walking with a limp.

I absorbed sunlight outside to magnify the energy flow and directed it to my injured knee. There was a growing sensation of warmth around the injured area. I visualized a volcano around this area, which magnified the sensation further. Finally, there was only light: The body, together with the self, had dissolved. When I came out of this transcendental state, I found the pain gone. I had healed myself—a tangible benefit that was verifiable to several people who knew about my injury.

On other occasions, vivid images appeared, spontaneously or directed at will. The virtual was experienced as the real. I came as close to willful hallucination as

I had ever. One unforgettable sequence was seeing myself being nailed on a cross, which was lying on the ground. I wanted it to be raised, so I could see things from a vertical perspective. I felt no physical pain, but intense feelings of pathos for the sufferings of humankind.

I felt what Jesus must have felt. (Please don't read this as "I believed I was Jesus.") All these came as close to a transformative, religious experience I have had in my life—up to now, that is. Another sequence was a transgender experience: turning myself into a woman, feeling and acting like one. It was educational, more powerful than any role-reversal game in psychotherapy. I also experienced androgyny, the yin and the yang, united in one body.

David Your phenomenological report serves as a means to glimpse into the mystical-transcendental. One concern I have is that the combined forces of heightened sensibility and intensified emotionality can be hazardous. You may be too easily fired up by ephemeral ideals and thus act impulsively. Or you may be overly attached to, and hence enslaved by, objects of pleasure or beauty.

The Buddhist attitude of nonattachment, however, may keep overattachment at bay: engaged and involved with worldly objects, without being possessive; letting go of fixations. It differs from detachment, which refers to emotional noninvolvement with and disengagement from the world. Where were all these experienced? Were others aware of how unusual they were? Were there differences among the episodes you have had? How did you come out of mania?

YF My unusual experiences occurred mostly at home, in private. Only a few people had intimate knowledge of them. So I didn't appear stranger than what I was already perceived to be. By the present episode, I had learned enough to anticipate what was coming and tried, though unsuccessfully, to avoid behaving publicly in ways that would cause unease in others.

Mania 1 surpassed previous episodes in intensity. But it also pushed me to new heights of artistic expression. Sleep held the key to recovery: I knew I would come out of it if only I could get enough sleep for a few days consecutively. Alas, I also feared that, having succeeded, self-torment and other negatives would return, along with normality.

David A psychoanalyst would say that in your case repression vanished. The unconscious became accessible. Nothing was unthinkable. Your mind functioned with holistic oneness, interconnected. This had the effect of enhancing your aesthetic, empathic, and cognitive capabilities. Retrieval of information and association of ideas were superefficient, so much so that you were overwhelmed

	by your own outpouring of creativity. You became obsessively attached to ideas and objects, including the self. You had no physically aggressive or destructive tendencies, although direct expressions of verbal aggressiveness sometimes exceeded your normal level.
YF	I have now greater insight into what mystical experiences are like. Here is a question to absorb the interest of those in search of enlightenment. How does one maintain optimal balance for extended periods between creative expressiveness and control? That is, exercise adequate control over impulses without the need for repression; get in and out of manic-like states at will.
David	The person who attains such balance would be sage-like, united in body, mind, and spirit; he lives his daily life in accordance with his inner wishes, and acts without transgression. Destructive forces having been harnessed to serve creative purposes, genuine harmony within the self is achieved. Mastery indeed!

I have not been able to duplicate the feats achieved during Mania 1, at least not as dramatically: self-healing, the completeness of the no-mind state of emptiness, or the willful visual hallucinations. The depth into which I had gone was proportional to the extent to which my social relations suffered. The greater the pain, the greater the gain? Can rare and precious experiences be gained without social and emotional costs? This is but one of the issues discernible recurrently in other episodes.

Loneliness and Anguish amid Exuberance

Social costs are incurred when we get carried away by our own intentions and desires, without sufficient regard for the feelings and reactions of others. So even an eccentric has to be mindful of how he is perceived by others. This point was made painfully clear to me in Mania 2. Early in the episode, I wrote in my diary (30 June 2007):

> I must preempt the extreme condition, sleep before I fall into the manic phase, keep the hyperactive sympathetic autonomic nervous system under control, learn to keep my behavior within the bounds of social acceptability.... Eros without thanatos, safe.

Clearly I was apprehensive about falling into "the manic phase"; the "hyperactive sympathetic autonomic nervous system" was the culprit; I thought there was safety in "eros without thanatos," that is, loving without destructiveness or aggressiveness. But I did not succeed in keeping my behavior "within the bounds of social acceptability." I sent out email messages that offended some people, and acted in ways that cost me dearly in occupational and interpersonal terms.

Disinhibition surpassed Mania 1. My words and deeds were expressed more directly, sometimes pointedly or aggressively, than I had before. I probably offended or alarmed quite a few people. However, there was at no point any violence, loss of impulse control, or disregard for the safety or well-being of others. From a positive perspective, I exhibited what Dance Movement therapists call "authentic movement," which I gather means unbridled movement stemming directly from the id without censorship. For the first time in my life, I danced (in private) as a totally uninhibited person, liberated from *all* feelings of shame. My judgment was compromised: I failed to consider adverse consequences that might follow my actions. For instance, I sent an email to my colleagues at work. The following is an excerpt:

> During the last few days, I have been in hiding.. ... For a good reason. I have achieved a quantum leap, self-transformation, at home.. ...Unproductive, random activities are unproductive. Consistently predictable chaos is incurable. Unethical practices here, as in the rest of HKU, must stop. Quality must be restored to qualitative research. (Remember, academic glory should not be measured in catties.) Boundaries, professional/organizational, if not maintained, is anathema to organizational psychology.

That was a dumb move. I miscalculated how the staff would react. "Self-transformation"? To them, it was more likely just another descent into madness. I minced no words in my criticisms of the research and professional work done in the center at the University of Hong Kong where I was working. Most of my colleagues shared my views, which they dared not express openly. My boss was miffed, and terminated my employment. This greatly upset the students I had been teaching.

The social cost to me was the highest among all my episodes. A few of my friends terminated their relationships with me. But what kind of friends were they, considering the fact that none suffered any harm other than embarrassment or apprehension consequential to my actions? They ended our friendship simply because they were bewildered by behaviors they could not, and did not, comprehend. Of course, that's my fault. An eccentric to begin with, I turned myself into an even odder person and in doing so invited others to perceive me in psychopathological terms.

I was humbled by my failure to keep this episode under control. I have yet to learn to modulate my actions to avoid damages to my social image, without dampening creativity and heightened sensibilities. After recovery, the same friend who wrote about my condition in Mania 1 sent me a message, an excerpt of which (translated from Chinese) is reproduced below.

> In your eyes, many people like us all think slow. You always say that your demands are not high; but even these not-so-high demands of yours make people feel they can't meet them. This perplexes you. . . . You lament that people are foolish, selfish; that you are always helping others, but others can't ever help you. . . . You want all academics to excel. So you get really put off when you see some academics you regard as basically incompetent proclaiming they are doing so-called research. . . . Because you are a person who has an extreme passion for living, your taste and demands are extremely high. . . . You are an extremely kind-hearted person; moreover, you treat people with extreme sincerity. That's why often you don't know how to protect yourself; you don't quite understand that sometimes you need to keep your inner thoughts private. Precisely because of your sincerity and trust toward people, you have brought forth a lot of unnecessary troubles. . . . As I said before, better to be your friend than to be your intimate companion by your side. . . .
>
> Your thinking is quick, with leaps and bounds. Your voice is sonorous. You talk primarily about things that you are interested in, not listening or unwilling to listen to others. . . . Regardless of whatever you say, I can feel that your mind is lucid, your thinking is normal. The way you deal with problems during the whole process is logical; however, your thinking is indeed too fast, making it difficult for people to accept you. You've got to know, because of this, you may have indeed given those jealous of you an excuse to make people who don't understand you to be awfully fearful of you. . . . Besides, you have such an unusual, distinct period annually, like a woman's menstrual periods. . . . I hope that you will learn to self-control your "cyclical periods of excessively quick, leaping thinking". . . . You mind is extremely lucid from beginning to end. By your strength of how to conduct your life, you are completely capable of mastering your own behavior, so other people wouldn't find your quick thinking unacceptable. You are completely capable of going up and down, left and right, really "acting according to your wishes." I pray that such a day will soon arrive.

These passages are consistent with my own assessment of my condition during the two manic episodes. I am amused by the analogy of "menstrual periods"; at least menopause is predictable, which is a comforting thought. It is reassuring to hear that my mind was lucid and that I was logical in the way I dealt with problems during the whole episode. But I must also mend some of my ways, such as "not listening or unwilling to listen to others."

My self-perceptions differ from others' perceptions of my mania: I find the experiences inspirational; people around me are worried, perhaps even petrified. This remains a contradiction I have to face. Attending to perceptions by other people about my behavior is no less important to effective social functioning than self-perceptions. The art of persuading without offending *unnecessarily* is what I have to acquire and perfect.

Above all, I must learn to master myself, to "act according to my wishes," without arousing fear and inviting rejection from others. When will such a day arrive? All my life, separations from or departures of friends often evoke transitory feelings of depression in me. I don't like saying good-bye. As I once wrote, "No beginning and no end; so whence the need to say good-bye?"

Mania 2 magnified those depressive feelings, adding to the high emotional costs I had to bear. Devoting most of my time to academic and professional pursuits, I seldom engaged in social activities, other than those involving my colleagues and friends at work. So being cut off from work was a great loss, in terms of not only occupation but also human contact. Living alone at the time rendered me even more socially isolated. My response was to spend a lot of time on telephone conversations, something I would normally not do. The episode was, in large measure, "mania via telephone."

It was time for emotional healing. Out of nostalgia, at the height of the episode, I went back to the Jesuit school for boys that I attended as a child. That visit was a watershed experience in my life. It evoked a lot of memories. One sadistic physical education teacher made me crawl between the legs of the entire class standing in line. I couldn't remember what I had done to deserve such humiliation, but I didn't feel at the time that I suffered any psychological damage, other than embarrassment.

But walking again, in my adulthood, on the sports ground where the incident took place brought forth strong emotions. Seeing that nobody was around, I took off my shoes, feeling the pain from walking on gravel. I cried like I had never cried before: total catharsis. I said to myself: "I have arrived."

Taking Concrete Actions of Caring and Generosity

This was also a time that I extended personal healing to loving thoughts and actions for humanity. I wrote in my diary (30 June 2007): "Return to my original face [nature], love." This theme stands out and reverberates in other episodes. It affirms two core values of spirituality: love and authenticity. Ironically, I am more ready in states of madness than of normality to take concrete actions of caring and generosity. Some examples are offering to pay for the dental expenses of a taxi driver, whose wife is a friend of mine; helping friends in financial need with large sums of money, without expecting repayment.

For a number of years, I had been contemplating the foundation of a philanthropic organization. I finally took action after Mania 2 ended. The organization, named Chizi Institute, was established. The name comes from the *Book of Mencius*, which refers to "the heart of a *chizi* (newborn babe)." The word *chi* means many things: red, bare, loyal, and empty. So the ancients of China used *chizi* to refer to the modern concept of authenticity. "Newborn" or "nascent" are the closest English translations of *chizi* I can think of. What better name could there be? It resonates with "return to my original face." The Institute is devoted primarily to advancing civic-environmental-health education. It supports projects and educational activities aimed at promoting civic values, environmental conservation, and holistic health.

Finally, I made good on the claim of being a world citizen. This is a milestone in my journey of spiritual discoveries. Why focus on civic virtues? Because spirituality is to be realized not just individually but also collectively, by being-in-the-world, no less than in the wilderness. Why environmental conservation? Because an aesthetic environment beautifies the spirit, and a beautified spirit will not pollute the environment. Why holistic health? Because health is holistic in nature, an integration of body-mind-spirit; it is not just the absence of illness or disease.

A Free Association

Incredibly, I have never been able to locate an actual transcript of free association in the psychiatric literature. So it is fortunate that I did a free association (see Appendix C). It was my first and, thus far, only attempt. It was written rather than uttered. Using my computer, I simply typed as fast as I could what came to mind, without attempting to make any corrections. The free association numbers 1,620 words. Here is an excerpt.

> **not** allowed to change a word anticompulsive traininguse this as illustration finally i know how to treat read on, all ye who suffer from sleepless nights cunning [not cunt please] go with the folw do not resist and you will fall asleep try it. . . . Now laugh those of you who are informed if you are indeed informed rm donald ? rumsfel you don't know what you don't know the most brillian man who ever lived now you are really offended right? Go with the flow don

not resist and every vally shall be exalted meaning that in case you don't know what i am talking about this treasure trove . . . enough is enough you have suffered long enough please suffer no more if you would only listen to you inner voice. . ..

i am really tired can't go on i am going to sleep my apology . . . but you see you have been tricked, i am not going to slppe because i don't whqt you to suffer sleepless not anymore read on because you get this opportunioty only one in your life time the see that falls on bareen soil will not grow be kind to yourself after you have been so creel to all your life read on i beg you sat guanranteed . . . not i am not sure i am SURE you have been tricked again and again i guarantee you innumberable time. . ..

i became enlightened have you ever been enlighted i bet you have ? i am not going to insult you yes i am goint o insult you to wak y up from you rslumber ylou have3 ben sleepijg long enough

The excerpt makes clear that I was "**not** allowed to change a single word," as "anticompulsive training." I was "really tired" but could not fall asleep; my strategy was to "go with the folw [flow]" and not to resist. I seemed to enjoy playing tricks on the imaginary reader with opposites, such as "i am not sure i am SURE you have been tricked again and again." Significantly, I told myself to "be kind to yourself after you have been so creel [cruel] to [yourself] all your life"; and I felt "i became enlightened."

Freud devised two avenues to the unconscious. The first, which he called "the royal road to the unconscious," was the interpretation of dreams. The second was free association, the fundamental rule of which is to say whatever comes to mind, regardless of how trivial, irrelevant, irrational, embarrassing, or painful it might be. Unfortunately, I have not been able to locate actual transcripts of free association by clients undergoing classical psychoanalysis. Free association is difficult to do; try it to discover how difficult it can be.

As I look at the entire free association later, it is perhaps more like an outpouring of a stream of consciousness than totally free association. Progressing from the beginning to the end, it becomes increasingly free; the outpouring becomes increasingly uncensored. Discursive thoughts, including flight of ideas, are rampant, and features characteristic of mania may be discerned. Still, the passages are intelligible, arguably more so than some of *Ulysses* by James Joyce (whom I alluded to). There is fragmentation and incoherence, but no confabulation or loss of contact with reality.

On the contrary, in the last sentence I wrote at that time, I showed a capacity to anticipate the reader's reaction: "NOW you must be really **confused** good for you i know it." I also had a playful attitude while reflecting on my writing style in this passage: "Let see who has the last aaugh notice why how already my stuyle changes no english professor can write like i do they will regret it you see highly competive people they don like to see others game of oneupmanship they jealos of their competitors no? i have offended you enough just kidding [i laughing this very moment]." I showed low regard for professors, but held students responsible for allowing their instructors to remain boring:

> Funny professor have been teaching all their life then were students once how come they have never learned to less boring just a little but you think i am curing professuions i was once a PROFESSOR a dime a dozen no i am cursing you the students who allo it to happen respoonsibility.

This is coupled with disdain for the counseling profession (not to be confused with disdain for counseling itself): Therapists "are a hopless bunch." I confessed that I never read a book in counseling "from cover to cover," implicating counseling texts as boring, intellectually bankrupt. I mentioned some negative aspects of American society: "Salemen in the United States those blasted psychopaths who sell thir mothers for a dime." George Bush is singled out for attack:

> He will come down a the worst p in US history asndnow the rest of the world is very very angry with you why becase you had the aufacity to elect an idiot you have only yours to bl American have short mem.

Animosity, however, was reserved for arrogant Brits: "Damn the brits arrogant SABs [SOBs] who not that long ago felt so superiot to americans." In all, I had critical-aggressive-hostile as well as lewd impulses: "cunt," "fucking shit [first time in my life, deep apoloty if i have offended you but i don't mind if i had indeed offended you]." I was aware of megalomania and acknowledged the explosion of creativity as I free associated: "Megalomanic this is what i m racing thoughts pass through my head a explosion of creativty." Toward the end, positive themes of struggle with compulsivity, self-transformation, and benefiting mankind appear: "Breakthoughtsd self-transformation . . . i really have struglle hard resis compulsity all my life 'i am dead tired but i can't let this these thoughts be lost forever without their benef mankind.'"

What have I learned about my unconscious? Not much, if anything, that I don't already know. I am not negating the value of free association. After years of self-analysis, and especially having gone through previous episodes, I have already gained ready access to my unconscious. Nonetheless, to me the free association is quite an achievement; in particular, never before have I expressed my lewd or hostile impulses so blatantly (in words, not deeds).

Aesthetic Sensibilities: Music, Art, Creative Writing

Music Comes to Life

Hypomania 1 had everything to do with music. In this respect, J. S. Bach was special. I listened to his music in a way I had never listened to before. The music came to life for me, evoking emotions that brought me to the lofty realm of spirituality. I wrote in my diary (12 Oct 1997):

> Great are the creators of music for all time. Second best are the creators for the moment. The third are the simulators, imitators who partake in the creation. The fourth is the audience. The last are the creators of non music.

I named the episode "The Conductor Who Couldn't Count." As I listened to music, I began to move—first my arms, then my whole body. I pretended to be a conductor. Conducting for the first time, I surprised myself. "Ah, I can do it. I can count!" This was a moment of rational exuberance. You see, I began taking violin lessons at age 16. I loved playing the violin, excited by the dream of being a performer. But I had trouble tuning it, and I couldn't count. I used a metronome. I practiced hard. But it didn't work. Finally, I gave up.

During Hypomania 1 my music appreciation took a quantum leap, even for pieces that I had listened to countless times. I noticed the sounds of different instruments; I sensed the beat, rhythm, tempo, intonation, and dynamics. I discovered that I have previously unknown capabilities. As I practiced more, I became more proficient, on the beat. Instead of following the music, I felt as if I were creating it. The more I immersed myself in the process, the less self-conscious I became and the more I enjoyed doing it.

Unlike passive listening, conducting is strenuous to an extreme. One can get exhausted after doing it for some 10 minutes. The conductors Arturo Toscanini, Bruno Waldheim, and Herbert Von Karajan lived long lives. Aside from the regular exercise, they benefited from the intense love of their work.

I strongly suspect, too, that music has intrinsic qualities (like rhythm) that are associated with longevity. Therefore, you don't need to look beyond conducting music for the elixir of leading a long and healthy life. In retrospect, I might not have been as hopeless as I thought. Perhaps my approach was flawed: too methodical and overly cognitive, not spontaneous. Now, immersing myself in the music and entering into a state of selfless-oblivion, I no longer have trouble. It is like entering into trance.

Actually, such altered states of consciousness are not that unusual, and may require no special training for experiencing them. (Witness how two lovers become totally absorbed in and by each other, oblivious to everything around them.) However, cultivating a habit of mind freed from overcontrol through some activity, such as simulated conducting, certainly helps.

Music figured prominently in other episodes as well. I would turn on my high-fidelity system, on which I have spent an extraordinary fortune, and listen to music all day and night—literally, I lived by music. Listening to Wagner evoked imageries of bedroom acrobatics; and J. S. Bach evoked invariably spiritual feelings. In Hypomania 3, I wrote in my diary (2 Nov 2003):

> Listened to *Rigaletto* [*Rigoletto*]. I never knew it's so beautiful. The story too. *Rigaletto*, loud, occupies my right brain, so I don't have to think, [would be interesting to have an] fMRI… cried, brief but extremely intense, father-daughter [evoked thoughts of relationships with my own daughters].

Expression of Aesthetic-Literary Impulses

The aesthetic-spiritual dimension cried out to be heard during Mania 2. I wrote in my diary (July 2007), "I have rediscovered everything (not quite everything) that the mystics of old knew." I was referring to aesthetic-spiritual experiences (e.g., heightened aesthetic sensibilities, depth of feelings, complete spontaneity). I told a friend, "I have never felt so good in my life." I recited poems repeatedly. Not only that—I moved my head and upper body in a circular motion, like the Chinese poets of old did. Poetry has to be not just read out loud, but read in unison with bodily movements. Try it, and you will see what I mean.

Increasingly, my literary impulses found expression during the episodes. In Hypomania 7, I wrote a "Chinese" poem in English. It began with going to Victoria Park in Hong Kong, an interesting place where one can find people doing all kinds of exercise or practicing martial arts. I had been spending too much time in isolation; going to the park opened my eyes to a new world. Walking around the circles in the park, I was inspired to write a poem (3 July 2009).

Walk like a Buddha

The Taiji circles go round and round,
Small, yet boundless, surrounded
By wooded enclaves, themselves surrounded
By concrete jungles that threaten
To engulf their existence.

Now walk like a Buddha in the circles,
Listen to the droning sound of cicadas,
Look up, see the rays that penetrate
The green leaves in ceaseless motion, and proclaim
That Heaven, Earth, and Man are One.

This was my first attempt to write a Chinese poem in English. In this connection, I am reminded of the evangelist John's extraordinary language in the Book of Revelation. Biblical scholars have noted that John breaks all sorts of grammatical rules. This is not due to incompetence, for he is capable of writing correct and powerful Greek. He seems to be echoing Hebrew constructions, perhaps to give a biblical feel to Revelation.

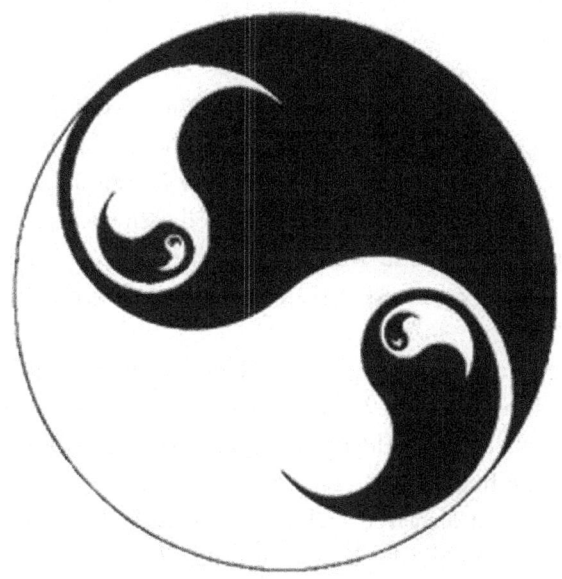

Figure 2.1. Taiji Symbol

I could not have written the poem had I not actually walked around the Taiji circles, listened to the sounds, and seen the light in their midst. The idea of walking like a Buddha came from a Buddhist retreat, where I followed the Vietnamese monk Thich Nhat Hanh and walked "like a Buddha" for days. It also came from the conquest of my poor posture several months earlier. Walk like a Buddha, stand like a Buddha, and sit like a Buddha: That's dignity. So, experience and knowledge are required for writing poetry, no less than for writing scholarly works. That much I understand.

Extraordinary Experiences: Audacity or the Courage-to-Be?

This theme underlies two episodes, Hypomania 2 and 4. In terms of duration, intensity, and extensiveness, Hypomania 2 exceeded the previous episode (Hypomania 1). Characteristically, I had trouble sleeping; toward the end of the episode, I was physically exhausted.

However, I felt that my motility was efficient, "with not a single movement wasted," as I wrote in my diary. Even my handwriting changed. The association of ideas was fast and rich. In my diary I also wrote, "The density and intensity of creative, new discoveries surprised even myself." Intense feelings, fluctuating between negative (loneliness, anguish) and positive (liberation, enlightenment), were constant companions.

Changes in my social behavior were pronounced and sometimes publicly noticed. I called friends and talked with them for hours. My behavioral changes caused great anxiety in my family and among my friends and colleagues. Some thought I was acting more strangely than expected even from an eccentric person like myself. Others undoubtedly thought I was mentally disturbed. Some of my colleagues in psychology pointed to their bible, the DSM, and made their diagnosis of mania.

What was the most outrageous thing I did or manifested? On one occasion, standing in front of a large class of undergraduates, I talked about the June Fourth massacre in Beijing. Suddenly, uncontrolled (not the same as uncontrollable) emotions took hold of me. Tears flowed from my eyes, visible to all. This was the first time I had displayed such emotions in public. Some students were disturbed, because my public display was incompatible with their image of a professor. I thought to myself, "This just goes to show that the Chinese are a people whose capacity for emotional expression has been truncated."

I felt no shame. More fundamentally, self-acceptance came at last. I saw myself as indeed an unusual person, kinder, more sensitive, perhaps even wiser than most other people. This gave me comfort that my self-perception had become more accurate and adaptive.

Self-acceptance did not result in arrogance. The thought of just being different calmed me. Still, could I ignore other people's perceptions of me for long? Being different has been an issue in my life, regardless of cultural context. It has haunted me from my student days in North America to my life back in East Asia. It underlies my loneliness, stemming largely from feelings of not being understood or accepted.

The overall tenor of Hypomania 4 was remarkably positive, despite my physical and mental exhaustion. Significantly, it occurred during my golden age. I wrote in my diary (23 June 2006), "Suppression of artistic impulses can be hazardous to your health." This realization would evolve into a cardinal drive in subsequent episodes. I felt more positive of my role as teacher-educator than I had ever felt before. For decades, my professional superego had been weighing on me heavily, haunted by the feeling that I was failing to live up to my ideals. I learned to treat myself more generously, as I wrote in my diary:

> I have been liberated from self-doubts. Now, I have the courage to be myself, an inspiring teacher, loved by students. Every class I conduct is an enjoyable experience, full of laughter. I have succeeded in touching the lives of many students in a positive way. I can now rightfully regard myself as an educator.

In the midst of this episode, I attended the graduation ceremony of a youngster in mainland China, whose education I had sponsored for a number of years. The location was the international secondary school he had been attending. It was an expensive school, attended mostly by children from families of China's privileged class, the rich and the powerful. Several on-site visits I made to the school, however, raised many disturbing questions about the school's educational philosophy, policies, and practices. In a nutshell, the school conformed to examination superstition: Examination results are everything.

During the ceremony, the school boasted of its achievements, such as the number of its graduates admitted into first-rate Chinese universities. One by one, dignitaries, teachers, and student representatives came onto the stage to read out prearranged scripts in a soulless manner. After a while, I couldn't stand it anymore. I went up on the stage and addressed the audience with a microphone. Here is a translation of what I said:

[Preliminary niceties. . . .] As the sponsor of one of your students and hence an honored guest, I feel obliged to share some of my thoughts with you. Weeks ago, during the time of the university entrance examination, parents could be seen near the examination sites, staying in hotels and giving support to their children. Today, hardly a parent has come to attend the graduation ceremony. What does this say about our educational priorities?

The school has listed many of its achievements. Student representatives come onto the stage and read out their scripts. I would appreciate their independent display of creativity much more. Why not let them speak their own minds?

This ceremony is prepared for only those who have done well in the examination. The higher the marks, the greater the glory. What about those who have not done so well? They can't hold their heads up high. Right now, they need the understanding and support of educators more than ever. Why, then, not a word for them has been uttered?

We teach by setting personal examples. The State Council of the Chinese government has urged the people to practice conservation. Yet, today, I see the doors of this assembly hall are open while air conditioning is running. Are educators concerned about wastage and damage to our environment?

At this point, the school principal stood up and spoke: "Are you here to stir up a fight?" I replied: "No, that's not my intention. I am responsible only for what I say. You have to be responsible for how you hear it." Then, several people approached me on stage and tried to grab the microphone from me. I surrendered it, walked down the stage, and left the assembly hall. After the ceremony, some teachers and students approached me stealthily and told me how much they appreciated my remarks.

The speech was impolite, even inappropriate, given the occasion. Lest misunderstanding may arise, I hasten to add that I had never done anything like that before. I wouldn't normally have the audacity. Hypomania gave me the courage to speak my mind publicly, on the ills of education in China I had been feeling very strongly for decades.

Having done it, I am proud of it. For at least once in my life, I have spoken, with conviction and fortitude, if inappropriately. So be it, if my inappropriate speech served the purpose of making a point for the good of education. Would my life be lesser lived, if I had not done the inappropriate? My evolution from audacity to courage-to-be is an essential part of my spiritual journey.

The Empty Mind: Gone with Repression and Overcontrol

In Mania 1, I experienced the selfless self, self-healing, and vanished repression. This theme is developed further here. I learned from Hypomania 1 more about how the mind is capable of performing amazing feats (e.g., simulating music conductors) when it is freed from conscious overcontrol.

In this connection, I recalled in the midst of the episode that I was once asked to be a simultaneous interpreter between Chinese and English at a technical conference. Not having performed simultaneous interpretation ever before, I had no clue about how it could be done. Not surprisingly, I made a mess of it in the beginning. I waited for the completion of a sentence in one language before translating it into another. That, of course, was a fatally flawed technique. The result was that I found myself hopelessly behind, not "simultaneous." I resigned myself to disastrous failure. I didn't care anymore. Suddenly I found that I could do it. I simply kept on translating continually. Utterances flowed from my lips with the ease of water flowing out of a tap. I called this *automatization*, a fundamental attribute of language performance.

Compulsivity and fear of losing specific thoughts are manifestations of overcontrol by the mind. These reemerged in two subsequent episodes, Hypomania 3 and 4. Hypomania 3 was marked by its brief duration of only a few days. I recorded that I "slept for 12 hours [and] completely recovered." So sleep held the key to recovery. There were no adverse effects on my occupational or social functioning in the least. For instance, I conducted a two-day workshop on depression and suicide prevention just before the onset (ironic, isn't it?). I attended court as an expert witness on the following day. However, at home I was struggling with fatigue, compulsivity, and disturbance of short-term memory. Hypomania 4, sandwiched between two manic episodes, was quite mild. It lasted less than a month.

Recollections or remembrances may throw fresh insights informative on brain functioning. The positive side was the creativity. Like boundaries between the conscious and the unconscious had vanished. The unconscious became accessible. Retrieval of information was superefficient. In addition, association of ideas was facilitated, fast, but I also felt overwhelmed by these endless associations. In the psychiatric literature, these are called flight of ideas.

Consumption of energy by the brain must have been extraordinarily high. The normal level of consumption is about 20 Watts. This led to some very disturbing states of brain functioning. I could not perform simple operations, such as simple arithmetic. I was completely forgetful. Immediately forgot where I had laid something down a moment ago. I had to walk around for some 20 minutes before I located the "lost" object. Similarly, I had to try to focus on one thought. While staying focused, a myriad associations appeared. The next moment, the memory of what I had just been thinking about was gone. Attempts to recall were usually futile.

I became obsessive about keeping memories from being lost. So I tried to record my thoughts on paper or in a computer file. Thus, brain fatigue may well be the mechanism for obsessive symptoms. I have also experienced this when the air conditioning is turned off. Mild cerebral anoxia. I don't want to say that this applies to all forms of obsessive phenomena. These obsessive phenomena I have described are qualitatively different from the psychoneurotic varieties described in the psychiatric literature.

Cumulative experiences eventually lead to insight. I have come to think of obsessive-compulsive overcontrol as "cerebral constipation." My antidote is No-Mind Therapy. It began during Hypomania 4 with my attempt to help a student who was cerebral to a fault. He sent a message to me that raised all kinds of questions about therapy. Here is my reply to him and his classmates.

> Your diligence is impressive. It could also be an impediment to enlightenment. Do nothing, no-think, for a while, and see what happens. Dialogic Action Therapy can be hazardous to those who use their brains too much. To treat the patient with the right kind of medicine, I use No-Mind Therapy (invented/created at this very moment; see, therapies can be a dime a dozen).
>
> Mindfulness is a misleading word that may lead many into tortured paths. It does not allow for the full strength of no-mind to run its course. If people from the West don't understand, they may be forgiven; it would be tragic if we don't. The adult is full of thoughts pure and impure. Therefore, to return to his natural state, he must focus his attention to reexperience the emptiness of mind.
>
> Focus, alas, implies conscious effort. For some, heroic effort, too much for a lazy person like myself. My path to the no-thought, selfless self is one of least resistance. Sorry, I can't tell you what it is. Each will have to discover it for himself. (Hint: music and poetry help.) You must read a poem aloud. Hear its beauty. Let your head, your whole body, move, like the bygone poets of China. Now, empty yourself of even the *idea* of emptiness. Simply embrace it, experience it. Therapy is poetry. Poetry is beauty. Therefore, mind and no-mind. Get it?

Mindfulness-based therapies are in vogue these days. I prefer the term *selfless mind* or *empty mind*, which comes closer to the Buddhist notions of selflessness and emptiness. A mind empty of ideas, cravings, even a sense of itself is the antithesis of overattachment, fixations, or rigidities. No-Mind Therapy accommodates much better the notion of vanished repression. What is there to repress in a mindless, empty mind? Two verses capture my thinking on what a true selfless self can do.

The Mindless Mind (20 Dec 2009)

A mindful mind is mindful of dust.
A mindless mind, mindless of the dust,
Minds nothing and everything all at once.
Full and empty, empty and full at will,
The selfless self acts without effort,
On target every time.

The Selfless Self (25 July 2010)

Without the self in the heart,
With feelings then reason flies.
Now ask the heavens, search
The earth, and penetrate
The cosmos' mysteries.

Caught Between the Challenges and Rewards of Hypomania

Now Get Physical: I Could Have Danced All Night

The idea that repression of artistic impulses can be hazardous to one's health evolved into a cardinal drive. Here, my body could be tired but still driven to perform. Music and dance figure prominently, especially during sleepless nights. I fall into an enchanted state, in which pieces of music I love have the power to grip my being and keep my body in motion. The lyrics in My Fair Lady, "I could have danced all night and could have begged for more," come to life, literally.

Recall in this context that in my youth I once went to a folk dance camp and danced for three days and nights, almost nonstop. But I know full well that the fountain of youth is not eternal. Be that as it may, music and dance in madness has informed me to grow professionally. Later, I created Dynamic Relaxation and Meditation, with music and dance as key components, as an avenue to enhance holistic health (see Chapter 3). In view of these, liberation from stagnation beginning from the body provides a natural thread that weaves various hypomanic episodes into a coherent story.

Hypomania 5 took place on board the *Queen Victoria* cruising around the Mediterranean. A confluence of circumstances and mishaps made joining the cruise physically and psychologically exhausting. Being traumatized at Heathrow Airport in London deserves special mention. Its Terminal 5 can only be described as a Terminal of Terror. The staff is positively unhelpful and rude. Understandably, security has to be tight, in view of the terrorist threats that Britain has been under. There is little excuse, however, for the security staff to yell "Take off your shoes," and scare the daylights out of passengers, including me, on transit.

By the time I saw the *Queen Victoria*, it was getting ready to set sail. The last gangway was about to be closed. I made it just in the nick of time. By then, having been deprived of a good rest for several days, I was in a state of exhaustion. What followed was a clinical tale of scary symptoms.

On board the *Queen Victoria*, I had a hard time recovering. There were lots of activities, and I could not fall asleep. Hypomania 5 differed from previous episodes in that the salient symptom was mental and physical depletion, rather than racing thoughts; however, elation of mood remained an important feature. On the fifth day, I finally went to consult the physician on board. This was the list of symptoms I described to him: constipation, insomnia, extreme fatigue, disturbance of executive functions; in addition, I had cognitive deficits and spells of shaking chills, which I had not experienced before.

My body, impervious to signs of exhaustion, was pushed to its limit. In fact, I was dancing almost nightly, which I enjoyed immensely. I surprised myself with how good I was. I entered into a state of selfless-oblivion with ease. That was the secret. For the first time, I was able to be spontaneous, to move without any inhibition, to enjoy myself, *in public*. Sometimes, when I danced alone, people on the dance floor would stop dancing and watch me.

My sociability, love of adventure, and aesthetic capacity were undiminished. I took the initiative to interact with passengers as well as staff on board. One night, I ventured into the grand theatre inside the *Queen Victoria*. No one was there. I took advantage of the occasion, walked onto the empty stage and danced, as if the theatre was full of people—thus to satisfy my aspiration, long frustrated, to be an artistic performer, at least for a while.

Unable to fall asleep, I went up to the upper decks of the ship early one morning to watch the sunrise. I discovered what "the majesty of the heavens" really meant. Above the horizon, brilliant golden rays penetrated a dark cloud, making a colossal sandwich of lights in the sky.

Sleeplessness, Fatigue, and Confusion: The Price of Feeling Too High

The cardinal symptom of Hypomania 6, as in Hypomania 5, was a prolonged low level of energy, punctuated with frequent bouts of depletion; racing thoughts or excessive talkativeness was secondary.

I became a better therapist during episodes on account of magnified empathic sensitivities, superefficiency in retrieving and integrating clinical data, and unhindered access to my own inner self. I remember I had a three-hour therapy session with a family, which involved nonverbal techniques demanding an enormous expenditure of energy. At the end of the session, I was so tired that I simply collapsed. Afterward, when I went to a restaurant for lunch, I had to conserve my energy with extreme measures, such as half shutting my eyes (a yoga technique) and avoiding all unnecessary talking or movements; I ate at the slowest pace ever. These I had not experienced before, not even in Hypomania 5.

The quest for holistic health and artistic self-expression marked Hypomania 6. It began in the physical realm. One of my blessings is good health, at least in relative terms, which I have enjoyed all my life. I've never had a major illness or been hospitalized, except for a nasal operation I had in my youth. However, posture had been a problem for decades: Spending hours in front of a computer monitor was an occupational hazard. My upper back had been slightly hunched, and my head used to stick out. I was not aware of how bad it looked until I saw some photographs in which I appeared with a "turtle neck." I had to do something: Fight back; exercise.

My massage chair was not a luxury, but a necessity to relieve the tightness around my neck and shoulders. While using the massage chair, I would move around in order to reach different parts of my body. This I did a lot, until finally my body was more relaxed than it had been for a long time. One day, while walking along, I noticed that my posture was completely upright. The hunchback had gone!

More significantly, I have been able to maintain the upright posture for years, especially during episodes, thus reinforcing my belief long held in body-mind-spirit interconnectedness. The human body is capable of doing extraordinary things when body-mind-spirit functions as an integral whole, as mystics, Buddhist monks, masters of Chinese medicine and martial arts have long discovered.

This physical breakthrough ignited a chain reaction in the psychological and spiritual realms. With heightened artistic-aesthetic sensibilities, I experimented with Chinese character writing for weeks. Deviating from standard writing, I used curved strokes to construct rounded characters, which suggest femininity, softness, and smoothness of emotions.

I also took up singing in German. This I informed a German-American friend of mine in a message. An excerpt:

> Two days ago, I was listening to some German opera arias, which I normally don't do. But the beauty of *O du, mein holder Abenstern* in Wagner's Tannhäuser gripped my being, and I started to sing. Now, I have never sung anything properly, least of all in German. After a lot of repeated practice, I finally succeeded in making myself a semblance of a baritone. I taught myself. Lacking in technicality, strength, *usw* [etc.], I made up with expression. I then went onto Schiller's ode *An die Freude* in Beethoven's choral symphony and Louis Spohr's Faust, immersing myself in these beauties.

It seems that working with the physical domain is easier and hence may be a recommended first step. In this episode, I gained health first through conquering poor posture and second through allowing myself full artistic self-expression, *without regard for how well or how poorly I performed.* Thus, art and health are intertwined. Isn't this a vindication of the claim that repression of artistic impulses can be hazardous to one's health?

Hypomania 7 was basically a continuation of the preceding episode. My level of physical activity was very high, spending a lot of time singing and practicing qigong and martial arts. But I was low on reserves, frequently overcome by both mental and physical fatigue. My energy level fluctuated dramatically; my condition was one of severe imbalance.

On one occasion, I suffered from acute cognitive dysfunction for about an hour. It was like a sudden attack of mental depletion (rather than confusion). I was simply mentally exhausted. I could not perform even simple tasks, such as making a telephone call. I also suffered from ejaculation retardation and even ejaculation incompetence for several weeks, something I had not experienced before.

Despite the physical imbalance, however, my mood was elated. I felt confident and self-assured. I felt a sense of mastery. Perhaps, finally, I have learned to reap the benefits of explosive creativity without incurring social costs. There was little or no indication that people with whom I interacted found my behavior out of bounds. To them, I was eager to learn, friendly, and jovial.

Years ago, when I was about to receive my PhD and then depart from the United States to return to Asia, I wanted to learn as much as possible about how to do hypnotherapy in the remaining months. I had private sessions lasting two hours every day, seven times a week, with a former professor of mine. Now, I was busy preparing for relocation to the United States in the midst of this episode. I became an apprentice again, in Hong Kong.

This time, I wanted to learn qigong and Taiji push-hands, an advanced Taiji exercise involving two persons "pushing hands" against each other. I took private lessons from two Taiji masters. Taiji is one of the "inner" schools of Chinese martial arts (as distinct from the "outer" schools, e.g., Shaolin gungfu). It is difficult to learn, far more than I had imagined. It demands strict adherence to an attitude in conformity with the Daoist idea of *wuwei* (nonaction, not inaction). The principle is to use your opponent's own forces to defeat him. This means suppressing common, instinctive tendencies and waiting for and capitalizing on the opponent's mistaken moves.

For months I had to learn, and relearn, the fundamental technique of moving my arms in "perfect" circles. My Taiji masters were impressive and convincing, capable of doing things to which verbal description can hardly do justice. Their forearms felt like rods of steel; they could push and move me off my feet at will, but I couldn't move them an inch. So immersed I was in the push-hands that when I awoke in the middle of the night, I would find my arms moving in circles.

Hypomania 8 took place in Southern California, after my relocation from Hong Kong in July 2009. It lasted for about three weeks. Familiar symptoms appeared, such as mental hyperactivity, mood elation, enhanced artistic sensibility, and aesthetic appreciation of ordinary objects (e.g., the root of a tree). I craved physical activity. I yearned to listen to music. Unfortunately, I noticed that my tolerance for volume diminished dramatically, and somehow the music didn't sound right; reminded of how brain trauma (e.g., concussion) may result in oversensitivity to noise, I thought that these were signs of a tired brain. There was, as usual, insomnia, but having severe, frequent shaking chills was a new experience.

What followed was a descent into a scary state of severe mental fatigue and confusion. It was so bad that I would get lost while taking a walk around my neighborhood. I dared not drive. However, even in this state the wisdom of the body could be discerned: I moved around and performed tasks without conscious deliberation, as if my movements were to a large extent automatized.

I consulted a physician. He ordered laboratory tests, none resulting in positive findings. Unable to sleep, my condition got worse. I took sleeping pills for a few nights and slept better, but that did nothing to stop the mental hyperactivity and fatigue. I was then desperate enough to go to a hospital on an emergency basis. All sorts of tests were done, again none resulting in positive findings. The attending doctor decided that hospitalization was not necessary. He prescribed risperidone, an antipsychotic drug, after I told him about how previously taking Risperdal (trade name for risperidone) helped to clear my hypomania. Taking the drug put me on the track of recovery. Predictably, as my mood elation disappeared, my mundane life resumed again.

A Hypomanic Episode in China

In May 2011, I was invited to serve as a Visiting Professor at one of the most prestigious tertiary institutions in mainland China. This was an opportunity I had long dreamed of. My social life was as rich as my material condition of living was poor. In a message to my daughters (6 June 2011), I wrote:

> I am doing very well in Beijing. The students are just wonderful. They are the cream of the cream. I have never seen so many super-intelligent people who are thoughtful and eager to learn in my life.... I am happier than I have been for a long time. I have found greater meaning in doing something good as an educator. Furthermore, my health has improved dramatically, largely through practicing martial arts/dancing. I feel much younger!

Soon after my arrival in China, I sensed a general elevation in my mood and energy level. Gone were the feelings of social isolation and depression I had following my relocation to the United States. My posture was upright. I felt healthy. I experienced an upsurge in mental, physical, and sexual energy. Putting physical inertia behind, I practiced martial arts and Dynamic Relaxation and Meditation (DRM). People were surprised when they learned of my advanced age. I had, in fact, entered into a state of hypomania.

This episode, Hypomania 9, was marked by multiple peaks of mood elevation during a period of about four months. I underwent a self-transformation and became more creative, more colorful, more adventurous, more generous, and more appreciative of all the good things in life. Most reassuring was the fact that, although I appeared strange to people around me, I didn't transgress the bounds of cultural acceptability. I thought to myself, "Finally, I have succeeded in reaping the fruits of madness, without being mad."

But all was not well, I suspect. After a month or so in China, disturbing prodromal symptoms appeared. One day, on my way to meet an appointment,

I got distracted by a book display for about an hour. I was immersed in books, oblivious to everything else, and nearly missed my appointment.

The amazing thing was that my distractibility was matched by my hyper-focused concentration on the books. However, such concentration was like tunnel vision. My distractibility could not be rationalized as behavior characteristic of absent-minded professors.

Also, I suffered from acute cognitive dysfunctions, such as being unable to recall my mobile phone number. For days, I was too mentally fatigued to do any work that required sustained concentration. Again, these were like attacks of mental depletion rather than confusion. I became very worried about my condition.

I put this question to a psychiatrist friend of mine, "Is it unusual for manic or hypomanic patients to suffer from mental fatigue?" The answer was no, which confirmed what I had been suspecting. It was reassuring, in the sense that I felt less atypical: "There are others who suffer the way I do. I'm not alone." Again, the key was sleep. Most of the time, I was able to sleep remarkably well. This enabled me to maintain my energy level and function adequately on a daily basis.

There were aspects that I had not experienced before, at least not as dramatically as in past episodes. I engaged in new, previously unimagined activities. I was able to enter into states of selfless-forgetfulness as naturally as breathing. For instance, I practiced "sitting down and forgetting everything."

This is an idea originating from Zhuangzi, "I smash up my limbs and body, drive out perception and intellect, cast off form, do away with understanding, and make myself identical with the Great Thoroughfare. This is what I mean by sitting down and forgetting everything." Actually, I didn't smash up my body and so forth. Rather, I practiced *literally* sitting down on a chair from a standing position and instantaneously entering into an altered state of consciousness. Through demonstrations, I taught some friends and students to experience what it was like.

Some nights I was too mentally active to sleep, though physically tired. Rather than trying to force myself to sleep, I got out of bed, moved around, and simply followed my natural inclinations. I found myself practicing a DRM technique that I had been trying to perfect, namely, moving both arms independently of each other. There is endless variation in this independence of left-right arm movements. For instance, one may draw a small circle rapidly with the right hand while drawing a large square slowly with the left. Soon, drawing figures turned into virtual calligraphy—writing Chinese characters in the air. I attempted to write with both hands simultaneously.

I practiced systematically, in steps of increasing difficulty. First, I wrote Chinese characters with only my right hand and then with only my left. Curiously, after practicing with my left for a while, I found it difficult to write with my right. This appears to be a phenomenon of neuro-hemispheric interference.

Second, I wrote the same characters with both hands in synchrony, following the same sequence of strokes.

Third, I altered the synchrony and sequence, so they became different for the two hands. I learned to follow these three steps with amazing speed.

Finally, I tried to write different characters with two hands, with or without variation in synchrony or sequence. This proved to be too difficult to be learned in one or two nights. As I practiced virtual calligraphy, I went deeply into an altered state of consciousness; and the deeper I went, the more I was able to perform feats beyond my wildest dream.

Writing characters in the air is a technique that some Chinese calligraphers use to perfect their art. This technique helps to solidify the mental representation of Chinese characters in their minds. Because each character has a prescribed sequence of strokes, the technique also strengthens the kinesthetic memory involved in writing. But this is to speak in the language of cognitive psychology. I speak in the language of Buddhist-Daoist psychology. Being right-handed,

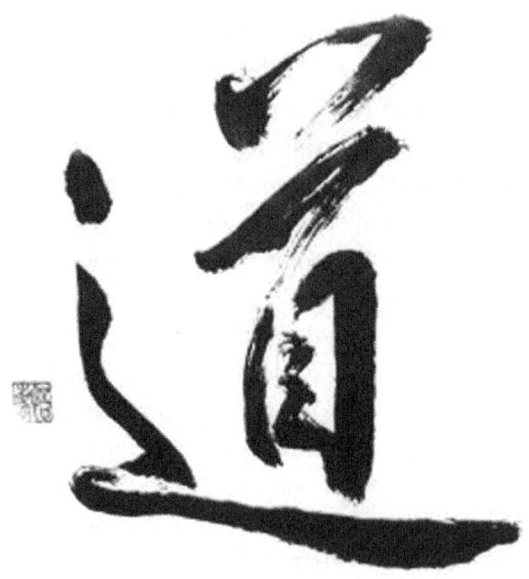

Figure 2.2. The Chinese Character Dao

I would find it difficult to write with my left. In a state of selfless-forgetfulness, however, many things become easier. My body, mind, and spirit become interconnected. When I stay still, I am totally still; when I move, my whole body—no, my whole being—moves with total commitment.

On one occasion, some students and I were having dinner in a restaurant. It was already quite late, and most of the customers had left, when I gave a public display of writing Chinese characters in the air with both hands. One of the students made a video recording of this "bizarre" event. Interestingly, the restaurant staffs were quite accommodating; apparently, none thought that I was crazy.

A Laowantong *(Aged-Naughty-Childlike) Professor*

The students were impressive! I've met the cream of the cream, the brightest of the bright, from China's population of more than a billion people. Quite a few shine through as geniuses. Some appeared to have encyclopedic knowledge. Most were well read and articulate. Like other Chinese students, they showed deferential regard toward teachers they respected. Faced with such lovely students, my affection toward them grew naturally. Unlike other Chinese teachers, I made no attempt to conceal my affection. A friend of mine once remarked, "Your likes and dislikes are written on your face." I am simply deficient in my ability or willingness to conceal my emotions.

The students were touched. One class sent me a card wishing me a Happy New Year (1 Jan 2012). On it were written these words (translated from Chinese):

> The happiest thing is to have spent such an interesting semester together with teacher Ho. We like your distinctive teaching style; we like your frankness and spontaneity—like that of a *laowantong* ["aged naughty child"]. You encourage us to doubt, to ask, to rebel, to practice. You are most unlike other teachers, also one we love the most. . ... We will always remember teacher Ho, the most loveable *laowantong*.

Messages like this lift me from despair that occasionally creeps into my life. The name *laowantong* is loaded with emotions; it captures not just my personal style but my being. I simply don't behave like a "normal" professor in China: Whatever I may gain from behaving like one wouldn't compensate for the loss of character I will suffer. I am aged, yet naughty and childlike. This ruffles people, especially those steeped in academia. But I want to keep it that way—to preserve my original face. Besides, I can't morph into what I'm not, even if I wanted to.

One of the students, whom I call Little Kitten, was most special. I met her briefly the year before, when I went to the university for a short visit. She wrote a message to me after I returned to the United States, expressing her desire to learn from me. I replied, as I normally would to messages from students or young colleagues asking for guidance. I didn't think I would meet her again. But I did meet up with her again when I reported for duty at the university. She and her boyfriend were about to receive their doctoral degrees.

Yuan (a Buddhist idea meaning predestined affinity) brought us together. A Chinese saying puts it this way:

With *yuan*, we come to meet from a thousand miles apart.
Without *yuan*, we pass each other by face to face.

Little Kitten is one of the brightest, if not the brightest, persons I have ever met. Her empathy is more impressive, surpassing even her intelligence. She has an uncanny ability to comprehend what goes on in my mind. She predicts my utterances before they are uttered. In particular, she helps me to adjust to life in mainland China, many aspects of which I find alien. She guides me through the intricate maze in which people think and act. She gives me sound advice on how to act in awkward situations or to deal with difficult people.

My fondness for Little Kitten grew into deep affection. After about a month of intensive interaction, I told her that I would like to have her as my goddaughter. She readily accepted me as her godfather. As was customary in China, we went through a formal ceremony, during which she offered me a cup of tea in the presence of friends—without having to kneel, as in the past.

Another one I am especially fond of is a graduate student in theoretical physics. He is the reincarnate of my youth, childlike and naive to a fault. He brings back memories of my days as a physics major in Canada. Curious about everything, his mind roams as quickly and widely as anyone I have encountered. Talented in musical composition, he set to music a poem I have written. His intellectual prowess is awesome, easily surpassing mine. What's more, he openly acknowledges his talents with neither immodesty nor arrogance. His unusual qualities, delightful to some but disconcerting to others, are apparent even to casual observers. In short, he surpasses me in being odd and atypical.

Once we walked around in Beijing for hours in the middle of the night. We were drawn to a littered flower bed, and as if our minds were interconnected, both of us spontaneously began picking up the litter. How could we bear to see natural beauty spoiled? He would sing in the streets, without being self-conscious or embarrassed. He ran around, back and forth, following his unbridled impulses. Except for his adult size, he was just like a child. It was nearly dawn by the time I arrived home, nearly exhausted but still savoring the time we had spent together.

He is not just my reincarnate. He represents what I wish to be, but cannot be. Through him, I fulfill my frustrated aspirations of being a music composer and a promising physicist. Psychologists call this vicarious satisfaction. Brilliant students tend to have psychological problems with atypical features. I can understand them better than others, given that I have had a fair measure of atypical problems myself.

I have helped troubled students with Dialogic Action Therapy (DAT), both verbal and nonverbal, not in an office setting but in everyday life. I don't practice DAT with professional intent; rather, therapy is interwoven with social interaction. This way, I have been able to help quite a few in a short time.

One outstanding case comes to mind. For about two months, I had intensive interactions with a student and his girlfriend. His problems were deep seated and many, among which was avoiding eye contact. His girlfriend wanted him to seek help from me. He refused, thus causing quarrels between them. You can't treat people who refuse treatment. So the trick I used was to avoid using words like *therapy* or *counseling*. Yet, therapy was in progress.

One day, I felt that the moment for decisive action was at hand. With his girlfriend by his side, I grabbed hold of his head with my hands and said to him, "Look at me, look into my eyes. Stop avoiding. I like you, so don't turn away. Look how I am smiling. I like you to smile back, smile *with* me...." I refused to let go of his head until he responded. We struggled together for a few minutes. Finally, he looked into my eyes and smiled a sweet smile. The eye contact avoidance was at least half gone. His condition improved as our interaction continued. This was my best gift to him and his girlfriend.

I was acting more like a mentor than a therapist. Casting aside all theories, I followed my feelings. There was no analysis, only intuition and raw emotions. My exuberance had an infectious effect on others around me. In a state of madness, I was able to personify therapy.

The Dark Side of Life: Alienation on an Unprecedented Scale

I must also talk about the dark side of life at the university. Walking around the campus, I noticed many students, especially those in large lecture rooms, dozing off, reading newspapers, playing computer games, or doing their own work, without paying the slightest attention what the lecturers were saying! The lecturers simply kept on talking, oblivious to the students' inattention. I have not seen such student behavior anywhere else, except in mainland China. Neither have I seen the lecturers' blasé attitude toward such disrespectful behavior elsewhere. Do the lecturers have self-respect? Apparently, the lecturers have not yet learned from the sayings of Chairman Mao:

> There are teachers who ramble on and on when they lecture; they should let their students doze off.... Rather than keeping your eyes open and listening to boring lectures, it is better to get some refreshing sleep. You don't have to listen to nonsense.

So, in actuality dozing off in class may have been prevalent for a long time. In large measure, students learn in spite of, not because of, their professors.

I have been visiting academic institutions in mainland China since 1971—just before the "ping-pong diplomacy" that led to a thaw in Sino-American relations. So I am a witness to dramatic changes that have taken place in China's academic institutions in response to the political climate within which they operate.

The controlled atmosphere is not confined to the classroom. Typically, during an academic or professional forum, the chairperson, who is more likely male, would begin by setting the tone and defining the perimeter of the ensuing discussion. The vice-chairperson, if present, would be the next to speak. After that, others would take turns to speak, according to an implicit order of authority or status. Participants who occupy a low status speak little or keep silent. Toward the end, the chairperson would summarize the main points and conclusions, if any, of the discussion. Clearly, the right to voice an opinion correlates closely with authority ranking.

In 1971, psychology was denounced as a bourgeois subject that has no place in a socialist society. Rooted in the ideology of collectivism, the negation of individuality and personal aspirations was total. The individual was obligated to place collective interests and needs above one's own and to follow the "centralized allocation" of job assignments by state bureaucracies after graduation. Considerations for personal career plans were attacked as "careerism."

During my visit in 1971, I found that cadres in educational institutions negated even the idea of individual differences in aptitude. By 1981, while teaching at a major university in Shanghai, I discerned a quiet ascendancy of individualism among students, as one put it to me in private: "To think of the state's needs is rather 'abstract.' We have to consider our own future."

On the first day of teaching, the whole class stood up in unison to salute my entrance. Totally unprepared for such an occasion, I was petrified instantaneously. The students seemed as determined as any I have encountered not to participate actively in the learning process. Some informed me quietly that it was considered impolite to ask questions in class. I found out that students have serious misgivings about boring classes. In many ways, the university reminded me of a *sishu* (private school) in past centuries. Now, decades later what in the world has the docile, obedient, and deferential Chinese student become?

And how do the professors relate with one another in the present day? Competitiveness, mistrust, and backstabbing define the world they live in. The lack of collegiality among professors seems endemic. Holed up in their offices, many professors live in oblivion of the social world outside. Some don't talk with each other. Some show a singular lack of basic courtesy to colleagues. In all, their behavior defies stereotypes (or romanticized Confucian ideals?) of the traditional scholar-teacher.

Academic governance is typically paternalistic and autocratic, as the reader would have guessed, given the concentration of authority in the "leader" (e.g., heads of departments) at different echelons. The leaders don't lead; they issue edicts. There is little to constrain them from practicing "management by terror."

I once mentioned to a department head that students were afraid of him. His reply was, "That's good. I want students to fearful of me, so they will be more obedient." I was taken aback because the head in question professed to be an expert in management. Factionalism is rampant. If the leader doesn't like you, you may find yourself being ostracized. It is not personal. The colleagues who shun your company simply want to avoid displeasing the leader. This is called "drawing the line." During the Great Cultural Revolution, you would have to "draw the line" even against your family members out of self-protection. This sends a chill down my spine.

Another open secret: BMWs line up to pick up female students in the performing arts in the evenings. Befuddled, I asked some of my students what was going on. The answer confirmed my suspicion: Access to high-class escorts is a special privilege of the rich and powerful in China. Language use reflects social realities. The term *xiaojie* (literally, little sister) used to refer a young, unmarried lady from a well-off family. Nowadays, it is a euphemism for fallen women. So be careful when you use it to address a woman lest she may be offended. From this, one can deduce how prevalent prostitution has become.

The dark side of life in the university I have described is a microcosm of the ills of Chinese society. The university is not an ivory tower. It cannot insulate itself against outside influences. Decades of communist indoctrination appear to have done little to cure the ills of China. Has it fallen on deaf ears, like "water passing over the back of a duck"? This is worthy of deep reflection.

Mainland China is communist in name, but Confucian deep down. Education is not indoctrination. It is integral to the fate of nations and humankind. I decry the education I received when I was a schoolboy. Now, as an educator I deplore what I have seen in a ranking university, and others, in China. I long for a creative synthesis of Eastern and Western learning. What I see is an indiscriminate, tasteless mixture in which the worst elements of both worlds are incorporated. Collective madness? I lament!

A spiritual wasteland best describes life there generally. I don't know how to put it more mildly. The campus is like a sanctuary, encroached from without. Outside, the first thing I notice is that laughter is rarely seen in public places. Workers go on with their business in a perfunctory way, joyless and burnt out. Interpersonal relationships are marked by guardedness and lack of trust.

In the name of development, concrete jungles have transformed much of the landscape beyond recognition. Chinese cities are no longer Chinese. Urbanites have largely lost touch with nature. Urban children see animals mostly in pictures rather than in real life. Air, water, and noise pollution threaten to lower the quality of life beyond human endurance. In sum, the symptoms of alienation and environmental disregard are manifest everywhere. The more materialistic values predominate, the less spirituality can be found. Anguish!

I mince no words to make my points strongly, at the risk of exaggeration or overgeneralization, in proportion to the depth of anguish I feel. Anguish, because I empathize with the human condition in mainland China. That's living psychohistory. It may take decades before the wounds of spiritual emptiness can be healed. In the meantime, I take comfort in the thought that I have sowed the seeds of spiritual awakening, no matter how humbly, among my students. Never before in human history has the word *spirituality* mattered so much to so many people.

A Living Buddha in a Schizophrenic City

Three of my episodes (Hypomania 10-12) took place, at least partly, in Macao. Of these, Hypomania 12 stands out in my mind. It lasted about two months, during which I conducted training workshops for counselors. Macao may be characterized as a schizophrenic city split between the casinos district and the rest; the money that changes hands daily dwarfs that of La Vegas. No wonder, Chinese people are notorious for their proclivity toward gambling. I was moved by the irony of my situation: What can I really do for the counselors attending my workshops to improve the quality of life in Macao? As I have felt throughout my professional life, mental health professionals are waging a hopeless battle against larger societal forces.

Personally, I have been involved in cases where families are wrecked by addictive gambling. Here is a typical heart-breaking account of the tragic consequences. The husband borrows money from a loan shark, loses the money in a casino, and is unable to repay his debt. The loan shark and his gang of psychopaths lock up the husband in a hotel room and make a threatening call to his family, "Come and pay back the money, or else . . . ." Unable to repay, the wife may be "borrowed" for a period time and forced into prostitution.

I don't know how to deal with psychopaths. In one case I worked on, the husband who owed money to a bunch of loan sharks related how an initiation process prepared his wife for prostitution: For a week, his wife was gang raped. Her identity as an innocent woman and wife was destroyed. After her release from prostitution, she tried to practice some of the sexual techniques she had "learned" from the initiation process with her husband. This accentuated the husband's difficulty accepting his wife again as a sexual partner. Subsequently, the marriage ended in divorce. At this point, the reader would have no difficulty in understanding why I have a revulsion against psychopaths in general and loan sharks in particular.

Once I decided to venture into a "casino nightclub," equipped a large pool where lustful men were there to pick a beauty out of some 20 lined up around. Some of the manual staff came from the poorest countries in Southeast Asia. They were treated like enslaved workers, constantly apprehensive of being watched by surveillance cameras everywhere and afraid of interaction with customers.

With a state of mind filled with compassion, I told a few Buddhist workers that I was a Living Buddha, there to make an appearance for their consolation. They seemed to have no trouble believing what I told them. Finally, I was appalled enough to cause an incident by lighting cigarettes repeatedly in urns in front of Buddhist statues, and was driven out by intimidating security guards. Looking back at my adventure now, I can still feel the same compassion I felt then.

On a sleepless night, I took a ferry from Macao to Hong Kong. At the port, several boisterous young men plus an unmistakable prostitute they had picked up were lining up at the immigration checkpoint. I asked them politely, "Please don't be so noisy." Soon I found myself in trouble in the embarkation perch, crowded with passengers: One of the men started to push me around, so hard that I almost hit a wall some ten feet away.

Actually, I was hopping away as a reflexive technique to minimize the force of the push. Avoiding a fight but fearless, I walked around the perch demonstrating my fighting skills in full sight of all. The passengers were appalled by the muscular man treating an elderly person in this manner, and the pusher had been restrained by his buddies from making a fool of himself. In a state of sanity now, I would not have the courage to do what I did.

After arriving in Hong Kong, I continued to practice Taiji Quan (an inner school of martial arts), of all places inside a subway train, by maintaining balance without holding onto anything. Of course, nobody took notice, except a woman smiling. She happened to be an advanced Taiji practitioner. We exchanged a few words before I got off the train. It was an improbable encounter, brief but memorable.

Later Hypomanic Episodes in America

By the time I returned to America, the benefit of cumulated learning from past experiences amounted to premonition. Prodromal signs appearing about two to three weeks before onset could be read: prolonged hiccups, unexplainable mental fatigue and confusion, fluctuations in energy level, heightened esthetic-literary sensitivities, and emotional responsiveness to music.

During Hypomania 13, mental fatigue prevented me from serious writing for several weeks. At the same time, various enchantments added to my distraction. I found myself enjoying the simple activities of daily life, including those that I normally resisted doing (e.g., brushing my teeth, and washing dishes). Not least among the enchantments was the music of Mozart, which put me readily into a mood of dancing to it. I thought to myself, "I don't have to be a genius like Mozart. All I need is to have enough sense to exploit the works of a genius to enrich my own life."

With humor, I found it easier to interact with difficult people. In social situations, I conducted myself with a renewed sense of self. Significantly, even close friends or relatives had little idea of what I was going through and did not notice any "abnormality," as I had gradually learned to better manage my social image. The episode ended after lasting for about a month.

Later episodes become increasingly mild, but characterized more and more by mental and physical fatigue. The demarcation between hypomanic and normal states has become blurred. This makes me very happy because, after sequential learning from one episode to the next, I may finally have found a way of harnessing the creative forces of madness without being damaged by it.

A Summation: Unanswered Questions

In all, my episodes are a goldmine of imbalances: ecstasy intermingling with anguish; maintaining a sense of psychophysical well-being while suffering from inability to fall asleep, physical exhaustion, and depletion of reserves; hyperactivity coexisting with mental fatigue and confusion; alterations between bursts of creativity and cognitive disturbances (e.g., extreme forgetfulness).

The chronology reveals that shaking chills have become progressively more severe. Yet, the benefits derived cannot be overemphasized: lowering of blood pressure, to the point where medication is no longer necessary; maintaining good posture, infused with *qi* (energy), and so forth.

Even in a state of severe mental fatigue and confusion, the wisdom of the body could be discerned: I moved around and performed tasks without conscious deliberation, as if my movements were to a large extent automatized. Intensive exercise sharpened my proprioceptive perception, enabling me to be sensitive to tightness or weakness, even mild injuries I had sustained years ago, throughout my whole body. My kinesthetic sense was enhanced in dancing, practicing martial arts, and so forth when I entered into a state of selfless-forgetfulness. The end result was a healed body, more relaxed than I had ever known—visible to those who had witnessed my dance performances.

Mania or hypomania is supposed to be a mood disorder. Yet, my description has been focused primarily on the psychophysical and cognitive, rather than affective, aspects of functioning. This is dictated by the reality of my firsthand experiences.

In the language of psychoanalysis, I had unhindered access to the unconscious and was able to record the workings of the id. Defenses had broken down so much so that I found myself in a psychotic state. Yet, the raw impulses of the id were never in danger of being acted out. Rather, they have served me well in my artistic and literary pursuits later through sublimation.

Finally, I must ask: At rock bottom, what is the nature of the conditions I "suffered" from? I was perplexed about my episodic experiences, especially in the beginning. They appeared alien to me, for I had not yet gotten used to them. So after Hypomania 1, I wrote a message to a psychologist, renowned for his studies of intelligence, hoping that he would provide me with some answer.

Recently I experienced something extremely unusual, which I would like to share with you. It relates to intelligence and creativity, I think; but I don't know if it has been intensively studied as a phenomenon.

For about a couple of weeks, my mind "exploded." All kinds of ideas came so fast that I could not put them down on paper, or into a computer, fast enough. Thoughts, ranging from cosmology to psychology, raced through my mind. They were entertaining thoughts, at least to me, so much so that I had difficulty sleeping (unusual for me).

What I experienced may be called mental hyperactivity, but it might be more than that. . . . The ideas were creative ideas: enough for a book that I would love to write. I also experienced flashes of insight. Somewhat like enlightenment! I noticed many things more sharply than before. For instance, I listened to music, and heard sounds in a way that I did not before. And I did many things for the first time in my life, such as dancing, entering into a trance, and so forth.

People around me say that I have become "strange"—or, more precisely, stranger. More expressive, for instance. I am not sure how these fit into current understanding of intelligence. Because of your research in human intelligence, you might be able to provide me with some answer.

Unfortunately, I did not receive a reply. My perplexity continued. Physical symptoms (e.g., insomnia, fatigue) were prominent during all episodes. Shaking chills appeared for the first time on board the *Queen Victoria* in Hypomania 5 and became severe in Hypomania 8. Experiencing cognitive deficits (e.g., extreme forgetfulness) and mental confusion (e.g., getting lost easily) really scared me in both of these episodes. No physician has yet proffered a medical explanation for these symptoms.

Are the physical symptoms a part of my madness? And what is the nature of this madness? What is the dynamics of positives (e.g., exuberance) coexisting with negatives (e.g., anguish) in terms of spirituality? These are crucial questions to be addressed in the following chapters.

I have learned to identify telltale prodromal signs that forebode the onset of an episode and to prevent it from developing into full-blown hypomania or mania. Preceding onset, there are times when I easily get tired and absent-minded, so much so that I can do hardly any work at all for weeks. At the same time, I become more emotional and sensitive. Tears would flow from my eyes when I hear music I love or contemplate about my life condition. I can just sense that something is brewing. Sure enough, an episode would follow.

But I admit to an unsettling thought: For how long will my madness last? I have a premonition that it will last for a long time to come. My parents had a long life. Physically I can do things that most other people of my age cannot do. I have discovered the elixir of longevity in my passion for music and dance. All these point to a long life. As I say, "I want to die young, but to delay it as long as possible." I look forward to seeing more madness in a man at age 100 or beyond! That would be legendary.

Again, the benefits give me consolation if I am indeed condemned to be mad unto the end of my days. One of the greatest benefits, obtained in Hypomania 8, was nothing short of a transformative religious experience on an Easter Sunday. Unlike previous religious experiences, which were experienced in private, this one took place in public, in front of an assembly. This experience will be described at the end of Chapter 6.

My episodes are characterized by imbalances in terms of extreme fluctuations in energy level, cognitive functioning, and mood. What happens to me when balance is restored? Life becomes mundane again. Inertia sets in: I become physically lazy. I succumb to one of the Seven Deadly Sins, sloth.

Moreover, I do many things better when I'm "imbalanced." I dance without being self-conscious; I don't question myself about accepting new challenges, like learning Taiji push-hands or writing Chinese poetry in English. Now that I'm "balanced," I've become more self-conscious, and I question myself. The greatest irony is that my transformation is characterized by sequential alterations between creativity and stagnation. Damnation!

I've caught myself for being harsh again. Nevertheless, I do recognize that I owe much to the episodes of madness for the creative ideas I have gained, "enough for a book that I would love to write."

3

Madness Has Enriched My Life

A life that has failed to harness the creative forces of madness is an impoverished life.

A body in motion invigorates the mind and uplifts the spirit; an invigorated mind makes the body healthier and pushes the spirit forward; an uplifted spirit gives the body calm and the mind serenity.

I have been a clinical psychologist for most of my working life, in Hong Kong as well as North America. Drummed into my head are the psychopathologies of various mental disorders. At one point, I thought to myself, "But there may be positive values to abnormality!"

An opportunity to witness how madness may enrich one's life came when I reached the age of 58. I experienced something I had never before experienced: an explosion of creativity, emotional reactivity to music, freedom from impulse inhibition, and the like.

At the time, I did not interpret these strange phenomena in psychiatric terms. Why should I? Since then, more episodes have occurred—all of exuberance, none of depression—spontaneously, unpredictably, and mysteriously. Bewildered, I am compelled to ask myself, "Am I mad, or enlightened?" In response to this question, I wrote a book *Enlightened or Mad? A Psychologist Glimpses into Mystical Magnanimity* published by Dignity Press in 2014.

A Self-Study of Unipolar Mania and Hypomania

The present undertaking is an assessment of madness in my life and, by extension, to madness in the lives of others. My contention is that, on balance, madness has enriched rather than damaged my life. I discuss the atypical nature, cultural context, and clinical implications of my case. My self-study casts doubt on the deficit model according to which mental disorders are viewed solely or primarily in pathological terms.

Extraordinary Experiences

Taking advantage of my specialty, I conduct a self-study of abnormality, acting as both "doctor" and "patient." The primary data consist of firsthand experiences I have gained from my episodes of "madness."

As expected, major symptoms include inflated self-confidence, talkativeness, and flight of ideas; less expected is the salience of inability to sleep; mental fatigue and confusion (unable to perform simple tasks, such as arithmetic calculations; at worst, unable to parse whole sentences, getting lost around my neighborhood). I was aware that my behavior sometimes went beyond the bounds of social acceptability, thus causing considerable anxiety in my family and among my friends and colleagues.

However, my mind retained its logicality and self-reflectiveness. Even in the depths of madness, I would monitor my thinking and behavior. This helped me greatly to maintain perspective and deflate my supreme self-confidence periodically. My impulse control was adequate. At no point was there any threat of my losing contact with reality or of acting in destructive or violent ways. My inflated self-confidence was nowhere near delusions of grandeur. I became a more colorful person, more empathic, generous, and loving during episodes. I struggled to harness the creative forces of madness without incurring unnecessary social costs.

Moreover, I had glimpses of enlightenment, a mystical state of magnanimity, tranquility, and freedom from inner turmoil. I say "glimpses of enlightenment" because they are exactly only glimpses that are unfortunately extinguished at the exit from an episode. However, they remain experiences to be treasured, acting as a beacon for the remainder of my journey through life.

The Mind Can Work in Wondrous Ways

Some of my experiences stand out as extraordinary. During episodes, everything seemed to have speeded up, in my thinking, talking, writing, responding to social cues, and so forth. During Hypomania 13, in a state of near mental exhaustion, I found myself unexpectedly able to recall the strategies of grand masters of *Weiqi* (*Go* in Japanese, *Baduk* in Korean) I had studied decades earlier, thus enabling me to compete with advanced players via the Internet. There were many other similar, although less dramatic, experiences in memory recall (e.g., of events long past, rapidly and in great detail, that were relevant to the immediate moment).

To me, all these were a convincing demonstration that the mind can work in wondrous ways during episodes. Superefficient retrieval of past learning and memory may occur. I asked myself: could this be an underlying mechanism for the explosions of creativity or enhanced empathy I had experienced?

Other extraordinary experiences were gained when I entered into a state of selfless self. I was able to achieve feats beyond my wildest imagination. While practicing "virtual calligraphy," I was able to write Chinese characters in the air with both hands simultaneously, differing in synchrony and stroke sequence.

On one occasion, in a state of no-mind emptiness, the self seemed to have vanished. I healed a seriously injured knee through magnifying and directing the energy flow within my body to it. This was verifiable by several people who knew about my injury.

On other occasions, I experienced hallucinations: vivid images appeared, spontaneously or directed at will (e.g., seeing myself being nailed on a cross and feeling intense pathos for the sufferings of humankind; experiencing androgyny, the yin and the yang, united in one body).

A Cosmic Experience of Being in a Coffin to Be Interred

One episode I have had (Hypomania 17) represents a high point of my spiritual journey. One night, I lied down in bed, assuming a "corpse" posture (a yoga technique for utmost relaxation). I then visualized myself lying in a coffin about to be interred. I could hear and feel nails being pounded as the cover of the coffin was closed, quickly. Then there was absolute darkness, silence, and nothingness. Yet I had no fear at all. Soon I sensed a faint shimmering of light, quite impossible to describe.

Yes, it was a cosmic experience. The cosmos is a boundless sphere, infinite beyond human imagination, I dimly sensed. What's the infinity of infinities? Not a question to be answered simply because rational thought was absent. The sense of time vanished too.

Definitely, there was no big bang. No fire, no volcanoes, and no nothing— implying a terminal state of deep freeze, eternal terror (based on my knowledge of cosmology and eschatology)? Then I fell asleep, probably more deeply than I ever had before. Upon waking up, I sensed that the episode had come to an end. I said to myself, at long last I have arrived!

I pray that henceforth what I have gained through extreme endurance will carry into my "normal" life. Then the demarcation between madness and normality may be undone. Under such circumstances, to experience rapturous delight requires no justification anymore.

A Life Enriched, Rather Than Damaged

Having had as many as 22 episodes provides me with ample opportunities for learning to cope. I have learned to read prodromal signs appearing about two to three weeks before onsets, such as unexplainable mental fatigue and confusion, fluctuations in energy level, heightened esthetic-literary sensitivities and emotional responsiveness to music. This enables me to take precautionary measures to better manage my behavior in public and avoid incurring unnecessary social costs or exposing myself to physical danger (e.g., driving in a state of mental confusion). Chronological trends across episodes may be discerned. Later episodes tend to be mild, although cognitive and psychophysical disturbances have become salient.

During episodes, I had to struggle with imbalances, such as anguish intermingling with ecstasy. A Chinese saying helped to put me in perspective: "There is no greater sadness than a heart made numb." Anguish did not incapacitate my daily functioning. On the contrary, it allowed me to be in touch with my deepest pains and anxieties. Real catharsis! I thought to myself: "The world has long wanted to expunge unhappiness from human consciousness. But I treasure the capacity for depth of feelings—in both positive and negative directions." I managed to maintain a sense of psychophysical well-being while suffering from an inability to fall asleep, physical exhaustion, and depletion of reserves. My hyperactivity often coexisted with mental or physical fatigue. My mind alternated between bursts of creative output and cognitive disturbances (e.g., extreme forgetfulness or confusion).

Looking back at the firsthand experiences I have gained, I would say that, on balance, my encounters with madness have enriched, rather than damaged, my life. The psychiatric symptoms have indeed incurred occupational and social costs. Still, if given a choice, I would rather absorb these costs for the gains in creativity, literary-artistic-esthetic sensibilities, and capacity to enjoy life; and in health, physical, mental, and spiritual (e.g., liberation from obsessive-compulsivity and self-condemnation). It would be hardly appropriate to characterize the overall picture solely in clinical terms.

On Being Strange in Normality as in Madness

This first-person account is exceptional in more ways than one. First, the presence of life-enhancing features, coupled with the absence of depression, run counter to commonly described mood disorders in psychiatry. Second, both the doctor and the patient (being the same person) are steeped in a bilingual-bicultural background. To my knowledge, a self-study of such an exceptional case has not been reported before. In the process of conducting the self-study, I have to remind myself: "Don't overgeneralize." I am also constantly challenged to reexamine my own thinking on abnormality, particularly the deficit model that views mental disorders solely in pathological terms.

Atypicality

I am aware that other people may view my madness differently from the way I do. To some of my colleagues, I fit into the profile of hypomania or mania, according to their psychiatric bible on diagnosis, the *Diagnostic and Statistical Manual of Mental Disorders* (see Chapter 8). This, I don't deny.

However, they have missed the significance of my atypicality. My firsthand experiences counter much of the psychiatric literature on mood disorders. The presumption of a shift in polarity between mania and depression is inherent in the use of the term *bipolar*. Having had 22 episodes of mood elevation and none of depression, I cannot be said to have suffered from a bipolar disorder at all. If so, a new diagnostic category has to be added: unipolar disorder with only hypomanic and/or manic episodes.

Moreover, there is no impairment serious enough to incapacitate occupational or daily functioning. Self-reflection and self-monitoring, both indicative of a sound mind at work, play a crucial role in maintaining my capacity to function: through helping me to deflate my supreme self-confidence, keep in touch with reality, and avoid causing more harm to myself or others. Most important are the positive features I have described, such as superefficiency in the recall of past learning and memory, creativity, and enhanced literary-artistic-esthetic sensibilities.

All these clinical features summate to a most atypical case. However, I am also atypical in a more general, nonclinical sense. All my life, I have found myself atypical in thought and action wherever I happen to be. So, I am strange in normality as in madness. The existentialist Sartre says that man is condemned to be free. Am I condemned to be atypical as well?

In madness, others perceive me as stranger than my usual self. Being stranger than the strange often invites ostracism, stigmatization, and even unconditional rejection. I am no stranger to these unpleasant experiences. For instance, when I decided to pursue a career in psychology, many of my Chinese friends and relatives thought I was half-mad.

Now, some of them may be convinced I am totally mad. On the other hand, I have other friends who find in me a more humorous, entertaining, and authentic person when I am mad. And these are ones I count as true friends.

My self-study casts doubt on the deficit model according to which mental disorders are viewed solely or primarily in pathological terms. Is it not possible that a life totally devoid of madness is an impoverished life? This then becomes my goal: to lead a dignified normal life enriched by madness.

Madness in Cultural Context

When I studied clinical psychology in the U.S. back in the 1960s, basically I was exposed to nothing but Western psychology. When I began introducing clinical psychology into Hong Kong society, I encountered formidable obstacles: There was little to support professional clinical psychology transplanted from the West into an alien context. To reeducate myself for professional development, I had to dig deep into my cultural roots, in order to achieve a creative synthesis of East-West learning. In particular, I was fascinated by the contrasting conceptions of selfhood between the East and the West.

In Western psychology, the healthy self is conceived as stable over time; it is a coherent, integrated, and unitary whole; in Eastern thought, Daoism and Buddhism in particular, the notion of selflessness is central to the conception of selfhood. Little did I know that later on in my career I would actually experience the selfless self in a *literal* sense. During madness, especially in the depths of mania, I did enter into states of transcendent consciousness. In such a state, cognition was suspended; the self was absent.

I would argue that to experience the selfless self or the empty mind is to go beyond, not supplant, the normal and healthy intact sense of self. In a similar vein, the achievement of impulse control is prerequisite to experiencing the extraordinary. In terms of psychodynamics, this implies overcoming repression and gaining access to the unconscious. If what comes out are unchecked rampant impulses and raw destructiveness, the result would be horror.

Digging deeply into my own self, I see a preponderance of positives (e.g., love of humanity) over the negatives (e.g., hateful violence), and I foresee no horror when impulses are expressed in magnified intensities. Early in my second manic episode, I wrote in my diary, "Eros without Thanatos, safe." However, a reversal of this preponderance raises the specter of madness wedded to evil.

Differences in the conceptions of selfhood between the East and the West have implications for how and when psychiatric diagnoses are applied (see Thematic Group 3): the need to guard against uncritical viewing extraordinary experiences (e.g., willful hallucinations, selfless self) in pathological terms. I would argue further that expanding our conceptions of selfhood opens more doors to life enrichment in the West as well.

Clinical Implications

My madness has been instrumental in my professional development, particularly in terms of seeing things from a patient's perspective. What I have learned about professional service delivery may be summarized as follows. First, as mental health professionals, we have to be more alert to atypical cases, or atypical features of a case, that do not have a good fit with established psychiatric thinking. Second, we need to exercise greater caution against making a diagnosis without regard for cultural context. Third, we need to think beyond the deficit model of psychopathology and look for positive features that may be exploited for therapeutic gains. For instance, I would encourage patients to exercise more self-monitoring and self-reflectiveness to the fullest extent of their capacity; and to find some meaning or value in madness wherever they can be found (without falling into the traps of denial or rationalization), rather than to dwell in misery.

My self-study has provided some evidence in support of my contention that madness can enhance a person's capacity to enjoy life, specifically in terms of health, creativity, literary-artistic-esthetic sensibilities, and spirituality. The psychiatric disturbances I have experienced may be monitored and rendered relatively harmless.

Sequential Learning and Coping: Practical Suggestions

Some readers may have had experiences similar to those of mine. How can this book be of service to them? An imaginary dialogue ensues.

> **David** What have you learned in terms of coping, now that you have had twenty bouts of madness already? What are some practical suggestions?

YF Bearing in mind that different cases vary, I don't want to offer definitive, formulaic answers in the form of do's and don'ts, or "An Idiot's Guide to. . .." Rather, I delight in respectful sharing with an intelligent audience. First and foremost, refrain from driving if at all possible, especially in the height of mania. Distractibility leads to reckless driving that can kill you. As in Hypomania 8, for a while I dared not drive, on account of mental fatigue and confusion—rather than of recklessness. I value my life too much to endanger it, in madness no less than in normality.

David In the midst of Hypomania 2, you wrote in your diary (Nov 1998), "Men are not stupid, except when they are bewitched by women." This reflects an awareness of the dangers of "falling in love" during spells of exuberance: An outpouring of emotions is characteristic and may be directed to a specific person.

YF Being self-bewitched is closer to the truth.

David Romantic entanglements established during madness may well rest on perilous grounds because perceptions may be distorted and judgment impaired. If the target person does not reciprocate, one may not read or discount the signals of rejection. As well, my cautionary remarks apply to depressive episodes, during which the sufferer may be more vulnerable to temptations of emotional support from someone he is attracted to.

YF Romantic relationships are, I suspect, of foremost interest to many readers. And I do want to come to the defense of romantic love. All my life, drummed into my head is the injunction, "Think before you leap." If I think too much, what would become of me? Paralyzed, I suspect. Plunge before you think: That's falling in love. The most important decisions in life are leaps of faith, not of thinking.

David But you don't want to leap too often either! You are an incurable romantic. Being overly enthusiastic, optimistic, and self-confident is another problem. You are probably running too far ahead of people around you. In the midst of a spell, your enthusiasm may be unshared by others; reality may be clouded with wishful thinking.

YF When I read my diaries now, I am dumbfounded by how my self-confidence was inflated and how difficult it would be for my wishes to be realized. That's why it is ill-advised to make major decisions when your mood is abnormally elevated. With greater familiarity of the symptoms, which are basically similar in my case, detection gets sequentially easier.

Early in Mania 2, I called a friend and said, "I feel that I am beginning to get overly excited, but I am clear about my physical condition. I will be all right after several days of good rest." Clearly, I was aware that I was about to enter into another period of unusual excitement.

As it turned out, however, I was overly optimistic about recovery. Similarly, in Hypomania 8, I could tell exactly when I first sensed trouble brewing: One day, while having lunch with relatives, I noticed a more-than-usual pressure toward being talkative. Early detection enabled me to take preventive actions. The lesson learned: Nip it in the bud when you sense that something has gone awry, physically or psychologically.

> **David** Maintaining contact with friends and relatives is important: Their feedback on your behavior may help to keep you on track. The trouble is, however, you may not want to listen to them when you are high. At the very least, be receptive to your own inner voices of caution. But what if your suffering is inflicted upon you by your friends and relatives?
>
> **YF** There is no point to self-inflict more suffering. As I wrote in Hypomania 5, "Let not the folly of others torture you. That's the Dao of remaining sane in an insane world." Sequential learning bore fruit. I took measures (consulting a physician and taking the medicine, including sleeping pills, he prescribed) in Hypomania 5 to take care of physical symptoms. Recovery was relatively fast and easy.

By the onset of Hypomania 6, I had probably learned enough to forestall a full-blown episode. I was determined to keep it under control, but I didn't want to kill it. My goal was to reap the benefits of creativity and heightened sensibilities, without costly social consequences. As in other episodes, the key factor was sleep: I knew that if I could fall asleep, I would be all right. That's exactly what happened. There was no insomnia. I was mostly able to control the madness myself, without taking medicine. It did not result in damage to my social image.

Hypomania 7 was kept under control early on. I took sleeping pills for two nights, enough to get rid of insomnia. But I knew that mental hyperactivity remained an underlying problem. Somehow, I managed to keep the spell dormant. So there were few overt hypomanic manifestations that might disturb others. Eventually, just before my departure for the United States, balance was restored, thus ending the episode.

My main concern in Hypomania 8 was not to scare my friends and relatives in America. I kept my manic-like manifestations secret successfully. As far as they were concerned, what I went through was an unexplained, mysterious medical condition.

> **David** But I am convinced that a psychological mechanism underlay Hypomania 8. The months following your relocation to the United States were the worst time in your life: You uprooted yourself from Hong Kong, where you had spent most of your life, and were feeling socially isolated; you had to adjust to life after retirement and to aging. Thus, the psychological mechanism may be thought of as counter depression.
>
> **YF** Yes, I was liberated from feelings of depression. And together with that liberation, creative-artistic impulses were unleashed. Rid of inertia, my body was propelled

to exercise. Counter depression was probably operative, to various degrees, during previous episodes also. It is as powerful as it is seductive. Who wants to be stuck in the depth of hellish feelings? And who doesn't want to be liberated from compulsivity and, even more, to have creative-artistic impulses unleashed?

David Acknowledging psychological mechanisms does not mean rejecting medical solutions. To take or not to take medicine for treating mental disorders is an important and difficult decision.

I generally prefer to let the body's own wisdom take care of itself, without medication. Sleep disturbances remain a big problem, however. During Mania 2, I was unable to fall asleep for about a month. Coincidentally, the apartment right above mine was undergoing renovation; loud sounds of hammers and electric drills made falling asleep doubly difficult. Staying at home most of the time, I learned to "tune out" these sounds with self-hypnosis; success was limited. I stubbornly resisted taking medicine. Eventually, I capitulated, for fatigue as a constant companion was too much to bear. For the first time, I took antipsychotic medicine (a low dosage, two Risperdal tablets, 1 mg each). I slept for several nights consecutively and came out of madness.

As to Hypomania 8, taking sleeping pills for a few nights didn't help much, but taking risperidone (generic name for Risperdal; also a small dosage, three tablets, 2 mg each) was definitive in ending the episode. Still, I was disconcerted by my capitulation because Risperdal is, after all, an antipsychotic medicine usually prescribed for severe psychiatric disorders, such as schizophrenia.

You would be more disconcerted to learn that Johnson and Johnson has been plagued by lawsuits over its marketing tactics involving Risperdal, one of the most commonly prescribed antipsychotic drugs. The healthcare giant is accused of having concealed Risperdal's many nasty side effects, some of which may be life-threatening. Here is a scary excerpt from the information sheet on risperidone provided by a well-known pharmacy.

> Drowsiness, dizziness, lightheadedness, drooling, nausea, weight gain, or tiredness may occur.... Tell your doctor immediately if you have any serious side effects, including: difficulty swallowing, muscle spasms, shaking (tremor), mental/mood changes (such as anxiety, restlessness), signs of infection (such as fever, persistent sore throat).... Tell your doctor immediately if you develop any unusual movements.... Get medical help right away if you have any of the following symptoms: fever, muscle stiffness/pain/tenderness/weakness, severe tiredness, severe confusion, sweating, fast/irregular heartbeat, dark urine, change in the amount of urine. Rarely, males may have a painful or prolonged erection lasting more than 4 hours. If this occurs, stop using this drug and get

medical help right away, or *permanent* problems could occur. . . . This is not a complete list of possible side effects. . . . [Italics added]

> YF   Scary side effects are by no means unusual. Aside from this issue, medication is inherently limited. Taking medicine alone is no solution to problems of living. It does not promote health, lead to new ways of relating or viewing the world. However, we have to balance the benefits against the costs. I am now more receptive to medication, on the basis of need. In particular, I accept that taking sleeping pills alone may not be enough; they do not address mood elation, mental hyperactivity, fatigue.
>
> David   We have now learned that being able to sleep is a necessary, but perhaps not sufficient, treatment of fatigue. Putting an end to mental hyperactivity is also necessary. Restoring balance, physical and mental, is essential to recovery. This is systemic thinking, on which Chinese medicine rests. In the long run, Chinese life-fostering practices such as qigong are preferable to medication; at least, they would reduce overreliance on medication. Balance holds the key: You will be a happy person if you can reap the benefits of creativity in madness, without costly adverse consequences.
>
> YF   I can testify to a success story. During one of my hypomanic episodes, I was able to lower my blood pressure to healthy levels without medication through intensive practice in martial arts and dance to music. Later, I told my physician what I had accomplished and asked him if I could stop taking or reduce the medicines he had prescribed for lowering my blood pressure. He was skeptical and said no. At that point, I decided not to adhere to his medical regimen.
>
> David   Frankly, what abhors me is the extent to which Americans rely on drugs to treat mental disorders, alleviate anxiety and depression, control hyperactive children, and so forth. Some even rely on psychedelic drugs, marijuana, and the like for "peak" experiences of spirituality, in denial of the perils of brain damage that these drugs may bring.
>
> FY   Immersing myself in peak experiences through music and dance entails no such perils. I go for self-intoxication, not intoxication by wine or any other means.

A Chinese proverb, rooted in the Buddhist conception of self-enchantment, puts it this way:

> Not wine, we intoxicate ourselves;
> Nor beauty, we enchant ourselves.

The proverb expresses the same basic idea, nearly word for word in translation, in what Shakespeare wrote:

> Not wine, men intoxicate themselves;
> Not vice, men entice themselves.

In all, the main lesson we have learned is to speak of solving problems and enriching life, rather than of curing a disease.

Body-Mind-Spirit Interconnectedness

What do my episodes of madness inform the reader about how the mind, body, and spirit are interconnected? Manic or hypomanic states are thought of as disturbances of mood. So I am particularly intrigued by the physical, flesh and blood changes I have described, such as fatigue, oversensitivity to noise, and energy flow within the body. Clearly, physical changes are concomitant, even integral, to changes in mind and spirit. What are some of the more dramatic changes?

> **YF** On several occasions, I had hiccups that lasted on and off for some five hours in the middle of the night. Bewildered, I consulted a Taiji master about what happened. She congratulated me, saying "It's a good thing." True enough, although the process was unpleasant, the end result was beneficial to my health. After the hiccups subsided, I felt a sense of extraordinary well-being; whatever gastrointestinal imbalances or disturbances I had previously were gone.

One particular feat I achieved in Hypomania 10 stands out in my memory. On a chilly morning, I practiced Taiji in a park. I did not follow a set sequence of movements, as most practitioners do; instead, I moved spontaneously, without constraints. I entered into a state of selfless-oblivion. Soon I felt a powerful flow of energy or *qi* within my body. I felt warm throughout, even though I was wearing little. My hands turned red, radiating heat that another person could feel at a distance of several inches.

> **David** This brings to mind Tibetan monks who are able, in a state of deep meditation, to generate enough bodily heat to produce steam effusing from blankets put over their bodies. Your body must have been burning up calories at an explosive pace, depleting reserves. This may explain why you have shaking chills during your episodes. A measure of "megalomania" may be essential to creative adventures and is, to that extent, healthy.
>
> **YF** Afterwards, I joined a couple of advanced Taiji practitioners and followed them in performing a set sequence which I had learned only as a beginner some years ago. To my surprise, I had no trouble at all. So it seems that my kinesthetic sense may be enhanced, in dancing as in practicing martial arts, when I am loosened from self-consciousness and enters into an alternate state of being.

There were also perceptual changes as well. Most dramatic of these was a supersensitive sense of smell. On one occasion, I was walking along the bank of an inland swamp. Incredibly, I was able to smell the unpleasant odors from the swamp more than a hundred feet away, even though there was a steady breeze blowing. I am positive that normally I would not have been able to do so. Was my sense of smell really enhanced? I don't think so. It was my mind made quiet that enabled me to read the odorous signals with my normal nose.

My time perception also changed. Eating a meal, for instance, might take hours—to my surprise when I looked at my watch. Simply, I had no awareness of how much time had passed. On one occasion, it took me some two hours to adjust a pair of new goggles, fumbling clumsily along. This exceeded by far the time I took to learn how to do it for the first time (an embarrassing 30 minutes or so), bearing testimony to my extraordinary inability to perform even simple tasks during episodes. I didn't know how long it took until I asked someone what time it was. Then it dawned on me that my time perception had altered.

In all, I am grateful that I have learned so much from the episodes of madness through groping and self-discovery, without the benefit of guidance from a master. But I don't think that I have really discovered anything new. I am only fortunate to have *experienced* what is already known to luminary masters of martial arts, qigong, or yoga, and thus to marvel at the hidden potentialities of the human body.

David   There is an irony. In Hypomania 8, you said that even in a state of severe mental fatigue and confusion, "The wisdom of the body could be discerned: I moved around and performed tasks without conscious deliberation, as if my movements were to a large extent automatized." This recapitulates what happened in Hypomania 2: "I was physically exhausted. However, I felt that my motility was efficient, 'with not a single movement wasted.' Even my handwriting changed." Wouldn't it be great if "the wisdom of the body" were to take its course in your normal life as well?

YF   The wisdom of the body reaches its pinnacle in what I would call Body-Mind-Spirit (BMS) interconnectedness. BMS health presupposes interconnectedness among the body, mind, and spirit. It is, above all, holistic: Changes in one domain lead to changes in other domains. A disconnect spells trouble, resulting in imbalances. Hence, balance is the hallmark of holistic health.

My episodes are a goldmine of imbalances: inability to fall asleep; physical and mental fatigue and even depletion of reserves, coexisting with mental hyperactivity; cognitive disturbances, such as extreme forgetfulness; alterations between compulsivity and bursts of creativity. Running through the episodes are recapitulations of what happened in Mania 1: "The body was near exhaustion, yet the mind remained active, running on fast time."

> **David** You focus too much on the negatives. You have experienced remarkable realizations of the human body's potentialities, particularly when you enter into the state of selfless-oblivion. I have been pondering another question in connection with BMS interconnectedness. Earlier, you thought that a hyperactive sympathetic autonomic nervous system (SANS) characterized the underlying physiology of Mania 2.

So the physical underlies the mental: Underlying mental hyperactivity is probably a hyperactive SANS. Two implications follow. One, physiological causation should be given more weight. Two, controlling or reducing SANS hyperactivity may hold a key to treatment; medication may be indicated. Of course, the mental also underlies the physical: Mental hyperactivity contributes to fatigue and is prodromal to mania.

> **YF** My libidinal drive tends to be stronger than usual during episodic spells. I strongly suspect that a hyperactive SANS has much to do with it.
>
> **David** Also your unbridled imagination and capacity to appreciate beauty! SANS is not the only culprit. "Pleasures of cloud and rain," a Chinese euphemism for sexual congress, sounds more abstract than "the birds and the bees." Both euphemisms are rooted in poetry. Samuel Coleridge wrote: "All nature seems at work. . ... The bees are stirring—birds are on the wing." Also, in English the term "cloud nine" refers to a state of blissful oblivion.
>
> **YF** In contrast, the Chinese idiom "whirling clouds, a blanket of rain" suggests the workings of considerable natural forces. Apparently, clouds in the sky evoke all kinds of fantasy on earth in different cultures.
>
> **David** To poetic minds, anything can. Revisiting Hypomania 5, you saw "a colossal sandwich of lights in the sky" on sunrise in the Mediterranean—brilliant sun rays penetrating a dark cloud. You felt overwhelmed by the majesty of the heavens. Now I read a deeper meaning into what you saw: the triumph of light over darkness. I bet you must have come close to a religious experience facilitated by madness.
>
> **YF** But I also see beauty in dark clouds. I would like to have nothing more than to remain in cloud nine in the midst of a cumulonimbus, a cumulus with a low dark base and fluffy towers that rise to great heights, portending the arrival of thunderstorms—and proclaiming the awesome power of the heavens.
>
> **David** Finally, we must spell out a major lesson learned from your experiences: Don't forget the body in any spiritual journey. Strategically, getting the body in shape is a good first step to take. The body suffused with libido produces

a mind that sees beauty everywhere, sublimating the spirit. That's BMS interconnectedness.

Now tell us more about how your encounters with madness have shaped your professional growth. In particular, using the lessons you have learned from these encounters to help others and enhance their mental health would be a fulfillment of generativity. You should mention two other contributions you have made in recent years: Dialogic Action Therapy (DAT) and Dynamic Relaxation and Meditation (DRM). A recurrent theme, in line with relational spirituality, in your approach to helping may be identified: Helping others is the best way to help oneself.

Dialogic Action Therapy

DAT integrates two cardinal ideas, dialogics and action, into a coherent framework for effective problem solving and effective living (see my book *Rewriting Psychology: An Abysmal Science?* http://www.universal-publishers.com/book.php?method=ISBN&book=1627347186). Both ideas are quintessential to defining what it means to be human. Dialogics refers to the study of all forms, aspects, and processes of dialogues. Virtually all therapeutic systems entail dialogues between persons, therapist, and client(s).

DAT stresses the importance of internal dialogues within persons as well. The therapist may exploit dialogues, both between and within persons, to achieve therapeutic gain (e.g., sharpening the client's thinking on the nature of his problems). But that is not enough. DAT promotes the unity of action and thought. It stresses that taking action is essential to successful therapy and therefore accords with the time-honored adage "Actions speak louder than words."

In DAT, the term *external dialogue* refers to an actual dialogue between persons. *Internal dialogue* (or *self-directed dialogue*) refers to a person "talking with oneself," that is, inner self-talk involving only one person, acting as both "speaker" and "listener." This self-talk may take the form of a dialogue between one's different (e.g., present and future) selves, or of an *imaginary* dialogue between oneself and another person.

Internal dialogue may be overt (spoken aloud) or covert (silent). In daily life, we shift back and forth between outer speech and inner self-talk (covert, to be discreet) when we converse with others. We fall into internal dialogic states, often without conscious effort, as naturally as we walk.

I make use of internal dialogues in normality as in madness. As an "absent-minded" professor, sometimes I may be seen talking with myself, dead serious in my quest for a solution to some intriguing problem. During my spells of exuberance, my proclivity toward internal dialogue increases. I am aware, however, that being seen to be talking with myself in public invites suspicion of madness. So I exercise caution to keep my internal dialogues covert, or I explain to others present that I am merely "thinking aloud." Even absent-minded professors have to suspend their self-absorption at some point and attend to external reality at hand. An imaginary dialogue ensues again.

> **YF** During bouts of madness, in particular, talking with myself preserves and even strengthens my sanity and gives me hope. I say to myself things like "Life is beautiful and precious, even when it descends into dark moments. There are value and meaning in suffering. Endurance gives me strength. . . .. You are too harsh on yourself. Be kind and forgiving to yourself."

Going beyond self-consolation, internal dialogue may serve as a guide and propellant for dialogic action: "You revel in your exuberance, but you must also pay attention to how other people perceive and react to your elation. Learn to harvest the benefits of madness, without incurring unnecessary social costs."

The fantastic experiences (e.g., vanished self, visual hallucinations) I had in Mania 1 were a treasure trove, which I later exploited for a useful purpose—to develop ideas of selfhood and identity in DAT. Assuming the identity of another person may be very powerful for enhancing interpersonal sensitivity and confronting prejudices. A therapist may invite clients, individually or in a group, to assume the identity of a member of the opposite sex, a minority group, a low-status group (e.g., domestic servants) or caste (e.g., untouchables in India), or a mentally or physically disabled group (e.g., people who are deaf or blind).

> **David** Yes, the self is dialogical in nature. It may be split into different selves, as in talking with oneself in everyday life or talking among our different selves in a dream. The very idea of self, moreover, sets psychology apart from the natural sciences: Unlike an atom, the self can investigate itself. Indeed, there are few ideas as pregnant with potentialities as the self.
>
> **YF** In DAT, the dialogic self engages in both internal and external dialogues, summates from its experiences, formulates and tests plans of action to solve problems. It participates in its self-transformation, even self-creation. Capable of healing itself, my dialogic self has helped me in my journey at every point.

DAT may be regarded as a general approach to effective and meaningful living, or as therapy for helping people in distress. Although articulated as therapy, DAT may be generalized to become a methodology that has universal applicability for problem solving, learning from experiences, and taking corrective actions in daily living.

> David   This marks DAT apart from dogged perseverance. To persevere without learning and without corrective actions is a fixation that runs the risk of energy squandered.
>
> YF   DAT is "Therapy for All Seasons." Haven't you already sensed the therapeutic effects on us at this very moment, when we are engaged in dialogue? And in the process of writing this book? Yes, the potency of DAT is awesome. I know because I have applied it to myself.

DAT has helped to take me out of egoism into greater union with others. Let me illustrate. I still get nervous sometimes when I have to give a presentation in front of a large audience, despite the fact that I have done it innumerable times. The technique I use is to reorient my attitude:

> You are here to perform for them, not for yourself. Uplift yourself from your egoistic concern over performance; instead, redirect your attention on how you may better communicate with the audience. Now be joyful, and delight in the delight that your presentation brings to them.

Next, I scan the audience with composure, paying special attention to those members who smile kindly. Once eye contact is established, my anxiety level drops to near zero instantaneously. I can then proceed with renewed spiritual energy. You see, you can "borrow" energy from people with whom you are in the process of forming a dialogical relationship.

The most effective way to reduce anxiety is to make others more comfortable in your presence. The best way to help oneself is to help others. I urge readers to be *committed* in applying the methods of DAT in their lives. What's the point of dwelling on how mistreated or miserable you have been? It is basically egotistic. Start to redirect your attention to making others around you happy. Now, empty your mind, unload the negatives, and be reborn.

Dynamic Relaxation and Meditation

I owe much to Hypomania 1. It gave me the idea of doing a self case study of madness. It enabled me to experience disinhibition; hence, spontaneity, flashes of insight, and selfless-oblivion. It was the first significant step toward the discovery of my artistic bent. My first love was music and dance, not psychology. My simulation of conducting music sowed the seeds for advancing art-aesthetics-psychology integration as a way of healthy living. Eventually, this integration was articulated in the idea of BMS interconnectedness. The imaginary dialogue continues.

> **David** Achieving BMS unity is the ultimate goal of holistic health: vigorous in body, tranquil in mind, uplifted in spirit. It is an essential part of my spiritual journey. Spirituality is integral to health, physical and mental; it cannot be reached without the participation of both the body and the mind. This thesis has been amply demonstrated in your episodic experiences.
>
> **YF** Mania 2 awakened me to the fact that my passion for the performing arts has remained undiminished. I would love nothing more than to put everything I have learned to advance BMS health. Finally, during Hypomania 16, I invested a small fortune to employ professional recorders to produce two DVD sets: Expressive Dance to Music and Living Safely and Well for Seniors. (Visit www.EasternTotalHealth.wordpress.com and see also Appendix D for explanatory notes on Expressive Dance to Music: A Royal Road to Holistic Health.)

I have learned many things in my life, *wushu* (martial arts), playing the violin, singing, dancing, fencing, meditation, yoga, qigong, none very well. Together, however, the whole is greater than the sum of its parts. Incorporating elements of all these together with hypnotherapy, I have created a unique approach to relaxation, stress management, and health enhancement. I call this approach Dynamic Relaxation and Meditation (DRM).

> **David** People usually think of meditation as being required to sit still, static.
>
> **YF** Therapists practice therapies that match their peculiarities, naturally, just as clients react favorably to therapies and therapists that match their needs. Given my disposition toward mental hyperactivity, the sit-still form of meditation doesn't work well for me. However, I enter a dynamic state of meditation with ease while moving or dancing to music.

While practicing DRM, I experience the body, mind, and spirit working as a unity. Adding a measure of madness, I enter into a state of complete selfless-oblivion, an altered state of consciousness, in precious moments. Repression is gone; primitive impulses animate creative self-expression. And DRM becomes poetry in motion, without words.

> **David** Some people may find it difficult to enter into a dynamic state of meditation, at least initially. Practice is required to progress from mere relaxation to

	meditation. Advanced meditative states of selfless-oblivion demand far more. What about DRM for beginners?
YF	DRM is suitable for men and women, adults and children. Practitioners do not have to know anything about hypnosis, meditation, music, or dancing; the only requirements are that they can communicate and move around. In short, DRM integrates self-expression and health. Its aim is to not only manage stress but also promote health in body, mind, and spirit. Above all, DRM is meant to be enjoyed.

DRM is applicable to the training of dancers, singers, actors, and other artists who take their chosen paths seriously. DRM may be done individually or in groups. In a group situation, verbal and especially nonverbal interaction among participants is emphasized. A therapeutic group is not just a collection of individuals; it is a dynamic field of forces acting on individuals-in-communion. The presence of others magnifies the therapeutic effects on each member of the group. Underlying this conception of the therapeutic group is, again, relational and ecumenical spirituality.

David	Could you point to specific techniques or practices that magnify therapeutic effects?
YF	A simple, but effective practice is Carnival of the Animals, named in honor of the French Romantic composer Camille Saint-Saëns. I ask participants each to imitate an animal of their choice. Naturally, children love it. So do adults when the music and movement bring forth the child hidden within their psyche.

Other techniques are as follows.

1. **Unloading of an Unwanted Baggage**: Each participant is asked to think of a specific negative (e.g., a persistent bad thought or habit), which need not be verbalized or made public, and to make a commitment to get rid of it upon passing through a door from one room symbolic of darkness to another symbolic of light. The process may be generalized to life outside: Participants are encouraged to get rid of at least one specific negative on a daily basis.
2. **Posture of Emotions**: I ask participants each to express through the language of the body a particular emotion, such as disgust, sadness, fear, anger, surprise, and happiness. They would soon learn the correspondence between emotion and posture. Identification and alteration of negative emotions may follow.

3. **Synergistic Energy Flow**: Participants sit or stand in a circle and join hands together in a meditative state induced by the therapist. Participants may be then induced through suggestive messages from the therapist to feel the flow of energy passing from one to another, first in a clockwise direction, followed by a counterclockwise direction. They may be asked each to activate their inner energy for self-healing. They may be encouraged to "borrow" energy from or to "lend" energy to other participants.
4. **Awakening of the Lotus**: Arising gradually from a prostrate position on the ground to a fully upright position, with both hands in the form of a lotus reaching for the sky. The process parallels those of growing up from babyhood to adulthood, from dejection to delight, or from ignorance to insight.

The symbolic meaning of the lotus has deep roots in Asian cultures and religions (Hinduism and Buddhism). Visualizing the image of Guanyin sitting on a lotus blossom is enough for me to forget, momentarily, all my troubles. Here is the Awakening of Lotus I have written (15 Jan 2014).

Awakening of the Sacred Lotus

What miracle of rebirth and longevity,
Save the Sacred Lotus,
Has a flower performed?
You are *the* survivor of all time:
A seed from the Sacred Lotus,
More than a thousand years old, spouts
Into life, undiminished
In her shining karma.

What other flower has inspired
Deeper, loftier spirituality?
See now the Goddess of Mercy
Sitting atop the Lotus blossom
And you too will be inspired.

What capability more advanced
Has another flower evolved to possess?
You generate heat to keep yourself warm
When the temperature around drops—
In triumph over adversity.

What other flower dares to embody
The noble virtues that mark your existence?
You remain immaculate, unstained
By the muck of the pond
From which you arise.
No glory in luxuriant adornment,
But in pure and simple dignity.

David   Looking at photographs of Chinese people taken a century or more ago, I am struck by their characteristic postures: stiff, rigid, lifeless. You would trace this to pervasive inhibition and impulse control rooted in Confucianism. What specific DRM techniques are suitable for loosening Chinese participants up?

YF   My own physical transformation may serve as a guide to treatment. My body was stiff and rigid too, though not lifeless, more so than I would like; this paralleled my mental rigidity, compulsivity, and obsessiveness. So you can imagine how overjoyed I was when I discovered the DRM route to undo oppressive inhibition and control: BMS interconnectedness. Suddenly my body becomes supple and expressive, more so than I could have imagined. I cried out loud in celebration, as if I had breathed life into Chinese civilization after centuries of suffocation. And for alleviating the sense of shame that I have described as "a shackle on the Chinese soul."

David   Posture of Emotions may be adapted to unshackle the sense of shame among Chinese participants. Invite participants each to express in posture and movements something *they feel* ashamed of (not the same as something to be ashamed of), only to find out that it is not so terrible after all. This technique is especially effective in the context of a therapeutic group because the presence of an audience, real, imagined, or assumed, is interwoven with how shame is experienced.

DRM cannot be understood fully in words. Experiential learning is essential. There are also nonverbal analogues of techniques like those used in DAT. For instance, physical distance may be used as an indication of psychological distance between individuals. One exercise is to ask two participants to engage in reciprocal movements, with one person advancing and the other retreating, and vice versa. A more advanced exercise is to approach synchronicity in body, mind, and spirit.

Witness Rudolf Nureyev and Margot Fonteyn, two of the greatest ballet dancers of all time, dancing with one body, one soul. That's ultimate synchronicity. The possibilities seem legion, limited by only the therapist's creativity. Therapy, however, is of no use if participants do not translate into action in their daily lives what they have learned in therapy sessions.

We spend an incredibly large portion of our lives on eating, though not as much as animals do. But we seldom devote time to reflect on how we eat. So let me illustrate how DRM may be extended to various realms of living with some (deceptively) simple advice on eating that are easy (but not really) to put into practice. They represent a distillate of insights derived from health psychology, Buddhist teachings, and the Christian tradition of the love-feast.

A Chinese idiom says, "The people regard eating as their heaven [primal want]." No wonder, the culture of eating and drinking has deep roots in China. You hardly see a person eating alone; but you see plenty families of three generations eating together. So having a meal is as much about eating as about sociality. But it is now threatened by the onslaught of fast-food chains, by the likes of McDonald and Kentucky Fried Chicken. Against this backdrop, I offer the following.

1. Get away from the desk where you do your work. (Eating at the same desk where you work is a bad habit. It is unhygienic, unsociable, and unhelpful to free your mind from thinking about work while you eat.)
2. Turn off the TV if you are eating at home. (This may be difficult to do in the face of opposition by members of your family. So it is essential to establish a norm. The implication is enormous: not to allow the TV to replace dialogues.)
3. Begin to regulate your pace. Sit down slowly, with your back upright.
4. Clear your mind. Rid yourself of negative thoughts, especially angry thoughts.
5. Close your eyes, breathe slowly, relax, and enter into a state of quiet calmness, if only for a brief moment. Then open your eyes with a sense of renewed life.
6. Reach out and hold hands together with your family or friends. (Remember Synergistic Energy Flow?)
7. Treasure the food in front of you and appreciate the labor that has gone into its preparation.
8. Eat slowly, allowing your mind to be fully present in the process of eating.
9. Don't go back to work immediately. Take a break, even if brief.

These are not meant to be just good habits, but habits of the heart. The whole process of preparing yourself for a meal takes no more than one minute or two. But your perception of time may change, as if the clock has slowed down and you will live long. I guarantee that you will discover the joys of eating you have not dreamed of before, prevent digestive problems from brewing, and in some cases restore balance to your disturbed gastrointestinal system—if, and only if, you adhere to the habits of the heart with persistence. You will then "eat like a Buddha."

Now why don't you take a break from reading this book, learn to practice DRM, and experience again the joy of the body, mind, and spirit working in unison?

Coping with Depression

A pressing question is how I cope with negative emotions that stubbornly refuse to go away and continue to wreak havoc within the psyche. Depression is by far more common than exuberance in the human experience. So we should talk more on "madness in the opposite direction of exuberance."

> **YF** People react in different ways to disaster, trauma, personal failure, serious illness, or loss of a significant other. Spiritual orientation makes a big difference; A negative orientation makes people more vulnerable; a positive orientation makes them more resilient.

Thus, some people remain bitter for life, feeling that the world owes them a better deal; others commit themselves to make the world a better place; still others, who have been treated with gross injustice by others, let go of their anger and forgive. Some plunge into depression out of despair; others prevail with hope. Some lack the energy to fight on and remain stagnant; others not only rebound but also grow psychologically and emerge from their ordeals better adjusted, stronger, healthier.

> **David** What are the strategies for facilitating fellow travelers to augment spiritual forces in their lives, especially in the face of adversity or in the depth of a depression? I must push you again, this time to share more of how you have coped with frustrations, despair, or spiritual emptiness.
>
> **YF** I offer four coping strategies to those who have soon to face or are already facing life's misfortunes: forbearance, forgiveness, hope, and meaning reconstruction. These strategies have pulled me out of black holes and restored me to spirituality. I would love nothing more than to see that they do the same for fellow travelers. (See Appendix B on how to apply these strategies in detail.)

Forbearance

First, forbearance is the capacity to endure pain, suffering, or ill fortune without complaint. The antithesis of forbearance is intolerance. In the present context, it refers to unwillingness or inability to endure frustration, pain, suffering, or ill fortune, coupled with a tendency to complain. A person with low frustration tolerance tends to be impatient, irritable, and prone to emotional outbursts; such a person is likely to make a habit of whining.

There is no point dwelling on how mistreated or miserable I have been. It's basically egoistic. Applying Dialogic Action Therapy (DAT), I try to redirect attention to heal others, and thus heal myself through them.

Besides, being Chinese, I have the capacity to endure pain, suffering, or ill fortune without complaint. Throughout Chinese history, forbearance is dictated by necessity: People fall victim to harsh socioeconomic or political realities beyond their control; they are hobbled by poverty, fearful of punishment or retaliation by the rich and powerful.

Forbearance may or may not entail fortitude—the moral courage to stand up for one's conviction in the face of threat or danger to oneself. Chinese people commonly regard self-cultivation as a great virtue. However, appeasement, placation, or conciliation motivated by fear is often mistaken to be self-cultivation.

Restraining oneself from getting angry in the face of provocation is the mark of a cultivated person. Of course, not showing anger externally is not to be confused with not getting angry internally. A Chinese idiom puts it this way, "Forbear insults and swallow sounds of protest": Exactly what I have observed many people do in response to humiliation, revealing a mixture of fear and repressed rage, all bottled up. So forbearance is not always a good thing.

Neither is uncontrolled rage that leads to fist fights, domestic violence, or in the extreme abominable mass shootings in America. American history is as short as Chinese history is long; its baggage from history is as light as the Chinese is heavy. Americans tend to be optimistic. They want to expunge unhappiness from their collective consciousness.

But true happiness includes the wisdom to embrace unhappiness as a part of life. Happiness comes more easily when we are no longer obsessed with pursuing it. It ensues naturally from taking actions aimed to make others around us happier and the world a better place.

The value of suffering is recognized in many religions. Take the Buddhist belief that suffering ceases through selflessness; the moral implication is that, likening others to oneself, one should reduce suffering in others. Its counterpart in

Christianity, though not identical, may be discerned. Suffering presents opportunities for acts of courage, forbearance, or kindness, as well as for strengthening one's faith. The exemplar is the suffering of Jesus for the salvation of all humankind. Thus, adding religiosity or spirituality to forbearance amplifies its potency.

Forgiveness

Forbearance in the face of natural calamities is difficult enough. It reaches a higher level when the deliberate acts of others inflict suffering on us. To forbear provocation, insults, oppression, and the like is probably the most demanding of all. This brings us to forgiveness, which has deep roots in religion and ethical traditions in diverse cultures.

Forgiveness takes two directions: To forgive someone, and to ask for forgiveness from someone. To forgive is to excuse someone from an offence, in thought and action. It does not entail negating the offender's responsibility for the offence: Forgive, but do not forget!

Full forgiveness is unconditional: It entails refusal to blame or to condescend, and letting go of resentment. Giving people a second chance is conditional and therefore does not qualify as full forgiveness. Granting a pardon is of a lesser degree; it may involve merely permitting the offender to go unpunished. Forgiveness reaches a pinnacle when it inspires the offender to be a better person.

Beyond the pinnacle is a magnanimous state of mind where the thought of forgiveness would not even arise: That's Buddhahood. I had a glimpse into this magnanimous state during moments of madness.

The antithesis of forgiveness takes two forms. Vengefulness: to harbor resentment or hatred, resort to personal vindictiveness, get even or seek revenge against the offender. Irresponsibility: to admit no responsibility for harm done to another, feel no remorse, and take no action that may undo at least in part the harm done.

Repentance is important because it means assuming responsibility for one's wrongdoings. It may be particularly effective for dealing with guilt, but not with shame, in which personal responsibility is not necessarily involved. Repentance may or may not be a prelude to ask for forgiveness: A person may feel remorse, contrition, or self-reproach, and yet take no *action* to ask for forgiveness or, better still, to make reparation or restitution as an attempt to undo, at least in part, the damage done.

We must also pay due attention to forgiving oneself, which stands in a dialogic relation with both forgiving someone and asking for forgiveness. Forgiving others and forgiving oneself are mutually reinforcing. But asking for forgiveness from others without forgiving oneself is incomplete forgiveness. And to forgive oneself without forgiving others is a mark of egocentrism; it negates the right to ask for forgiveness.

> **YF** The trouble is that I don't find it difficult to forgive others or to ask for forgiveness from others, but I do find it very difficult to forgive myself. My superego weighs heavily on my psyche with feelings of guilt and shame, as psychoanalysts would say. After years of self-therapy, I find much relief from this burden. Applying DAT gives me further relief. It is the madness of exuberance, however, that gives me total relief.

Now I have tamed my superego; I am getting nearer my goal of being "shameless." I have learned to be kinder to myself. Shame is not in the lexicon of the enlightened, I would imagine. Indeed, the consequence of refusing to self-forgive is to lead a life loaded with guilt and self-blame.

> **David** One point has to be emphasized. There is nothing worse than an insincere or half-hearted apology. So don't apologize unless it comes from the heart. Asking for forgiveness, which goes beyond apologizing, is especially difficult for the proud and mighty. The moral-therapeutic route beginning from denial to acknowledgment of responsibility is difficult enough; taking corrective action, including asking for forgiveness, may be even more so.

I must also question the basic premise that forgiveness is always possible. Some crimes against humanity are so heinous that they make it very hard for us to contemplate forgiving their perpetrators. What readily comes to mind are the Holocaust, the self-genocide of Cambodia, systematic rape as an instrument of ethnic cleansing, and so forth.

Are the perpetrators of such crimes forgivable? Even for lesser crimes, not all victims are willing or ready to forgive. Thus imposing forgiveness on victims may add conflict, pressure, even guilt to the trauma they have already suffered. Forgiveness cannot be done by religious decree.

> **YF** "I forgive not, at least not yet. But life goes on, and I will not allow bitterness and vindictiveness to lessen the value of my life": Forgiveness is not mandatory and is not a necessary condition for moving forward. For many, this may be a more realistic solution that may circumvent the moral dilemma entailed in asking people to forgive. The solution puts the emphasis on letting go of fixations (e.g., on past traumas, revenge), an idea rooted in Buddhism and Daoism.

David In line with what you have stated, forgiveness does not preclude anger. Prophets get angry, even Jesus. Those who cannot experience anger (not the same as hatred) cannot love.

Hope

I wish more people would experience righteous indignation over social injustice that might lead to corrective actions and ignite hope. However, defiant actions against injustice may lead to retaliation and more oppression, as the histories of China and other countries have shown. That's why hope can be a dangerous idea. Once ignited, hope propels people to defend themselves even when their chances of success—of survival—are grim. Beware: The path of hope may lead to the grave.

Be that as it may, I sent out a festive message on hope to friends and relatives in December 2005, a few months after Mania 1 ended.

> **Hope** is the mother of life: It gives us reason to live, to endure the unendurable.
> Hope is the archenemy of despair: That there is a way out and that all is not lost.
> Hope orients toward the future: What is bad will pass and what is good will be restored.
> Hope impacts the present: It activates action for change and holds despair at bay.
> Hope is not rationalization, denial, or self-deception: Authentic hope perceives reality accurately and accepts the present as it truly is.
> Hope is no mere optimism: The future will be better than what it is now, even in the face of calamity.
> Hope is a dangerous idea: It impels us to take action that may imperil our lives.
> Hope is also a hopeful idea: For the great peril is to take no action at all.
> Let hope triumph over despair, especially for all those who have endured enough.

Hope should be differentiated from rationalization, denial, and other forms of self-deception. Authentic hope is devoid of self-deception and distortions of reality; it is predicated on perceiving objective conditions accurately, and accepting the present as it truly is.

Despair is the archenemy of hope. It is extreme pessimism, believing that all is lost and that there is no way out of a present predicament or misfortune. It derives from exaggerations of fatalism, feelings of total abandonment, or prolonged learned helplessness.

Hope goes beyond forbearance: With forbearance, I shall endure; given hope, I say, "I shall prevail." I have maintained hope even in my darkest moments. In Mania 2, I plunged into a "Black Hole" out of deep feelings of loneliness, not despair. I have had only fleeting moments of despair—as of enlightenment. So I do have strong immunity against despair. I strengthen my psychological immune system further when I view my life as a spiritual journey of discoveries.

Meaning Reconstruction

David What exactly have you discovered? We do not presume to know in advance where or, more significantly, what a spiritual pilgrimage will lead us to. In your case, you weren't even cognizant that you had embarked on a pilgrimage in the beginning. You certainly do not conceive of a pilgrim's destination in terms of a geographical location of religious significance. In fact, you reject the idea of a final destination. For you, a pilgrimage is a lifelong process of discovery, in which the direction toward destination and even the nature of the destination itself have to be discovered.

YF This question brings us to the fourth strategy, meaning reconstruction. Meaning reconstruction drives the spiritual self to find its place in society, nature, and the cosmos. My spiritual journey is not about discovering something "out there," like a treasure island. It is about the search for meaning; the treasures to be found are in the meaning that emerges from reconstruction.

The recognition of profound ignorance is the first step toward discovery. There are times when I find myself in a state of ignorance or, worse, directionlessness. Indeed, my spiritual advancement is a history of discovering greater depths of ignorance than what I had previously acknowledged.

David In the extreme, your situation may be likened to a person searching for something, the nature of which he is ignorant, in the dark, or to a detective dealing with a case in which there are no clues to permit even formulating an initial hypothesis as a starting point.

YF I cannot claim to know what exactly I am searching for or what the final goals to be reached are. Without trodden paths or procedures to follow, there is only a global, undifferentiated notion of the goal to be reached, which is subject to change as I proceed. I do not even presume to know what questions should be asked, let alone the answers. That is, I admit not only that I do not know, but also that I do not know what I need to know.

In short, much of the time I have been groping in the dark. What else can I do but to embrace humility imposed upon me by the recognition of such ignorance?

Together with hope, humility uplifts me from the terror that might come when I grope in the dark.

The dynamic process of constructing meanings is what our dialogue is about. We are now engaged in DAT at this very moment. The will to meaning is uniquely human. But some may still ask, "Why should we bother to engage in meaning reconstruction?"

Because unwillingness or inability to find new meanings or purpose leaves old constructions untouched. Entrenchment of mental conservatism, fixation, or rigidity sets in and further inhibits meaning reconstruction. A life so entrenched is impoverished; it has no creativity.

YF Speaking for myself: A life that fails to harness the fecundity of madness is a life that throws away its opportunities for enrichment. It is not in love with all of itself.

David Sadly too many people fall into the trap of entrenchment, the negation of meaning reconstruction, as their option for life. One reason is that reconstruction can be painful and demanding. Remember how painful your own reconstruction of self-identity was; you had to perform a kind of "psychological surgery" to cleanse your soul of the pernicious influences of your own mother.

Meaning reconstruction can also be hazardous, as when the reconstructed meanings are acerbic and deleterious. Many a person may react to betrayal by a trusted friend in this way: "The more I think about it, the bitterer I become. I used to be suspicious; now I am convinced I can trust no one, ever." Affirmation of spiritual values comes to the rescue, as in other instances of impasse along our journey.

And reconstruction can hardly be achieved without prior deconstruction, which requires examining and altering previous constructions. However, it would be irresponsible to leave people already suffering from loss of meaning to suffer further from unended or, worse, unending deconstruction. An implication for therapy is that closure has to be achieved.

In some cases, closure may be achieved rather quickly and without pain. Let me give a specific example. Recall that my mother assigned a servant to accompany me to primary school every day? Ironically, this did not protect me from being sexually abused by a male physical education teacher who was very fond of me.

On one or two occasions he took me into his office, where his coworker was present, and kissed me. I was then about nine years old, and unsurprisingly I did not know what child sexual abuse was. I noticed his breath smelled bad because of his heavy smoking. I did not tell my mother because I was afraid she would get upset and cause a row in the school. Then I would be really embarrassed and be worse off, and the teacher might be punished.

The meaning I construed was: "That's his way of showing his affection for me, but I feel uncomfortable about the way he does it." That was the end of it. There was no deconstruction or reconstruction and no need for them. To this day, I do not consider that I have suffered psychological damage in the least.

Actually, I have been reluctant to disclose this private experience. The thought that it may be useful to others who have had similar experiences overcomes my reluctance. My example demonstrates that the way in which meaning is constructed has a decisive effect on outcomes. Psychological traumas, child sexual abuse included, do not necessarily lead to psychopathology and do not have to block the path of a pilgrimage.

Historically, the coping strategies I have described have been anchored more in religion and ethics than in therapy. But their place in therapy has to be recognized. Used within the framework of DAT and augmented with spiritual purposes, the coping strategies realize their potential to the fullest.

When the dialogic self constructs meaning and purpose, it entertains possibilities of what it may become—what it has never experienced before—in the future; it renders new forms of thought and action possible. It engages in internal dialogues and participates in its own re-creation. That is, the dialogic self has self-transformational capabilities. The result is the best outcome of coping: self-transformation, rare and precious.

Self-transformation is more than growth; it amounts to a quantum leap. It entails not only quantitative but also qualitative change and not only alterations of previously observed patterns but also new or emergent patterns that were previously dormant or unobserved. A self-transformed person thinks and acts like a new person, visibly to others.

Life as a Playful Journey: Intercultural Encounters

A spiritual quest does not have to be a journey of solemn, staid drudgery, but of dedication intermingled with playfulness. An imaginary dialogue ensues.

> **David** You were born in the Year of the Rabbit, according to the Chinese zodiac. What do rabbits do? They leap about and frolic in merriment. So naturally life to you is a gambol.

	Recall in this context that Hypomania 5 took place in a luxurious setting, on board the *Queen Victoria* and land excursions around the Mediterranean. The experiences you gained could fill a travelogue. They illustrate your worldviews as a world citizen. They serve to redirect attention from abnormality to the rich diversity of normality, in which madness may be embedded. More important, they demonstrate that spiritual journeys can indeed be playful.
YF	Life on board the *Queen Victoria* was anything but boring. One day, the captain broadcasted an announcement about security measures against terrorism, while crew members went around checking for hidden bombs. The announcement went something like this: "We take terrorist threats seriously. . ... So take note and report to the authorities if you see someone who looks suspicious, or if you see someone who does not look suspicious but has been seen in the company of people, among some of whom might have been seen together with someone who does look suspicious."

Double-O-Seven Reporting to Double-O-Six

YF	Upon hearing this, I blurted out, "Ridiculous!" Whereupon, an Englishman nearby was sufficiently amused to initiate conversation with me. I introduced myself as "Double-O-Seven"; he introduced himself as "Double-O-Six." Thus, both of us were working for Her Majesty's government, in search of potential terrorists on board. Later, he introduced me to his wife. I ran into his wife over breakfast one morning but failed to recognize her. She was visibly peeved. I thought to myself, "Now you know what it's like not to be recognized by people who ought to have recognized you. I have had plenty of experiences of not being recognized, intentionally or unintentionally, by Westerners."
David	Ah, don't all Orientals look alike?
YF	Mentally settled a moment later, I took corrective action and went over to the table where she and her husband were sitting. I said to her husband, "Double-O-Seven reporting to Double-O-Six." I then asked his wife not to take to heart behaviors natural to secret agents that probably look unnatural to normal people. This seemed to have placated her.

The English couple were curious about my occupation. I said, "You mean besides being a secret agent. You may ask me any question, to which I am bound to give a truthful answer. You have five guesses." I did give truthful answers, but with nuances calculated to mislead. I talked about various occupations with authority, coupled with counter questions to suggest that I knew a lot more than I actually did.

> **David**   This comes naturally to you after years of teaching practice: The art of teaching is not to conceal the teacher's ignorance, or to show his knowledge, but to demonstrate how knowledge may be generated through dialogue.
>
> **YF**   The Englishman came close but missed the target. Finally, I told the couple that I was a professor of psychology. His wife professed disbelief. She asked in a sarcastic tone, "You have a certificate to prove it?" She then took another good look at me and noticed the Gucci shoes I was wearing. "Ah, I believe you. Those expensive shoes befit a professor."

At that moment, I didn't know whether I was amused or vexed. I have seldom bought expensive items for myself. I bought the Gucci shoes so I could dance, not to impress people.

> **David**   Apparently, the Chinese saying "Respect the person's attire, before respecting the person" is not confined to Chinese people. Such great regard for worldly concerns is symptomatic of spiritual emptiness. Sadly, to many, materialistic pursuits offer more attraction than spiritual quests.

Linguistic Surprises

Nonetheless, I was very pleased to have met the English couple. Both thought that English was my mother tongue! For the first time in my life, I passed the test of being a native speaker. Nothing made me happier.

Another linguistic encounter was a surprise. After talking with a hairstylist for a while, I asked her what her native tongue was. She replied, "English." This answer instantly embarrassed me, for having possibly embarrassed her. Fortunately, she wasn't. She explained that, being Scottish, she was used to not being understood by the English. It took me a while to get used to her accent. I still remember the way she pronounced *but*, which sounded very strange to my ears.

Accent was certainly no barrier to communication. I sensed that there was something troubling her. After discovering that I was a psychologist, she wanted to talk with me about that something. We had a heart-to-heart talk for about 30 minutes and got to the bottom of it. It turned out that she was concerned about her relationship with her boyfriend's mother, who she felt was rather possessive of her son.

> **David**   So the classic antipathy between mothers-in-law and daughters-in-law is not unique to the Chinese.

YF   I felt gratified that we had both transcended our backgrounds. Indeed, kindred souls countenance no linguistic or cultural barriers to communication.

Active-Aggressive Westerners and Passive-Aggressive Chinese

Displayed inside the ship's gallery were photographs of passengers dressed in utmost elegance. A Chinese couple were looking at some of the photographs, and the lady aimed her camera at one. A staff member dashed in front of the couple and bawled out a pointed threat with an Australian accent: "These photos are copyrighted. If I see you doing this again, I'm going to confiscate your camera."

David   Typical Western active-aggressiveness!
YF   She had a build that dwarfed the Chinese lady. Standing nearby, I could imagine how the Chinese woman reacted, and I approached her to see if I could help. She explained that she didn't really intend to take a photograph of the photograph on display. I said that I would talk with the staff member concerned. In a typical Chinese fashion, she said, "Never mind."

I saw an opportunity to be an agent of intercultural understanding in action. In a typically atypical Chinese fashion, I approached the staff member and relayed to her what the Chinese lady said. The staff member explained: "You know, some people actually steal photographs from the gallery. We have to protect our copyrights." I replied, "I understand. However, the couple feel offended. You could have explained to them in a nicer way." She then went over to the couple and apologized for her ill manners.

Later, I talked to some Chinese passengers about the incident. One reacted: "I'll intentionally take photographs of photographs in the gallery, just to vex them." I thought to myself: Typical Chinese passive-aggressiveness! I was witness and intervener to numerous similar incidents of intercultural strain during the entire cruise.

Neither Eastern nor Western I had found myself, but a supracultural agent of understanding.

Serendipitous Field Research

So I treated the *Queen Victoria* as a perfect place for conducting field research on intercultural communication, organizational behavior, customer relations, and so forth. Too busy enjoying myself, I did nothing by design. Still, a generalization forced its way into my scientific consciousness: There was an inverse relation between status and friendliness or pleasantness among the staff.

> **YF** The high-status staff were typically European and fluent speakers of English. Some displayed condescending attitudes toward passengers who didn't speak English. The low-status staff came from the Philippines, India, or other third-world countries. Some had substandard proficiency in English. One waiter asked, for instance, "Are you all right?"
>
> **David** When what he meant was, "Is the food all right?"
>
> **YF** I discovered to my amazement, however, that those who came from Mauritius were articulate in multiple languages, although they had completed only secondary education. This would put Hong Kong to shame.

I found out that the low-status staff were not as well paid as one would imagine. This meant that I had paid less for the cruise on their account. Almost without exception, they were helpful and friendly. To repay them in a small measure, I would hoard chocolates given only to passengers and redistribute them among the staff. They showed grateful delight, far beyond the chocolates' value.

> **David** Without loving actions in the concrete, talks of universal love in the abstract sound hollow.
>
> **YF** Part of the cruise involved land excursions in Egypt and Italy. I visited the world renowned Library of Alexandria, where I saw groups of Egyptian schoolchildren on tour with their teachers. Like schoolchildren elsewhere, they were fun-loving, noisy, and not as attentive as demanded.

Their teachers, mostly men, watched over them like hawks over chickens. They had no hesitation in delivering a hefty blow to the head of a child whom they considered to be out of line. I followed the children around for a while. Occasionally, I caught their attention by making funny faces to reflect how scary the teachers were. They were greatly amused.

> **David** You had to be cautious, for nothing would infuriate teachers, in Egypt or elsewhere, more than someone who succeeded in distracting students from the crutch of their authority.
>
> **YF** In Italy, I saw an entirely different pattern of teacher-student relationships. Groups of schoolchildren were led by their teachers around to tour galleries and museums. The children were jovial and showed no fear of their teachers. I saw students and teachers joking around together, enjoying each other's company.
>
> **David** All your life, you have had a special interest in the socialization of children in different cultures. Here was socialization observed in person. You have often

said: The destiny of a nation is conditioned by the manner in which its children are socialized. Remember, even as a child, you thought that traditional Chinese upbringing "produces enslaved nations."

Ambassadors of Communion Between Two Ancient Civilizations

I saw busloads of tourists on their way to the Egyptian Museum in Cairo. Most of them seemed to show more interest in Egypt's antiquity than in its modern history, more fascination with dead mummies than with the living. Few showed understanding of, let alone empathy toward, life outside the museum. I noticed, however, that the squalid conditions under which teeming masses of people lived did not seem to have taken the spirit out of them. Everywhere I went, people responded cheerfully to gestures of goodwill.

YF	I asked someone to write down on a piece of paper the equivalent of "Greetings, and thank you for your help" in Egyptian Arabic. All I had to do was to show it to people around when I got lost (sometimes in pretense) and they would come to my aid.
David	That piece of paper is a passport to pleasant and meaningful intercultural interactions. Serendipitous encounters tend to be the most interesting when you travel in another country.
YF	Inside the museum, I took a special interest in the death mask of King Tutankhamun, particularly the hieroglyphics inscribed on it. A young Egyptian woman appeared unexpectedly and asked, "Would you like some help?" It turned out she was a university student majoring in history. She could read the hieroglyphics, which she translated into English for my benefit! She then took my hand and gave me a personal guided tour around the museum. Pointing to a statue of a cat, she explained that it was crying with tears because it wanted another "man." Perplexed, I endeavored to discover the mystery behind such feline desire. It then dawned on me that she meant "meal."

Her name was Amany. Her stature was as diminutive as her charm was immense. Her head was covered with a hijab, which did nothing to conceal her facial expressiveness. Her large, enchanting eyes, like a pair of black pearls, would move even the most unmovable Bodhisattva. She taught me to write my name in hieroglyphics, and I showed her how to write hers in Chinese.

When it was time to depart, I took out a banknote of 20 euros and gave it to her. She asked me to write my Chinese name on it, which I did. "I will treasure this for the rest of my life," she said. At that moment, I felt what began as a casual contact had turned into a communion between two ancient civilizations, of which we were ambassadors.

David   A woman in a Muslim country taking initiative to approach a man in public? And taking his hand to go around? This defies the stereotype of heterosexual relations in Muslim societies.

YF   I remember my visit years ago to Mindanao State University in the Autonomous Region in Muslim Mindanao of the Philippines. On the way there, my travel companion, a Christian, warned me repeatedly: "Don't ever touch any woman, not even accidentally. Otherwise, dire consequences will follow!" However, Amany showed no unease and must have felt that her behavior was perfectly acceptable. As a matter of fact, nobody around paid much attention to our interaction. She provided a living demonstration of how misleading stereotypes can be.

David   The Muslim world is not monolithic. It is far more heterogeneous than is acknowledged by most outsiders.

YF   More fundamentally, my past encounters in diverse cultures give me little or no reason to be surprised: Everywhere women governed by strict codes of conduct will, nonetheless, find ways to express their humanity.

Be Yourself, Mad or Sane

Manuals in the form of do's and don'ts written for tourists often perform a disservice: They reinforce common ethnic or cultural stereotypes and put tourists too much on guard.

David   Now you have published many scholarly papers on transcultural psychology. Are you guided by your extensive knowledge of how people from different cultures interact when you travel to foreign lands?

YF   Having traveled around the world three times, I can say that attitude matters much more than academic knowledge. People all over the world appreciate gestures of good will. Ultimately, I have only one basic principle: Be yourself, whether you are living in your own country or traveling abroad.

David   Are saying, in effect, that there is no distinction to be made between traveling as a tourist for pleasure and traveling as a pilgrim for spiritual fulfillment? If so, you have taken a radical stance, in conformity with your identity as a world citizen. But "be yourself" also means being occasionally mad. Did you scare anyone around the Mediterranean?

YF   Being myself, I was playful. Not surprisingly, my playfulness was amplified by a measure of madness. Significantly, none of the local people I interacted with thought I was mad. So, it is possible to control or conceal my madness during episodes.

The Journey Continues in Search of New Meanings and Directions

I have provided some evidence that madness may enrich a person's life, given that the right conditions are met; and that it is possible to retain a measure of dignity in madness as well as to exploit madness for enhancing dignified living.

Whoops, we must not forget to make a transition to the following chapters. Madness has enriched and added color to my life. This questions the traditional stance in psychiatry that views mental disorders solely in terms of psychopathology and pays little attention to the positive values they may bring to a patient's life.

Has my madness facilitated enlightenment or detracted from it? How are madness and enlightenment to be differentiated? Have I been just mad, or mad and enlightened? A deep sense of loneliness and being atypical permeates my life, prompting me to search for spirituality-in-communion.

4

From Psychiatry to Spirituality

> *The attainment of spirituality is a dynamic process in which struggle, change, and self-transformation are central. There are no shortcuts to attainment, such as taking psychedelic drugs.*

What is the nature of my episodes of madness? Many perplexities remain unresolved. For instance, reflecting on Hypomania 5 in the preceding, I raised the question: What condition was I suffering from? My answer was: "To this day, I am not sure"; brain fatigue appeared to be the salient feature. I now turn to the larger picture of my case as a whole. More questions are raised. What mental disorder, if any, did I suffer from? What is the diagnosis?

Actually, I have already made a thorough self-diagnosis once before. As a graduate student in clinical psychology, I went through intensive training in psychodiagnostics. Back in the 1960s, students spent a great deal of time in psychological testing, probably more than present-day students do. I was required to submit case studies, each involving a case history and a battery of psychological tests, as assignments. I used myself as a subject for one: I wrote reports on my functioning and diagnosed myself. So it was a self case study. Little could I foresee that I would do it for a second time years later. After graduation, I engaged my former professor for didactic psychoanalytic therapy for several months, as intensive as having two-hour sessions daily for seven days a week. The most memorable experience was having my Rorschach protocol interpreted while I was under hypnosis. Thus, I may claim to have a fair degree of self-understanding.

A diagnosis should be based on adequate evidence. Already I have amassed considerable materials on my case. In Chapter 1, I presented my life history. Clinical descriptions of my episodes are given in Chapter 2. Chapter 3 documents how I have derived personal and professional benefits from sequential learning in the process of coping with madness. In the present chapter, I add excerpts of self-reports submitted as assignments. Together, these materials cover diverse areas of my life history and psychological functioning; they provide the evidence for making a diagnosis.

An Early Case Study of and by My Own Self

Digging out my old self-reports turned out to be a revealing search for the early stages of my spiritual development. Decades later, I can see my former self containing the buds of my present self clearly in the responses to various psychological tests. A number of themes were already present in responses to the Incomplete Sentence Blank.

1. I want to know: sufficiently about the universe and man's part in it.
2. I can't: fight against the entire historic background under which I grew.
3. My mind: is a complex phenomenon which reflects the cultures of the East and the West today.
4. When I was a child: I became aware of things that other children were not aware of.
5. My nerves: are sometimes extremely excited.
6. Sometimes: I feel the ecstasy of life, sometimes its sorrow.
7. I secretly: cherish thoughts that society does not accept in general.
8. I: am a being—unique in my own ways.

Here we find themes like being caught in history and between cultures, being different, nonconformity, struggle, wanting to know man's part in the universe, extremely excited nerves, ecstasy and sorrow.

The Thematic Apperception Test is a well-known projective technique, in the sense that the subject projects his inner drives, emotions, and complexes onto outer stimuli of varying degrees of ambiguity; the more ambiguous the stimuli, the more projective the test. The subject is asked to tell a story in response to each of a series of pictures presented. The test manual claims that "as a rule the subject leaves the test happily unaware that he has presented to the psychologist with what amounts to an X-Ray picture of his inner self." An exaggeration?

No matter. Here are excerpts (with keywords appearing in italics) from some of the stories I gave and, where suitable, from my TAT report submitted as an assignment (following the word *Interpretation*—in other words, my own interpretation of the stories I told about the pictures). The serial number of the picture is given within parentheses (B for young boys, G for young girls, M for men over age 14; F for women over age 14).

1. (3 BM) ... This picture seems to be symbolic of the misery many boys in the world face, and of the hardships they have to overcome to realize a bright future. The last picture was also symbolic: of *artistry*; but this one is symbolic of *pathos*, which is *universal*.
2. (7 BM) A father is talking to his son... [who] has lost *faith* in goodness... the young man will regain some of his faith in man. [Pause] Gradually and surely. It looks like they are both philosophers.
3. (12 M) Here is a boy lying in bed. He is asleep. He has been sick. Now this man is putting his hand on his forehead, and is lifting it. He has great *spiritual* powers. Symbolically, it is like faith. With faith, the boy will get well again. Perhaps this is what the artist is trying to depict in this picture. (*Interpretation*. The Subject qualifies his acceptance of spiritual healing at two levels: it is symbolic, and it is only a picture of an artist.... By being impersonal (using qualifications), the Subject in essence says that he has not abandoned his faith in logic or reason either.)
4. (12 F) This is a picture of two women, one young and beautiful, the other old and ugly—a striking contrast. The artist illustrates the inevitable course of human development; nothing human is *everlasting*. There is an end to everything, including beauty and youth. Also the young woman is calm, but the old woman seems to be afraid and worried, perhaps of approaching death. What is lasting? The art of capturing fate in a painting. That is everlasting. (*Interpretation*. Actually there is no story told to this card, but an interpretation of a painting perceived by the Subject.... The response is rich in description, both in relation to the stimulus and its symbolic significance as the Subject defines it. The subject's interpretation shows that he tends to think in terms of generalities.... As in [a previous story], there is an intense awareness of the natural forces beyond man's

power, and to which man must submit and accept. But it is not true that man can do nothing about his fate: At least he can capture it in art. . ..)
5. (14) A young man is looking from his window in his room. . ... His head is held up high, as if he is full of *hope*. Here he is surveying the town from his window. He can see many things other people cannot see. With hope and conviction, he will go out and make his hopes and aspirations come true.
6. (17 BM) This is a man climbing a rope. He looks very strong, but how can he measure against infinity! Halfway in between heaven and earth, what can he do? . . . Man against *infinity*; it's impossible. (*Interpretation.* The mode of response is much like that to 12 F. The card is only a painting by some artist, conveying symbolically the impossibility of measuring against the infinite. This is therefore a concept-driven response. Again, the Subject shows his intense awareness of man's helplessness against nature, insofar as his ability of completely transcending it [is concerned]. He readily resigns himself to this fate and accepts his *limitations* as a human being.)

In these stories, even in fragments, I cannot help noticing the words *artistry, pathos, universal, faith, spiritual, everlasting, hope,* and *infinity*. These words would be found in a book on spirituality. Thus they presage the present undertaking. The idea that nothing is everlasting, in particular, is akin to the Buddhist notion of impermanence—nothing is, everything becomes—although I knew next to nothing about Buddhism in my student days.

Thinking in abstractions or symbolic terms is clearly characteristic of my cognitive style. The feeling of distinction ("seeing things other people cannot see") reverberates with another response in the Incomplete Sentence Blank ("When I was a child: I became aware of things that other children were not aware of"). Optimism, backed by conviction, comes through clearly. Yet, human limitations and acceptance of the inevitable are recurrent themes.

What began as an intellectual attitude in my youth has evolved into spiritual experiences of humility and acceptance later in my life. In the midst of Mania 1, I felt a deep sense of humility: "The more I knew, the more I became aware of my profound ignorance. Knowledge and humility were like twins." Themes of human limitation and humility reemerge in epigrams I have written in the last decades. Some of these echo the theme of not knowing what one does not know and the dangers of absolutistic self-conviction; others wonder about the nature of knowledge itself. Reading these epigrams again, I note that self-reflective thought and the sense of humility in the face of human limitation come through loud and clear, amounting to what has prevented me from descending into greater despair.

1. To know what one does not know is the beginning of new knowledge. For some people, this knowing is never grasped. (25 Aug 2006)
2. The scholar labors to know the unknown. The fool strives to know the unknowable. But where is the boundary between the unknown and the unknowable? Upon this question rests the verdict of whether you are the scholar or the fool. (6 Aug 2006)
3. Knowledge is power. Absolutistic knowledge is tyrannical power. (29 Dec 2007)
4. If you think you are always right, you are a very dangerous person, especially if indeed you are. (6 June 2008)
5. Someone says: "If I think I am right, I will continue to think I am right, regardless of what others might say; and if I think I am wrong, it is only because I think I am indeed wrong." Is this borne of conviction, or tyranny of the mind? (8 June 2008)
6. Knowledge is the sum total of information required to render it impossible for any sentient being to distinguish truth from falsehood, or reality from virtual reality, anytime, anywhere in the cosmos and beyond. In other words, to deceive a being like you or me cocooned in a virtual world into believing that it is reality. Who is the deceiver? A super mathematician called God. (1 Jan 2014)

The Rorschach test is the best-known projective technique. The subject is asked to look at 10 inkblot cards, one at a time. He is to say what the inkblot represents or looks like to him, what comes to his mind. My initial reaction to the Rorschach was skepticism. As I went deeper, skepticism turned into amazement, of how much one can learn about the psychology of personality in general and individual persons in particular.

Around the time I was completing my doctoral training in the United States, I went to one of my professors whose specialty was hypnotherapy. The professor interpreted my Rorschach protocol, which was unusual in many respects, while I was under hypnosis. The protocol contained some 200 responses, an exceptionally large number. The examiner (i.e., myself) recorded a remark I made during testing: "All kinds of ideas come to my mind so fast; sometimes I can't tell you fast enough." Even though I was by no means experiencing a flight of ideas, my experience with the Rorschach test was similar to the bouts of madness that occurred later in my life.

Along with responses indicative of obsessive-compulsivity (e.g., small details) were those of creative imagination, just as obsessive-compulsivity and creativity have been the dual aspects of my personality. These aspects are like antagonistic twins engaged in a continual battle within my psyche. Winning this battle would be momentous for not only my mental health but also my spiritual fulfillment. It amounts to freedom from fixation and liberation from self-imprisonment.

One of the percepts I identified in the Rorschach test was a devil, followed by a spontaneous remark, "The best defense is mockery, for the devil fears nothing more than your laughter." Indeed. The significant point is that the usual direction of fear is reversed: I am in control; it is the devil who fears my mockery. As a matter of fact, I have never been afraid of devils, vampires, or ghosts. Once I went to a cemetery alone in the middle of the night, hoping to obtain a glimpse of these beings. I didn't; instead, I saw for the first time the beauty of the bright moonlight shining on tombstones and angels made of white marble all over the cemetery.

When I was about 10 years old, someone told me that beautiful ghosts of banana trees would come out at night. So I went to the backyard of the house where I dwelled, alone at night, because it was full of banana trees. I waited and waited under the trees. I saw nothing but a snake. Could the snake be that beautiful female demon who assumed human form, according to the Chinese legend of the white snake, before her transfiguration? Another percept was a butterfly, to which I alluded in a poem I wrote many years later (1 Aug 2005).

Who's Dreaming?

Awakened from my slumber, still
Enchanted by the butterfly,
Flying happily in Zhuangzi's dream,
Dreaming about the philosopher.

"A wish forbidden to be fulfilled,
In a dreamer's wet dream," Sigmund declares.
Zhuangzi retorts: "What's forbidden?
The Dao is all embracing!"

"Oh, Sigmund, trying to analyze the Daoist?"
"The royal road to the unconscious leads nowhere.

I'm lost in this Daoist labyrinth.
Hermann, you give it a try."
"Please tell me more about the butterfly."
"As dainty as Dame Margot, as serene as Guanyin,
Emulating varied floral coloration,
Metamorphosing itself into a flying orchid."
"Metaphoric, combining movement, color and its nuances:

A rare percept indeed!" Hermann mumbles
To himself. "Now, which part of the inkblot
Looks like the butterfly?"

The butterfly flies away, leaving behind
The smoke of Sigmund's cigar.

This is really weird. Who's dreaming
Another dreamer's dream,
Privy to others' inner thoughts?

I calm myself: "Don't worry. *You* are only dreaming."
But then, this means I'm still *in* the dream.
"So, when will I wake up, to know
I'm awake, or dreaming I'm awake?"

Still perplexed.

> *Note.* The personalities that "appear" in the dream are Zhuangzi (Daoist philosopher), Sigmund Freud, Hermann Rorschach (Swiss psychiatrist who invented the inkblot test), Guanyin (Chinese goddess of mercy), and Margot Fonteyn (one of the greatest classical ballet dancers of all time). The poem is inspired by the famous tale of Zhuangzi's dream of the butterfly.

To this day, I still feel the *presence* of the butterfly. Empathy and emotional reactivity are evident in my test responses as in real life. In Hypomania 2, I wept in front of a class of students when talking about the June Fourth massacre in Beijing. Even when I am normal, tears sometimes flow from my eyes in poignant moments. On occasion, watching starving children in Africa on television can overwhelm me.

Empathic and emotional responsiveness in the extreme may have negative consequences. Being as sensitive as a *living* Rorschach inkblot enables me to be a good psychologist; it can also tax my emotional life. Sympathy, empathic sensitivity, kind-heartedness, and the like are admirable attributes; in the extreme, however, they can be hazardous to mental health. A person who experiences all the pain of battered women, the homeless, the enslaved, and so forth—like Mother Teresa carrying the woes of humankind on her shoulders—would be loaded to the extreme.

I value my capacity to experience pain, as well as delight, as an attribute of psychological health. But I also know that there is a limit to that capacity. Moreover, the natural tendency is to defend myself from emotional overloading. The danger, by which I have been threatened, is that I may become callous: There are times when I succumb to the pressures of life, become indifferent to the pain and suffering of others, and descend into spiritual emptiness.

This leads me to interpret callousness as a defensive reaction against emotional overloading, at least among individuals who have the capacity for empathic sensitivity. Balance holds a key for spiritual fulfillment, as it does for the interconnectedness of Body-Mind-Spirit (BMS).

The conclusions of two particular self-reports are informative. One, the case history concluded that I was "quite well adjusted on a psychosocial level, but at the expense of a great deal of psychic energy"; that I had "serious internal conflicts"; and that the symptomatology pointed to "a compulsive personality, even neurosis." Two, the integrative report on all test results gave a similar clinical picture. It depicted me as a driven person who viewed his life as "an intense struggle"; my personality is "extremely complicated," and "seems to include extremes." Strengths and potentialities were also mentioned: a strong ego; highly motivated, with a fighting spirit in the face of adversity; intelligence and language facility; reality bound, yet imaginative; empathic capacity; emotional responsiveness.

In retrospect, I have no quarrel with these conclusions. They contain nothing inconsistent with my life history or with the sentiments I expressed in diaries and correspondence with friends and relatives written during my student days in North America. The germs of my spiritual quest can be discerned; so can the theme of liberation from compulsivity and the realization of creative potential. But I now must ask: Does a spiritual quest or liberation have to be an intense struggle?

One critical point is that there was no clear indication of a mood disorder. Moreover, the strengths mentioned would predict against the occurrence of severe mental disorders in the future. Thus, in the light of the early case study, the episodic madness later in life comes as a surprise.

The most significant issues to be addressed concern two of the atypical features of my madness. One is that the episodes occur late in my life. Why?

I frankly don't know. Two, all of the episodes are spells of exuberance, none of depression. Thus, my mood disorders are rather odd, unipolar instead of being typically bipolar. Why? The early case study provides a clue: Having "a fighting spirit in the face of adversity" is a potent antidote to depression.

Observing the Workings of the Mind

Now, observing the workings of the mind is tricky business. For, in principle, they cannot be directly observed. We have no idea, for instance, of how we arrive at the answer to a simple arithmetic problem or how we generate our thoughts. All we know is that the products of the mind's workings flow as naturally as water out of a tap. Once in a while, however, extraordinary circumstances provide opportunities to come close to observing the workings, the mechanisms and processes themselves. Brain researcher Jill Bolte Taylor had a massive stroke and witnessed her brain functions, motion, speech, and self-awareness shut down one by one. Eventually, she recovered to tell her amazing story. Interested readers may visit www.ted.com/talks/view/id/229 and watch a video about Taylor's experiences, *My Stroke of Insight*.

Self-Observations

Cruising around the Mediterranean on board the *Queen Victoria* during Hypomania 5 afforded me an opportunity to glimpse into the workings of my own mind. I gained firsthand experiences of cognitive processes at work. The following is a fairly accurate verbal report I gave to the physician I consulted on board the *Queen Victoria*.

> I know my body is giving me a warning. It has run out of reserve. So I would conserve energy when I am alone. When I am with other people, during dinner for example, I switch on again. So they don't know how depleted I really am. In my stateroom, I have spells of feeling cold. My body would shiver. I have to lie in bed and cover myself with a blanket. The spells last for 10 to 15 minutes.
>
> I have trouble performing even the simplest task. For example, to use a lift, I would push a sign with a number on it, instead of the correct button. I then wondered why there was no reaction. This happened several times. At the same time, however, I was aware of how stupid I had become. Getting oriented inside the *Queen Victoria*, which is not easy in any case, has been more difficult than what I would normally expect. Not so much a lack of visual-motor coordination

or spatial orientation as what I would call a disturbance of executive function for task completion.

For several days, I have had cognitive dysfunctions. I have great trouble comprehending what I read. Single words are all right. But I have great difficulty comprehending whole sentences. Oral speech is less of a problem, except for occasional difficulties with articulation or finding the right word. My memory fails me, especially about specifics, such as numbers and people's names. Sometimes, I get confused easily. Never before have I experienced such cognitive deficits. The thought that they might be irreversible, if only in part, really scares me.

My brain is like a battery running low, and not recharging properly. However, my reflective faculty is intact. I am aware of my situation and people around me. For instance, I am aware that, right now, far from being confused, I am coherent and able to give a detailed account of my condition. Would you please tell me what the shaking chills and cognitive dysfunctions, two symptoms which worry me the most, are about?

The physician's diagnosis was "acute stress/constipation." He didn't satisfy my curiosity about the two symptoms. He prescribed some medicine, which took care of my constipation and insomnia in two days. I began to recover physically, but the mood elation lingered. The cognitive dysfunctions were more severe than the "brain fatigue" I had during previous episodes.

My verbal report was not in the least indicative of a disordered mind. On the contrary, it was detailed, informative, and self-reflective—the kind that clinicians would like to obtain from their patients. In particular, it gave an experiential demonstration of how cognitively demanding linguistic functioning, especially syntax parsing (e.g., dealing with whole sentences), really is.

Self-Enchantment

Additionally, a special feature of my case concerns a syndrome commonly known in China as *zouhuorumo*, which translates as "catching fire, entering demon." This syndrome is found among qigong practitioners thought to have gone astray (literally, qigong means "breath work," and may be translated as "vital energy work"). It is different from the demon possession syndrome, the causation of which is thought of as exogenous.

One essential feature of *zouhuorumo* is a loss of cognitive control and reality testing; transient psychotic-like or bizarre behaviors may manifest. Not being an advanced qigong practitioner, I am sure I did not enter into *zouhuorumo*. At no point were there psychotic-like or bizarre behaviors. But I was self-enchanted all right, resulting in a blurring between the virtual and the real. Fortunately, metacognition saved me from being captured by the allure of virtual pleasures.

Here I am reminded of Satan's temptation of Jesus and Mara's temptation of Gautama, the founder of Buddhism. (Mara involved his three daughters to tempt Gautama—surely a depraved, if not an ultimate, scheme.) Surely, metacognition played a part in their triumph over satanic forces.

During Mania 2, I said to myself: "I don't want to be a Buddha." In other words, giving up sexual pleasure was too much even for supreme enlightenment. I want to celebrate life, not to be celibate. I wonder if Gautama might have given up his quest for enlightenment had his sexual drive been amplified tenfold. The rest had better be left to the imagination (but not too much imagination, because there was in fact nothing to whet the appetite of voyeurs).

I'm keeping some of my most private experiences private. By now, readers might be envious of my privileged experiences. In any case, I don't want to be guilty of inducing anyone into *zouhuorumo*. There is nothing in the idea of Body-Mind-Spirit (BMS) interconnectedness to negate sexuality. On the contrary, sexuality is inherent in all three BMS domains. It is the most intense of physical pleasures; it adds passion to love; it energizes spiritual feelings. This will reassure our fellow travelers in quest of spirituality. However, severe imbalances may disrupt the interconnectedness. And disconnected sexuality may debase, rather than enrich, life.

Mania, Superefficiency in Memory Retrieval, and Creativity

My firsthand experiences lend support to the linkage between mania and creativity. During madness, I experienced disinhibition like I had never experienced before. I became spontaneous, liberated. My mind exploded. Creative thoughts and flashes of insight rained down fast. I had supreme confidence, with a touch of "megalomania," enabling me to write without inhibition or self-doubt. I could become self-enchanted, captured by the allure of my own runaway thoughts. Inspired, I yearned to share my creative insights with others. These are favorable conditions for productions of inspirational creativity.

My superefficiency in memory recall during madness illustrates the mind's awesome capability to retrieve information it has stored and to make remote semantic or conceptual associations (see "The High Costs of Cognitive Superefficiency" in Chapter 8). From a psychoanalytic viewpoint, with repression vanished, the unconscious became accessible; my mind functioned with holistic oneness, interconnected.

Superefficiency in memory retrieval and ideational association may then result from undoing or bypassing repression with ease, thus enabling me to gain unhindered, direct access to the unconscious, a condition for creativity as postulated in psychoanalytic theory. In this way, superefficiency has the effect of enhancing my aesthetic, empathic, and cognitive capabilities.

Spiritual Fulfillment Versus Spiritual Emptiness: A Dynamic Process

Still, intriguing diagnostic questions remain. My writing in the midst of madness was not the product of a disordered mind. Rather, it was a self-reflective mind, supersensitive, audacious, experimental, intent on a transcendental-spiritual quest. Christ-like pathos for humanity—that is, love—triumphs over hate. Aside from diagnosis, the data I have assembled from diverse sources yield a composite picture of my thoughts and actions as I go through my life journey. They give me plenty to reflect on the joys and tribulations of my life.

As I look back, it dawns on me how fortunate I have been, with so many inviting tales to tell. Often, the happenings do not result from a deliberate search on my part; rather, they are serendipitous. I simply seize the opportunity to create meaning and revel in narration when they occur. It also seems clear that I have gone into different directions. In the end, what unifies my activities is spiritual meaning. A dialogue between David and YF ensues.

> **David** Unfortunately, the DSM-IV is silent here; in fact, it discounts positive features, especially when they are outside the normal range of human experience. We have to go beyond its scope.
>
> **YF** More than that: My case serves to reveal how deficient psychiatric diagnosis, based on the DSM-IV or otherwise, can be. Psychiatry tends to locate disorders within individuals; it pays insufficient attention to the interpersonal dimension underlying disorders. It lacks a dynamic conception to appreciate the coexistence of positive and negative forces. It is silent on how conditions that merely resemble a mental disorder but are fundamentally positive in nature may be distinguished from those that are truly pathological.

I refer to extraordinary religious-spiritual experiences of numerous people (e.g., mystics), historical and contemporary, in diverse cultures. Abnormality comes in great varieties; witness the vast number of diagnostic categories in the psychiatric literature. Why should normality be more impoverished in diversity? Religious-spiritual experiences can be highly problematic to a person's life—not being understood, or worse, misunderstood by family, friends, and yes, psychiatrists. I bring this up only to illustrate once again how inadequate psychiatric diagnosis can be. Here is all that the DSM-IV has to say about Religious or Spiritual Problem:

> This category can be used when the focus of clinical attention is a religious or spiritual problem. Examples include distressing experiences that involve loss or questioning of faith, problems associated with conversion to a new faith, or questioning of spiritual values that may not necessarily be related to an organized church or religious institution.

Why is the focus of attention "clinical"? This is disingenuous, inasmuch as Religious or Spiritual Problem, the DSM-IV makes clear, is not a mental disorder. Obviously, we have to move beyond psychiatry toward spirituality.

David It is rather ironic that these scathing remarks come from the mouth of a person who has taught psychiatric and psychological diagnosis for most of his professional life. You must have seen the light, to come up with such an anti-establishment argument. I'm sure there are readers who have suffered from mental aberrations. The usual course of development is psychiatric diagnosis followed by treatment (psychotherapy and/or medication). The diagnostic label (e.g., schizophrenia, literally "split mind") can be scary and lead to stigmatization; treatment can be worse than the disorder.

Rarely is there an attempt to help the patient understand his disorder in a larger context, as an existential quest for meaning. That's why your insistence that madness may be a part of one's spiritual journey is refreshing and reassuring. Others can benefit from your experience. What perspective, beyond psychiatric diagnosis, promises to shed light on a fuller understanding of your journey?

YF A dynamic conception of the struggle between spiritual fulfillment and spiritual emptiness cries out to be heard (see Chapter 18).

The attainment of spirituality is a dynamic process in which struggle, change, and self-transformation are central. Speaking from personal experience, the process may be described as a movement, back and forth, from disorientation-alienation to reconstruction-reorganization. Spirituality and spiritual emptiness have coexisted, alternating at different moments, in my lifetime. Certainly, my journey in search of spirituality has not been easy, peaceful sailing.

What Is a Spiritual Journey Like?

A spiritual journey can be lonely and hazardous. Lonely because it is intensely personal; segments of it, at least, have to be taken without accompaniment; feelings of being different or distant from others may appear. Hazardous because the traveler may go astray, wander into the path of evil cults or be overcome by madness. It is especially hazardous for those who have gone far enough to experience ecstasy, the mystical, and the like; for it is not uncommon for these advanced travelers to be viewed as weird, abnormal, or exceeding the bounds of social acceptability.

Spiritual journeys make no promises. There are no shortcuts, like taking drugs; that's fundamental. And if the traveler finally succeeds in reaching enlightenment, he would have a hard time making himself fully understood by fellow humans, not having experienced his experiences, about his state of being. Only a Buddha knows a Buddha, so to speak.

David Why bother with spiritual journeys if they are arduous, lonely, full of hazards and predicaments? Some might ask.

YF Because spiritual fulfillment is like a lighthouse, alluring and drawing the lost, the empty toward it. A journey can be fundamentally rewarding in itself, adding color to all aspects of life. And because failure to embark on one will eventually result in spiritual emptiness: Life becomes stagnant, unfulfilled. I would go as far as to say spirituality is built into human nature: We really have no choice but to seek it out; failure to do so violates our being. The trouble is that deep self-reflection and immense effort are required. Not surprisingly, inertia often gets the better of us, like a dead weight inside our psyche. At every turn, we may see plenty of people who want to be spoon-fed ready-made answers on questions of faith, religion, or spirituality.

David How many of us dare to take the journey? I suspect that genuine spirituality may not be easily found. Rather, spiritual emptiness is the norm; its symptoms may be discerned everywhere. We lead our lives with complacency, perhaps even numbness. We lack courage to make commitments, and we avoid taking risks for a fundamental change in direction. We may even be unaware of, and hence do not reflect upon, the empty state of our existence.

Of course, failure to take risks is the greatest risk of all. Sometimes, however, critical incidents or alterations in our life condition occur: bankruptcy, financial or social; inspired by a trusted mentor; cheating death to be given a new lease on life. They wake us from our complacency. Even spontaneous awakenings may occur.

YF As long as there is the will to struggle, there may be torment, anguish, despair—but not spiritual emptiness. Struggle confers meaning on life and thus negates spiritual emptiness; it has in itself positive value, even when success is not assured. But struggle is not enough; one must be committed and take action. Hardly anything is more uninviting than to be caught in perennial struggle. Action leads to change, perhaps eventual self-transformation. A self-transformed person experiences the joys of spiritual fulfillment and realizes his potential.

Herein lies the answer to why some people are willing to take the journey: The goal of spiritual fulfillment is seductive, and the process itself is exciting. Besides, failure to take the journey is decidedly unattractive. When a person gives up struggling, spiritual emptiness sets in: He becomes passive, withdrawn, self-absorbed, fixated, stagnant, and eventually embittered.

If this sounds too grave, let me hasten to add that the dynamic struggle between spiritual fulfillment and spiritual emptiness does not have to be as intense as I have described it. However, the struggle is relevant to a person's life regardless of his mental condition, normal or abnormal. It may be openly recognized or latent in your life. But it can no more be avoided than you can by burying your head in the sand. I have simply articulated a central nature of human life. And if it sounds too abstract, let me reassure the reader that everything I have said I have experienced in fresh and blood.

Spirituality and religiosity are distinct ideas. Religiosity puts the emphasis on personal salvation, deliverance from punishment in the present life or afterlife, and the promise of everlasting life. Often it is driven by insecurity, anxiety, and fear of punishment, hell, God. In contrast, spiritual pursuits are growth oriented, not driven by fear; they demand intense personal effort, soul searching. What is crucial is to seek some higher goal in life and principles that serve as a guide to leading the good life.

The Positives and Negatives of Madness

David Why not apply the dynamic conception to your own case? A fruitful way to proceed is to spell out the positive as well as negative forces of your madness.

YF The positives were many. Positive feelings (e.g., love of humanity, "Life is wonderful," "Eros triumphs over Thanatos") predominated. I was aware of my aggressive-hostile impulses, of course, but they did not threaten to be acted out in unchecked, destructive forms. The capacity for depth of feelings, both pleasant and painful, was magnified. I experienced heightened artistic-esthetic sensibilities (e.g., "The world is beautiful"); empathy and compassion; creativity and linguistic fluency. I was freed from obsessive-compulsivity, self-doubt, and shame.

The spells of exuberance afforded me precious opportunities to gain unhindered access to the unconscious, experience the extraordinary, and glimpse into the mystical-transcendental state of enlightenment. Among the most dramatic, memorable, and inspirational of my experiences were those gained in Mania 1.

These included experiencing myself as bodily vanished, empty; self-healing of an injured knee while I was in the state of emptiness; coexistence of yin and yang in an androgynous body; willful visual hallucinations, in which I saw myself vividly on a cross and, likening myself to Jesus, felt great pathos for the sufferings of humankind. With repression gone, access to the unconscious was total.

> **David** There's another positive that deserves to be mentioned: Madness adds color to your spiritual journey. The child in you comes out during your madness; you return to your "original face." You become more spontaneous, playful, humorous—also naughty, adventurous, audacious. Your creative potential is realized.

The great irony is that, in so many ways, I am a more attractive person when I am mad than when I am normal. My interactions with friends are full of laughter. People respond to me positively—as long as I keep my behavior within bounds. Is that the reason why I have so many bouts of madness?

Why can't spiritual journeys be playful and joyous? This is an important point, because too many people think of the pursuit of spirituality as a grave and staid undertaking, in which playfulness has no place. Struggle is essential, but spiritual journeys don't have to be based on viewing life, in my student days, as "an intense struggle."

The pursuit of spirituality is more sustainable if it is made attractive, as when playfulness intermingles with dedication. Spiritual journeys can be fun, especially when the spice of madness is added.

> **YF** Actually I have made quite a career of entertaining people. As a schoolboy, I cracked jokes that often made the entire class, already bored to death by boring teachers, burst into laughter. While I was an undergraduate, I had a summer job as an orderly at a hospital for French Canadians. My job was to prepare patients for surgery. Why not entertain them as well, I thought. And I did. The fact that I spoke little or no French did not diminish my ability to make the patients laugh. I wrote in my diary, "I cannot control myself not to be funny." One of the patients who had undergone abdominal surgery

David	Now, what about the negatives?
YF	At times, I have felt alienated and enslaved by work. I have been too much of a workaholic. Academic and professional pursuits have brought me prestige, not happiness; they might even be detours or, worse, escapes from my quest for spirituality. Achievement is important, but not nearly as important as happiness, which comes only with the participation of others.

laughed so heartily that I became concerned about his belly bursting open. I had to control myself. Years later, in my golden age, I succeeded in combining entertainment and education in the classroom, one of the secrets of being an effective teacher.

With this understanding, I will recount my search for communion in the next chapter. Have I felt spiritually empty? Rarely, only in my darkest hours. I have never felt that life is meaningless or purposeless, although I have experienced a loss of direction sometimes. If anything, I tend to be overcommitted to too many goals, but I take action toward reaching some of them. And I don't run away from struggle.

David	Thinking about important questions concerning life characterized by metacognitive, reflective thought, as in your case, would involve doubt or struggle. It does not fall back automatically on stereotyped or superstitious beliefs, blind faith, religious dogmas, doctrinaire beliefs for ready answers.
YF	Depth of feelings, both positive and negative, marks my madness. I experienced fluctuations between exuberance and anguish in different episodes, but never psychic numbing, the incapacity to feel happiness or sadness. Heightened aesthetic sensibilities were prominent: I had the capacity to experience simple, unabashed delight in ordinary things (e.g., the root of a tree, the droning sound of cicadas). I experienced serenity and inner peace, but also inner turmoil. In the self-report on my case history submitted as an assignment, I wrote: "I am all alone, in a new country; and, for the first time in my life, I experience loneliness and emptiness. . . .. Well, this is what really makes an existentialist: he has to create his own values, from the beginning of despair."

Decades later, I woke up suddenly one night in the midst of Mania 2, feeling I was the loneliest person in the world, understood by none and fighting lonely battles all my life. As expressed in a famous line by a renowned Chinese writer of bygone age: "All earthlings are intoxicated. I alone am sober."

It is never easy to remain sober while all others are intoxicated. So underneath the mania was a deep sense of anguish, loneliness, and yearning for human contact, expressed in a poem I sent out to friends (5 July 2007).

Black Hole

Into a Black Hole I plunge,
From which nothing can ever escape.
Its center singularity I reach,
Where Loneliness Eternal dwells.

I ask the Physicist,
"Is there really no exit?"
"If there is, you might continue
Your journey from one universe
To another—but never
To return to your home."
My body droops, my eyes downcast,
On the ground I prostrate,
As Loneliness turns into Despair.

I turn to the Philosopher. He says:
"The Dao is ONE, omnipresent, timeless.
Nothing is. Everything becomes.
Everything connects with everything else,
With itself, with the whole Multiverse."
Enfleshed in my body,
Hope drives Despair away.

The Physicist jumps in:
"Ah, Theory of Everything. Wait!
The topology of the Klein bottle suggests
Black holes can connect
To the universe as a whole."
As a child, I did think:
An atom is a universe
Unto itself; our universe is but an atom
In a larger universe. So each atom contains,
And is contained by, an infinity
Of universes up and down.

I turn to the Poet. He says:
"Now the language of science surpasses
The language of idle words, in connecting
Sentients throughout the Multiverse,
WhereverWhenever they may be."

A whispering voice says:
"Haven't you heard of *Karma Invariance*?
You are gone, truly gone.
You are here, here with us:
Just as our karma lives
In your consciousness,
Your karma lives
In ours, and continues
To work out its effects on our lives."

I see myself smiling back to bring
A smile on your face again.

Relational and Ecumenical Spirituality

To be eternally cut off from humanity: What greater horror can there be? But I am an incurable optimist. That's why I wrote at the end of the poem, "I see myself smiling back to bring / A smile on your face again." That's relational spirituality.

> **David** You view the self in a larger context: Spirituality is reached through transcending egocentrism and moving toward universal love. Transcendence is relational spirituality, reached through transcending egocentrism. Relationships are integral to one's meaning and purpose in life. The antithesis of transcendence is self-encapsulation, in which the self derives meaning and purpose solely or primarily from its own individual existence, without reference to a larger context. Self-encapsulation is a form of egoism or self-contained individualism (see Chapter 11, Chapter 18).
>
> **YF** Ironically, at the time I wrote the poem, I had warm relationships with quite a few friends and fellow workers. In my madness, I feel greater warmth toward people. I become more generous, more loving, more prosocial in words and deeds.

By nature, I enjoy having a good time with other people. I shun solitary recreation and I dread social isolation. So being gregarious does not save me from having lonely feelings. Intermittent tension between closeness and distance underlies my relations with other people. In Hypomania 7, I wrote, "At every turn, I encounter people with fixated mentalities who want to be spoon fed on how to 'grow psychologically.' They don't see what is in front of their eyes, or hear voices that should be loud and clear to them." And, "As I grow wiser, so too the distance increases between myself and others."

> **David**   As you grower wiser, other-acceptance becomes commensurate with self-acceptance. You would view people with greater understanding and acceptance, particularly of how they differ from you. Alternating between solitude and companionship is all right. There are times when we wish to retreat into our private selves, undisturbed by others, and there are times when we feel the need for human contact. The ideals are solitude without loneliness and companionship without loss of individuality.

We must talk more about the interpersonal dimension of spiritual journeys. Up to now, we have been talking about the quest for spirituality mostly as if it were an individual undertaking without the involvement of others. This dawns on me as we are engaged in the present dialogue. No, I say to myself, this is not meant to be. The quest should be a much more rewarding search for spirituality-in-partnership.

> **YF**   A great irony is that taking a spiritual journey may indeed increase the distance between the traveler and others. As the traveler becomes more advanced in his journey, he is likely to become more atypical, more unlike other people. This has been largely my experience. The question arises, How does becoming more atypical affect the traveler's relationships with his significant others?

Siddhartha Gautama, we may recall, went to the extreme of abandoning his family, parents, wife, and newborn son. Among my Buddhist friends, some have renounced marital life in their search for enlightenment. In these cases, the spiritual journey is taken individually, devoid of the participation of significant others.

What about journeys taken by intimate partners together? Ah, finding a suitable partner is as difficult as looking for a needle in a haystack, and more challenges await the traveler who succeeds in finding one. A journey taken by a single person is trying enough; a journey taken together with others, especially significant others, will tax all to the limit.

To me, however, the idea of spirituality-in-isolation has little or no appeal; spirituality-in-partnership is attractive enough to take on whatever challenge it presents. The whole is greater than the sum of its parts. Emergent relational properties, unique to the partners involved, arise from two travelers coming together in an intimate relationship. The partners transform, and are transformed by, their relationship: This is spirituality-in-partnership.

An operatic love duet provides a beautiful analogy. The opera depicts the individual character of the lovers in the duet. Yet the opera on the printed page is dead music. It becomes alive only when the musical notes, each and all, are articulated and the lyrics are sung by the performing artists. The performance of each singer acts as a powerful stimulus to the other. The "chemistry" between them gives life to the duet, resulting in a performance that cannot be reduced to a summation of individual artistic qualities.

Synchronicity holds the key to having a happy spiritual journey together, as it does to sustain intimate relationships in general. Consider the case of a dyadic relationship. Change in one partner acts as catalyst for change in the other, and vice versa; this leads to change in the nature of their relationship, such as greater trust, affection, and complementarity. This invigorated relationship, in turn, sets the stage for further changes within each partner. In sum, together the partners grow spiritually. On the other hand, an asynchronous journey, in terms of pace, direction, determination, and so forth, can be hazardous. It may increase the distance between the partners and tear their relationship apart. Both partners may be wonderful people, but both may suffer terribly.

But there is an absolute limit to companionship or partnership in any spiritual journey. Ultimately pivotal decisions and commitments in life must be made alone. Just as we come into the world alone, so shall we leave the world alone—unaccompanied. In between the coming and the leaving is when we may choose our companions wisely.

However, in a sense relationships do not end when a person dies: His karma continues to live in the consciousness of other people, such as colleagues, friends, and relatives, unrestricted by space or time.

My conceptualization is also ecumenical in orientation, not biased toward or anchored in a particular Christian denomination, or even in a particular religion. By ecumenicity, I mean universality, more than merely transcending denominational or religious boundaries.

Universal love is the lodestone of ecumenicity. It finds expression in the Greek idea of agape, the Confucian idea of *ren* (benevolence), the Buddhist idea of *daai* (great love), the Christian ideas of *caritas* and love feast. At root, it champions the intrinsic value of human life and cherishing care for one's fellow human beings. Buddhism extends the regard for life to all living creatures. Daoism views human life as person-in-cosmos; the regard for mother earth and nature follows.

"Within the four seas, all men are brothers." This Chinese saying expresses an embracing, ecumenical sentiment. In a modernized version, it might read: "In our global village, we are all sisters and brothers." This is an expression of ecumenicity: All members of humankind are welcome to embark on a spiritual pilgrimage; no one is excluded.

In keeping with pluralism, ecumenicity allows for, even welcomes, cultural or religious diversity. For instance, the value of suffering is recognized in Buddhism, Christianity, as well as other religions. Ecumenicity affirms the spiritual value of suffering but leaves open what that value may entail. Closely allied with ecumenicity is equifinality, the idea that the same ultimate goal may be reached from different paths. A fellow traveler is at liberty to define his own chosen path for spiritual fulfillment. In principle, there may be as many paths as there are travelers.

David No stranger to suffering, especially in your age of turbulence, you appreciate its value, although you do not profess to be Buddhist or Christian. You reaffirm your belief in "the dignity of each and every person, without exceptions"; "cultural uprooting" is an extreme that marks the path you have chosen.

Your intercultural interests and experiences may enrich our understanding of ecumenical spirituality. Ours is both principled and tolerant. Ecumenicity without tolerance succumbs to absolutism; unprincipled ecumenicity absorbs unwanted elements and risks becoming tainted. The tension between principled discernment and tolerance drives its further development—in a process much like the "creative synthesis" of the East and the West you have described.

YF Spirituality is being-in-the-world—a far cry from the practice of the hermit. It includes political activism for peace and justice, anywhere; it is not just an abstract idea.

Witnessing My Ineptitude and Decline: Acceptance

By all counts, among the negatives ineptitude in mechanical or practical things are the most salient. They make an in-your-face mockery of my intellectual prowess. My ineptitude manifests itself in different episodes: I experience great difficulty locating "lost" objects or recalling "lost" ideas, comprehending what I read, making a phone call, performing a simple arithmetic calculation, or finding my way around in my neighborhood. The list goes on and on.

But ineptitude is nothing new: All my life, I have found that many things other people find easy to do make me feel incompetent. (Equally, many things difficult for others seem so easy to me that I have great trouble, emotionally if not intellectually, understanding how they can be found difficult.) Once I took a U.S. Army's test of mechanical aptitude, during a mass induction exercise. I scored in the "idiot's range," prompting the sergeant who administered the test to suspect that I was faking.

I suffer from computer phobia, especially when I receive an invitation to be a "friend" on Facebook or the like. I have trouble with surfing the Internet, registration, user names, passwords, and so forth. Isn't living in this technological age overloading our memory capacity? Once, in the midst of Hypomania 7, I wrote the following message to my friends and colleagues, confessing how inept I felt.

> My apology to you for having sent multiple messages. My CSQ (Computer-Savvy Quotient), mechanical, clerical aptitude, etc. is in the imbecile range. Nothing irritates me like a temperamental computer does.
>
> I'm just not cut out for modern gadgets, and hereby swear on the Altar of the Almighty that I shall continue to refrain from using cell phones to avoid being enslaved by them. I have never owned one, because I don't want people to locate me when I don't want them to. People in Hong Kong think I am old fashioned. They can't comprehend why I refuse to have one, unaware how they themselves have been enslaved by modern consumerism, commercials targeting women on how to lose weight, etc.
>
> Oh no, I'm beginning to sound like Andy Rooney, the octogenarian who has become an institution in 60 Minutes. I concede, however, that he does have a knack for saying things that both entertain and instruct, especially to the ears of a nonnative speaker of English like myself.

Another confession I have to make: Having moved to the United States later on, I agreed to get a cell phone for safety reasons.

David   Ineptitude takes many forms. I imagine your daily life is a gold mine reinforcing the stereotype of an absent-minded professor.

YF   Yes, I make silly mistakes, like dialing the wrong telephone number, forgetting where I had put my things and then looking for them in frustration, and so forth. One of my techniques in teaching is to transform my weakness into strength, and thus to amuse my students. During lessons, my mind sometimes raced so much faster than my tongue that I would say one thing when I meant another. Thus, I unintentionally uttered a novel nominal construction: Xi Zedong, which collapsed Xi Tele (the Chinese name for Hitler) and Mao Zedong. (I hasten to add that I didn't mean to imply Mao and Hitler were the same.)

I forewarned my students: "Once in a while, I might say things that are false or misleading, just to see if you would jot them down in your notebook." An example: "There are three kinds of logic, deductive, inductive, and seductive." Most of my students dutifully recorded that utterance.

> **David**   This is not to deny the linguistic-logical-creative prowess you possess. Abstract, logical, systematic thought has never been a problem, except in the sense that it can sometimes make you overly conscious of conundrums, paradoxes, and inconsistencies in utterances or writings by yourself or by others. Such overconsciousness, or perfectionism, can make students uncomfortable and put them on guard.
>
> **YF**   It can also cause writer's paralysis, especially with regard to academic writing, from which I have long suffered. To avoid the task at hand, I would run around, looking for other things to do. Typically, the torment would last for about two weeks, after which I would settle down to write. Creative writing frees me from compulsivity, though not from perfectionism, and is in this sense truly creative. And during bouts of madness, I enjoy freedom from perfectionism. Better to be imperfect and remain human, as our maker's creation, than to be perfect and equal to our maker.

But now, I am confronted by something far more formidable than ineptitude: No question about it, I am witnessing my own decline. One day, I took my three-year-old grandson, hand in hand, for a walk along a country road. I drew his attention to something lying on the ground, "See this dead animal, poor thing." Whereupon, the three-year-old injected, "It's a lizard." My inner reactions were twofold. One, what grandfather wouldn't find delight in being bested by his grandchildren? Two, actually I was fumbling to find the right word *lizard* in my mind. Unable to do so fast enough, I used *animal* as a poor substitute. Such is the evidence compelling me to accept that my brain is aging.

> **David**   This is a far cry from what Confucius said: At age seventy, he acted according to his heart's wishes. As you age, your working memory is not as efficient as before. You have trouble remembering telephone numbers, names of people newly introduced, and the like; performing simple clerical or computational tasks cannot be completed easily and error free; processing information requires longer time periods. In short, your relative weaknesses, in what psychologists call fluid intelligence, have been exacerbated as a function of aging.
>
> The difficulty seems to be confined to registration and storage of new information. As of this moment, retrieval of old learning presents no problem whatsoever. My prowess in remote associations, retrieving, and synthesizing knowledge, undiminished in the least, continues to sometimes overwhelm

myself: I can't write down my thoughts as fast as they come. Perhaps I am getting even stronger in what psychologists call crystallized intelligence. So my decline in cognitive abilities has caused me no more than inconveniences and embarrassments.

YF I am grateful for what I still possess and not mourn what I have lost. Eventually, however, cognitive decline may reach a point where spirituality in the fullest sense can no longer be sustained. What then? I'm not going to get away from facing a question that no spiritual traveler can avoid. I pray that I will still be able to express and receive affection by whatever means unto my last breath.

David Isn't acceptance of the inevitable, and of what cannot be changed, wisdom to be attained in any spiritual journey? To make a stronger point, such acceptance is a basic value essential to spiritual fulfillment.

Remember the timeless wisdom of the Serenity Prayer?

God, grant me the serenity
To accept the things I cannot change,
The courage to change the things I can,
And wisdom to know the difference.

Shantideva, a Buddhist scholar of Nalanda University in India, expressed the attitude of acceptance in the eighth century as follows:

If there is remedy when trouble strikes,
What reason is there for dejection?
And if there is none,
Of what use is there in being glum?

The Jewish philosopher Solomon ibn Gabirol expressed a similar thought in the 11th century:

And they said: At the head of all understanding is realizing what is and what cannot be, and the consoling of what is not in our power to change.

YF I would also enlarge the scope of acceptance. Many things can be changed, but there is no moral necessity for changing them. For instance, take my being atypical, different from other people. If I try hard enough, I suppose I might succeed in being more like others and perhaps gain greater social acceptance; I would then lead an easier life.

But what is the point and at what cost? I suspect that the color in my life would be subdued. Gaining self-acceptance is part and parcel of my spiritual journey. I have struggled to arrive at a point where I value the way I am and feel "at home in the cosmos." So rather than trying to be what I am not, I would spend my energy on more worthwhile endeavors, such as helping our fellow travelers.

David The irony is that you seem to accept yourself more when you are mad than when you are not. Moreover, your firsthand experiences of madness have been instrumental to obtaining a deeper understanding of spirituality, and in particular to the development of the Multidimensional Evaluations of Spirituality (MES, see Appendix A).

The MES derives from your knowledge of comparative religion, Eastern and Western intellectual and religious traditions, clinical experiences in multicultural settings, and personal insights.

What is intriguing is that I have applied the MES, an instrument of my creation, to myself. In doing so, I have presented a convincing case for moving beyond psychiatry to spirituality.

I urge readers to make good use of the MES most earnestly. For them, this may be a pivotal step toward tipping the balance from spiritual emptiness toward spiritual fulfillment.

5

Glimpses of Enlightenment on the Midst of Madness

Spirituality without a measure of madness is devoid of energy; madness without spirituality loses its redeeming value.

This chapter goes to the heart of my journey in search of spirituality, punctuated by episodes of madness. It depicts my glimpses into enlightenment during episodes of madness. It confronts the central issue of how spirituality may interact with madness. In doing so, I will have to clarify the complex meanings of madness, creativity, religiosity, spirituality, and enlightenment. My extraordinary experiences during the episodes of madness provide an avenue for exploring the hypothetical nature of enlightenment, through extrapolation from a glimpse to the fully developed state. I say "hypothetical" to underscore our limited understanding of enlightenment. These glimpses of enlightenment are the raw materials that have given me insights on the interaction between madness and enlightenment.

Fleeting Experiences of Enlightenment

What can I share with fellow travelers? Strategies of coping with depression and life's misfortunes that I have found useful in my own journey? How can one fall in love with madness? How do poetry and spirituality drive each other? To answer these questions, an internal dialogue between YF and David ensues.

> **YF** There are times when I can say to myself, "I have arrived." I act according to my wishes, without inhibition or paralyzing inner conflicts. I feel a sense of supreme self-confidence, even self-mastery. My capacity for keen perception, appreciation, and humor is immense. I delight in things, large and small, complex and simple, and I proclaim, "The world is a wondrous place."

I enter into a mystical state of serenity and magnanimity, free from anxiety or inner turmoil. Guilt, shame, self-rejection, and self-mortification are minimized. I feel connected with people, at home in society, nature, and the cosmos. All the good things are present, in enhanced magnitudes. Gone are the fixations, prejudices, obsessions. Life is sweet, meaningful, and fulfilling.

Above all, the enlargement of love dominates my being and leads me to act in selfless ways for the betterment of humankind. Vivid willful hallucinations and the selfless self may be experienced, more readily than usual. In short, enlightenment is an extremely pleasant state to be in; it touches a person to the core of his being.

So even a fleeting experiencing of enlightenment is to be cherished as a beacon for the rest of my life. So I feel privileged. Like others who have experienced mania, I would prefer, if given the choice, to live my life without being deprived of manic exuberance.

> **David** Direct experiences of enlightenment or of the transcendent are inherently solitary. You may experience them together with someone else, but that someone else can't experience them for you *directly*. Moreover, they may be perilously close to madness when we fail to respect the distinction between subjective experiencing and reality. I would tread, therefore, with great caution and perhaps trepidation in the unknown territory of the transcendent.
>
> **YF** Not all of my experiences are enlightened or enlightening. They include, for instance, aggressive or hostile elements. However, most of the time, hatred, embitterment, and aggression are gone. More critically, my experiences include both positive and negative feelings. I experienced pain, pathos, and anguish intensely; I cried. But these negatives were also positive in a sense: From the crying came total catharsis, which has a powerful healing effect. I don't know if these emotions can still be found in the final state of enlightenment.
>
> **David** The capability for deep spiritual experiences is not the same as enlightenment. Some people have this capability but are not necessarily wise and may lead disorganized lives. Mozart comes to mind as an example. His music bears

testimony to his inward spirituality, yet his biography is a case study of a disorganized life.

On the other hand, wisdom does not necessarily include spirituality. There are wise persons who are not known for being particularly spiritual. Enlightenment is the summit: It includes both wisdom and the capacity for deep spiritual feelings, such as compassion; madness is excluded, however.

I don't think of enlightenment as a place or physical destination to reach. I describe enlightenment as a state of serenity and magnanimity hypothetically. My conception is based on an extrapolation of fleeting experiences—an admission of incomplete knowledge.

However, the value of firsthand experiences cannot be overstated, to the experiencing person as well as people with whom they are shared. But we must examine further the nature of firsthand experiences and the difficulties they present to sharing.

In this book are disclosures of my private experiences, at different stages of development from childhood to adulthood. These include intercultural encounters, some inspirational and some painful; encounters with madness as well as spirituality. Of these, the most difficult to recount are those of spirituality in the depths of madness.

> **YF** Spiritual experiences are privately experienced; they are highly personal, not easily revealed to or understood by others. Fortunately, these private experiences do not have to remain entirely private; they can be shared meaningfully with others.

Mystical experiences, transcendent consciousness, enlightenment, and the like present even greater difficulties. Like my fleeting experiences of enlightenment, they hover around the summit of spirituality. They are not only private but also unfamiliar, even inaccessible, to most of us. They cannot be publicly demonstrated.

> **David** Here we encounter what appears to be an insurmountable barrier to communication or external observation. However, physiological correlates (e.g., alterations in brain waves) of these experiences are publicly demonstrable. The experiences may be reported to a public audience, as you have done in this book. Their effects on the lives of people who experience them are observable; in some cases, the effects are dramatic and transformative.

The idea that "only a Buddha knows a Buddha" suggests a plausible approach to observation: comparing notes among advanced travelers who claim to have experienced enlightenment; or, better still, examination of an advanced traveler by a panel of other travelers, equally or more advanced.

This approach may render public what would otherwise be open only to private experiential verification: The authenticity of heightened, unusual spiritual experiences claimed by an individual may be subject to examination by a panel of judges whose qualifications are publicly acknowledged. Thus, the difficulties of communicating, observing, and verifying one's private experiences of enlightenment are not entirely insurmountable.

This is a happy thought: My private experiences of enlightenment and the like can be shared meaningfully with others and are, to some extent, accessible and understandable by others. I don't mind being examined by travelers more advanced than I, if it helps the sharing. Besides, I can learn from them.

The mind of a lesser order is incapable of understanding fully that of a higher order, just as humans are inherently limited in their comprehension of divine beings. God is unknowable. The absence of God, however, can be apprehended: It can be seen everywhere, in all the foolish things that people do, especially when they speak and act in God's name.

So to understand the mind of a Buddha, prophet, or saint is a formidable, if not impossible, task. However, we are not totally helpless. Reading the autobiographies, journals, or confessions of religious luminaries (such as George Fox and St. Augustine) is a good starting point. They can be a gold mine of madness, no less than of spirituality.

Ultimately, however, enlightenment has to be experienced; it cannot be known by other means. Presumably, enlightenment is the destination of a religious or spiritual journey. Is enlightenment like being in Heaven? And madness like being in Hell?

Madness and Hell both conjure imageries of a burning inferno, volcano explosion, and cauldron of untamed impulses like the Freudian id, as I wrote in this poem (circa January 2010):

Thus Speaks Lucifer

Cast into a lake of fire and brimstone,
Tormented day and night for ever
And ever, this is the mother of all tortures!
Hoping against hope that never comes,
Down and down we descend,
Layer upon layers of the Inferno,
Into the vast abyss

That knows not where to end.
No heavenly angels sing;
We hear only the Devil's Trill.
Lure and lust red hot inflame
Burning desire unconsumed.
O what sadist has invented Hell!

It is tempting to associate madness with Hell. However, madness has no necessary connection with evil. Hell has the connection, because it is where the evil are punished in everlasting agony, according to traditional Christian as well as Islamic theology.

Perhaps the most extreme of hellish torments is that desires are not extinct, but there is no possibility for their consummation—too much of a predicament for contemplation. Hell must be a human, not divine, invention, for it is hard to contemplate that divine beings are capable of such extreme sadism. I prefer, therefore, to think of Hell as a state of mind, especially about human relationships. Hell is other people, as the existentialist Sartre says.

Like Hell, Heaven is not a literal place, but a state of mind. What is it like to be in Heaven? The New Testament's Book of Revelation (21:4) gives an image of Heaven: "And God shall wipe away all tears from their eyes; and there shall be no more death, neither sorrow, nor crying, neither shall there be any more pain: for the former things are passed away."

No tears, no death, no sorrow, no crying, no pain—and no need for memory. Eternal peace, eternal boredom! What can one do with angels? Could Hell be more attractive, with its collection of fallen angels and the likes of Salome, still dancing her Dance of the Seven Veils? My vision of enlightenment differs from the Christian imagery of Heaven. It is anything but boring.

Dialectics Between Spirituality and Madness

In Western psychology, the healthy self is conceived as stable over time; it is a coherent, integrated, and unitary whole. I have no dispute with this conception. To experience the selfless self or empty mind, as in Dynamic Relaxation and Meditation, is to go beyond, not supplant, the normal and healthy. In a similar vein, the achievement of impulse control is prerequisite to experiencing the extraordinary, which implies overcoming repression and gaining access to the unconscious. If what comes out are unchecked rampant impulses and raw destructiveness, the result would be horror. Therefore, experiencing the extraordinary in the absence of adequate control is not to be recommended for all. How would one know if and when it is safe? This is a question that must be answered in order to understand how spirituality and madness may be intertwined.

> **David** You didn't actively seek extraordinary experiences, through drugs, meditation, or other means. They occurred spontaneously. In fact, even now you don't know how to switch them on or off at will. But we must consider the horror of this possibility: Your extraordinary experiences could be pathological and destructive through and through, without the redeeming value of the positives. Do you have any assurance that your extraordinary experiences are, or will be, positive when they do occur?
>
> **YF** I have of course pondered this question. And I can give you some assurance, but not an infallible prediction. To enter into a state of selfless self *safely* presupposes a developed, healthy self already in existence. In terms of development, the achievement of a healthy self is a prerequisite for experiencing its disappearance. The state of selfless self must be distinguished from nonexistence of self.

There are no shortcuts to the accumulation of experiences under normal and abnormal circumstances. Digging deeply into my own experiences, I see a preponderance of positives (e.g., love of humanity) over the negatives (e.g., aggressiveness), and I foresee no horror when they come out in magnified intensities. In Mania 2, for instance, the free association was replete with aggressive or hostile impulses, which I never acted on.

> **David** An idea that comes to mind is germane to our discussion at hand: In some cases, religiosity takes on a life of its own, coexisting with madness, and transforms the person's life. We should develop this idea further. Can we not contemplate the possibility that, in transforming the person, religiosity may also be instrumental in severing madness from the person's life eventually?
>
> **YF** In this context, I prefer to speak of spirituality, rather than religiosity, because of its closer conceptual linkage with enlightenment. Also, I don't think in terms of severance, but of harnessing or mastering.
>
> **David** Even before your encounter with mania, you made this very point (30 July 1996).

Harnessing Madness

Madness unharnessed is great peril;
Sanity devoid of Madness is boredom.
Madness,
O Madness, if only
I can control you, switch

You on and off at will,
Then I shall have
Not only sanity,
But also tranquility.

> YF The secret is to develop a master switch that can control madness. This has proven to be extremely difficult to do. Time and time again, I thought I had learned enough to keep my hypomania or mania under control, only to realize later that my optimism was premature.

However, what I want to achieve is clear: to reap the benefits of my extraordinary, mystical experiences, without having to incur the social costs. That means I have to pay more attention to the perceptions of others, including their views of my behavior, and adjust to the distance between myself and others. For instance, during episodes, my mind runs too fast, and I need to slow down for other people. I tend to forget that other people may not be as enthusiastic, fired up, as I am about my ideals, and I have to learn not to expect too much, or be disappointed afterwards. In short, I must learn to master myself, to "act according to my wishes," without arousing fear and inviting rejection from others.

The idea of harnessing goes beyond coexisting with madness. Coexistence with madness is like living at the foot of an active volcano, and you don't know when it will explode. Harnessing madness is more radical: *The creative forces of madness are made subservient to spirituality and drive its further development. The healing forces of spirituality temper the volatility of madness and keep it from causing harm or destruction.*

In this way spirituality and madness are not just in peaceful coexistence with each other. Rather, they exist in a dialectical relation. Spirituality without a measure of madness is devoid of energy; madness without spirituality loses its redeeming value. Spirituality derives creative energy from madness to reach new heights; madness receives the healing, calming effects of spirituality to become benign. This conception means that madness may continue to be intertwined with spirituality, not something I have to get rid of.

A dialectical relation between madness and spirituality entails tension and conflict. Many people, including psychologists, tend to regard inner conflicts as negative and self-consistency as positive for mental health. However, the notion of self-consistency may lead to a sterile conception of human functioning in which conflicts have no place. Conflicts are, however, a part of life—a source for change, adaptation, and creativity in the process of their resolution.

David Your own self case study, conducted when you were a graduate student in clinical psychology, is a convincing demonstration of how conflicts drive human development! I sense the positive attachment you have toward madness. You say madness becomes benign under the effects of spirituality. This is a critical point. But what does benign madness mean?

YF Elevated and expansive mood; hyperactive mental activity, flight of ideas, and racing thoughts; inflated self-esteem; and touches of grandiosity are all symptoms of madness I have experienced. So I know they can cause a great deal of trouble. They cannot be expunged from the mind, in the fashion of extirpating a tumor from the body. But they can be kept under control and rendered harmless.

It is important to distinguish between thoughts, words, and deeds in terms of impulse control. This is especially important when repression vanishes, as in my case, and access to the unconscious is unhindered. Impulses are harmless as long as they remain in the domain of thought. Nothing is unthinkable, for in themselves thoughts are innocent—a person cannot be found guilty for just having "bad" thoughts.

And when nothing is unthinkable, there is no boundary to creativity. However, not all impulses should be expressed in words, and even fewer should be in deeds. We may keep all our thoughts, be creative, and be all right, as long as we exercise adequate control over the expression of our impulses in words or in deeds. In this sense, madness may become benign.

Adequate control is not easy to achieve. People are always looking for shortcuts to Heaven. You bet technologies are already being developed, claiming to bring people closer to the dream of being able to erase unpleasant and unwanted memories from their minds selectively.

David A lot of people may think: Wouldn't it be wonderful if you can forget what you want to forget, simply by taking a wonder drug, like a "forgetfulness pill"? Remember the Christian image of Heaven: "No tears, no death, no sorrow, no crying, no pain—and no need for memory"?

YF No thanks. Such a pill, if available, may turn a dream into a nightmare. Every memory loss alters my identity, my being. What kind of a being would I be if I have only pleasant memories?

Unpleasant and unwanted memories are not to be extirpated, in the fashion of deleting junk files from a computer. Rather, they coexist with pleasant memories to define and enrich human nature. But we mustn't allow unpleasant memories to continue to do their destructive work. Healing is an essential part of any spiritual journey in which the past does not determine the present or future.

As spiritual forces prevail, unpleasant memories lose their destructiveness and madness becomes more benign. Eventfully, spirituality triumphs over madness, not so much by vanquishing it as by dissolving it into the total being of the person. When the ultimate goal of enlightenment is reached, destructive thoughts are extinct, and the mind is completely healed. Then, finally, madness is dissolved into the total being of the person, and can be found as a distinct part of it no longer. Such a goal draws us toward it like a magnet, even if it is beyond the reach of most of us. In this regard, I have had only limited success: experiencing moments of serenity, most ironically, during episodic madness. The success is less limited when spiritual forces augmented during madness carry into normal times.

David We have clarified the key issue of how spirituality may interact with madness, which goes to the core of what this book is about. Still, the reader would demand an answer to the question: Are you enlightened or mad? Everything we have discussed points to one conclusion: You are spiritual but not enlightened, at least not yet; you still have touches of madness, albeit quiescent during normality. So, the answer cannot be given in the form of an either/or statement.

YF I have to modify your conclusion. I have been mad, not just a few times: That's beyond debate. Enlightened? That's better for the reader to decide. We have more to say about this question in the Epilogue.

In Love with Madness

I may be self-transforming, but I can't say I have self-transformed. I have indeed done something I didn't have the courage to do before, such as giving the "impolite speech" at a graduation ceremony in Hypomania 4, and when I am normal I shall go on doing more things I have never done before. It is better to think of self-transformation as an ongoing process, not a terminal outcome—as part of a spiritual pilgrimage.

My entire journey is a dynamic process of constructing, deconstructing, and reconstructing meanings. In response to adverse life events, I make sense of what appears to be unfair or, worse, senseless. Even after 22 episodes, which are considerable, madness still appears alien to me. It should not be a part of my life. But it is, and I am compelled to face it. What can be more challenging than to make sense out of madness?

The constructed meaning: Madness is a welcome stranger, refreshing and joyous. She has brought me many gifts, extraordinary experiences never before experienced. Deconstructed, madness is a harbinger of many troubles. She gives me sleepless nights; she makes me plunge into a Black Hole, unsettle people around me and invite stigmatization. Reconstructed, madness is a companion in my journey, coexisting with spirituality. She can be rendered benign; furthermore, her creative energy can be harnessed to serve spiritual ends. Like being in love with life, even if mad? What greater force can there be?

> **David** I note a subtlety in your use of the pronoun *she*: Madness is female; she can be troublesome. She is also your spiritual companion and a source of creative energy. It's no wonder why you're so much in love with madness!?
>
> **YF** I'm not sure if my mind was conscious of such seductive, twisted logic. The word *she* just effused from my mouth.

Is there anything more lovable, yet troublesome, than the female in all of God's creation? She personifies both beauty and allure. The word *lunacy* reflects Western folklore that the Moon induces insanity. Most people think of the Moon, an object of fascination since time immemorial, as being female. And thus the feminine mystique is part of madness. I now better understand my state of mind when I wrote a poem on Chang E, the Chinese goddess of the Moon, on 29 April 2003.

Chang E

The *Mistress of the Moon* appears
To beguile mankind, in the guise
Of Chang E in the distant East.

She relays messages of amour
Across the heavenly expanse—to sow
The seeds of lunacy on earth.

She smiles like the crescent Moon.
Facing the Inferno, death by eclipse;
A moment passes, rebirth by light.

Behind the cloud she hides,
Invisible, almost—but for whom?
Enigma is her true name.

Daoists use female imageries extensively for cosmic and human fecundity. The Daoist philosopher Laozi is the first to enshrine the feminine mystique in words. In his *Classic of Virtue and the Dao* (see Ho, 2023, for an English translation and a psychological study), we find these lines:

> The Valley Spirit never dies.
> It is named the Mystic Female.
> The gateway of this Mystic Female
> Is the root from which Heaven and Earth (springs to life).

Daoist and Buddhist ideas have also inspired me to write this poem (15 Jan 2014).

Ode to Floral Beauties East and West

> What greater pride than the rose
> Has a flower ever possessed?
> What higher glory than your luxuriance
> Has a flower brought to its creator?
> What stronger passion than your sensuality
> Has a flower aroused
> In the man endowed to love?
>
> Enchanted, I swoon, I pluck, I bleed.
> The rose is a thorny lady indeed!
> Better to admire afar than to suffer
> The pain of possession.
>
> The lotus is as elegant
> As the rose is sultry.
> So shall I compare you not
> To a summer rose,
> But to the lotus of all seasons?
>
> The elements sustain your life:
> Rooted in mother Earth,
> You slumber in the season of Water,
> Only to blossom in the season of Fire,
> Then proudly stand your stalks upright in the Air.
> Your buds reach for the Sun,
> Your leaves shoot toward the sky.
> Each bud unfurls into a chalice
> And lets in glimpses

Of your exquisite beauty.

What other flower speaks
The language of enduring love?
Break your rhizome into halves we may,
Only to see lingering threads of silk
Connecting still the disconnected lovers.

In all the kingdoms of living things,
What other sorority surpasses
The Water Nymph of the West
And the Sacred Lotus of the East,
Each vying for attention, yet thriving
Together in the same amicable pond?

Discombobulated, the swains
Can't tell the beauties apart!
What greater folly can there be
Than a beauty contest, to judge
Who is the fairest of them all?
East is West, and West is East—
Beauty is peace; peace, beauty.

David   I can't but note that you used the name "Water Nymph," instead of "Water Lily." More poetic perhaps, especially when the flower names are capitalized to suggest impersonation. In abnormal psychology, the term *nymphomania* derives from the coinage of nymph and mania. . . ..

YF   Interesting, the Chinese equivalent is flower mania. The irony is that men enchanted by women may suffer from this condition more than women do!

David   Further evidence of your being in love with madness, discombobulated?

YF   Why not focus more on "Beauty is peace, peace beauty"? Remember the question I asked, "Where have all the flower babies [in mainland China] gone?" The fecundity of the Sacred Lotus brings it up again. The lotus flower produces a fruit in the shape of a shower head containing lotus seeds, which may be prepared for eating in many ways.

The sweetened lotus seeds prepared for the Chinese Lunar New Year, called *tanglianzi* (literally, sugar-lotus-seed), have an important symbolic meaning: *lian* (lotus) sounds close to *nian* (year) and *zi* may mean seed or son. So a lot of sweetened lotus seeds are consumed. Traditionally, one of the most common greetings exchanged is, *"Nian sheng guizi"*: In translation, "[May you be blessed with] a precious son each year." How about two boys in exchange for one girl in future if the outlandish disparity in the sex ratio (i.e., having many more boys than girls) among newborns continues in mainland China?

Poetry and Spirituality Drive Each Other

Bilingual proficiency is essential to bicultural competence, which is an asset of special importance to a world citizen. It would be instructive for me to say something about my bilingual experiences, including my flair for linguistic playfulness. Although I am a native speaker of Chinese (Cantonese), I have been using mostly English to express my thoughts in academic discourse. English has become my dominant language. What effect does that have on my cognition?

In a way, I have been permanently altered by the English language-tool I use. It has left its indelible mark on my cognition-being. Such is the awesome power of language-tools to transform their users. A frightful thought? Fear not. I now feel I have more than one tool at my disposal. Goethe goes further, "Those who know nothing of foreign languages know nothing of their own."

Can thinking transcend language? I think yes. Ultimately, any thought can be articulated in any language, in poetry or prose, in speech or writing, in logical-mathematical or ordinary language. I would include nonverbal language as well. The question is who is the master, the language-tool or its user? No trifling question, because I have seen language users enslaved by language-tools, especially among academics.

I would like to allude to a "linguistic experiment," which refers to experimenting with telegraphic styles of writing with relaxed grammatical constraints. It has nothing to do with shorthand text messaging with acronyms. I have been experimenting with constructing English sentences using Chinese grammar. Take, for instance, *I have not seen you for a long time* translates into *long time haven't seen*.

Typically, Chinese grammatical constructions take fewer words than English constructions. They satisfy a key principle of good writing, namely, economy of expression: The fewer the number of words, the better. Not a single word is superfluous, especially for poetry or poetic prose.

David Poetry is the ultimate mastery of the language-tool. You like to write poetry, mostly in a language not your own. Tell us something about your travail and delight.

YF My initial exposure to English poetry, in my first year in college, was utter bewilderment. Most of the time, I had little idea what the professor was talking about. But the sound of Chaucer's *Canterbury Tales* I heard for the first time got imprinted into my brain: It was pleasant to the ears, even when the connection between sound and meaning eluded my grasp. See, poetry is music in words.

Many years later, as a novice I visited websites for poets, aspiring and established. I even dared to submit a few of my poems for critique, one of which is reproduced here.

Virtual Realities

About my bedside the bright moonbeam spreads.
Surmise it is the frost upon the floor.
Lifting my head, I gaze at the bright moon;
Drooping my head, I long for my hometown.

Before my desktop images keep dancing.
They parody reality, and mock
Their maker, self-estranged. I ape these creatures,
So ill designed, and yearn for the real things.

The first verse is my translation of a famous poem by the Tang poet Li Bai (701–762 CE). The second echoes the first. This was my very first attempt to write a poem in pentameter. That took several months to complete, after what seemed to be endless experimentation. In the process, my head was filled with the sound, tempo, rhythm of words. I could be seen talking to myself while walking around. Never before had I consumed that much brain energy on a single task. The path to poetry led to lexicophilia, an incurable condition.

Critique was brutal. A seasoned poet, witness to how different versions of the poem evolved, had this to say about my "final" product: "I think the new version is metrical. Whether it's a decent poem or not is, however, a very different question."

One authority in English poetry who knew I was nonnative wrote, "Your inability to *hear* the modulating, shifting stress levels is just bringing you to grief." I should add that he also pours scorn on educators who believe in teaching self-esteem rather than grammar. He has a point. Devastated for a while, I continue to write poems and turn grief into joy.

David   Here you can see dialogic self-healing at work. Action *precedes* emotional change. The action is purposive, to meet a challenge head on. It has saved you from being devastated for good. I discern spiritual sentiments in many of your poems. Empathy advances when you rewrite the Golden Rule as "Do unto others as what *others* would have *you* do unto them." The spirit of ecumenism and world citizenship inheres in "East is West, and West is East: The world will be a better place." All these are ingredients of a spiritual journey.

YF I'm not sure if I have been conscious, especially in the beginning, of how much writing poetry has to do with our spiritual journey. I was simply too absorbed with learning and experimenting on how to do it. As time goes on, it becomes clear that the process is more important than the end product. I don't have to be an accomplished poet. I am well aware of my limitations. All I need is to delight in the delight of writing poetry that has enriched my spirituality.

David Poetry and spirituality drive each other: Poetry is a marvelous way to give spirituality concrete expression; spirituality opens the soul to poetic creation. To recapitulate, you have stated the conditions under which extraordinary experiences may be experienced safely: adequate impulse control and a healthy self. You find relief from your punitive superego through self-therapy, DAT in particular, and total relief from guilt and shame during madness. You have learned to forgive and be kinder to yourself. Given hope, you feel you shall prevail; you strengthen your psychological immunity when you view your life as a spiritual journey.

Above all, I have learned to harness, even if partially, the creative potential of madness in my spiritual development. The repression of artistic and literary impulses is no longer a hazard to my health. However, my journey has been one of spirituality-in-isolation, in which loneliness is a constant companion. This remains *the* problem I have to face.

6

In Search of Transcultural Spirituality-in-Commuion

Do unto others as others would have you do unto them.
—The Golden Rule restated.

Agency without communion is solitary individualism; communion without agency is but a plain life anchored in conformity.

The ideas on spirituality I have mentioned thus far derive largely from the West. Now I have to push myself to say more about how intellectual traditions from the East have informed my pilgrimage. In this chapter, my journey continues in search of spirituality-in-communion, while I share my karma with fellow spiritual travelers. I speak of my life in two worlds, the East and the West, and of being a world citizen. A creative synthesis embodies the best elements from both worlds. I now ask: In what ways can this creative synthesis enlighten a traveler taking a spiritual journey? But first, to speak of creative synthesis of the East and the West demands a better understanding of what each has to offer. Yet another glaring lacuna in our discourse is demanding to be filled, as the reader might have come to realize.

Insights from the East: Psychological Decentering

Selfhood and Identity

An East-West comparison of conceptions of selfhood and identity would help us grasp the idea of psychological decentering (see the extensive coverage of self psychology, especially selfhood and identity in Confucianism, Daoism, Buddhism, and Hinduism in *Rewriting Cultural Psychology: Transcend Your Ethnic Roots and Redefine Your Identity*).

Let me briefly characterize conceptions in the West. Of course, Western conceptions, as are the Eastern, are rich in diversity. Still, it is possible to distillate the core common to prevailing Western conceptions. What emerges is an individualistic self that is intensely aware of itself, its uniqueness, sense of direction, purpose, and volition. It is a center of awareness, at the core of the individual's psychological universe. The self is at center stage, and the world is perceived by and through it.

Self and nonself are sharply demarcated: The self is an entity distinct from other selves and all other entities. The self "belongs" to the individual and to no other person. The individual feels that he has complete and sole ownership of his self, which has an identity unique to the individual. The self is sovereign, or at least should have a sense of mastery, in its own household. Having a sense of personal control is essential to selfhood. In a healthy state, the self is stable over time; it is a coherent, integrated, and unitary whole. It is individual, not dividual. Rooted firmly in individualism, the Western self is in short the measure of all things.

In contrast, the Eastern self is not the measure of all things and is not at center stage. It is rooted in the relational character of human existence. Identity is defined relationally, in terms of the position that a person occupies in his social network. The self is not sovereign, but selfless and humble. Take a look at Chinese paintings, especially the Daoist-inspired, and you see the insignificance of the individual against the cosmic scale—in contrast to the dominant, triumphant individual in Western paintings, such as those by the Italian Renaissance artist Raphael.

These Eastern and Western conceptions form the dialectical tension for expanding our understanding of selfhood. I believe the formation of a healthy self is a precondition for the emergence of selflessness. To put it differently, the healthy self is the womb within which selflessness is nurtured. At the same time, selflessness makes the healthy self healthier. This is one playful way to arrive at a synthesis of East-West conceptions.

The Golden Rule, East and West

Eastern perspectives on communicating and relating cannot be characterized by anything short of psychological decentering. They suggest different approaches to decentering, a key to confront the problem of egoistic predicament and thus to rid oneself of prejudices. In Confucianism, the principle is to extend the consideration for oneself to the consideration for others, in the self-to-other direction; likewise, others are expected to extend their consideration to oneself, in the other-to-self direction. This I call the bidirectional principle of self-to-other and other-to-self reciprocity, or reciprocity for short. The Confucian Golden Rule states:

> The humane man, wishing to establish himself, seeks to establish others; wishing to be prominent himself, he helps others to be prominent. To be able to judge others by what is near to ourselves may be called the method of realizing humanity.

The negative form states: "Do not do to others what you would not want done to yourself."

Much like the Golden Rule in Judaism, as expressed by Hillel: "What is hateful to you, do not do to your neighbor." Reciprocity should be distinguished from empathy. In reciprocity, the consideration for others is based on the consideration for oneself. In empathy, it is based on a perception of others' consideration for themselves; the consideration for oneself is suspended. Reciprocity is an extension of one's own self-understanding to understand others. Empathy is understanding others through perceiving the self-understanding of others.

I'm afraid all these may sound awfully complicated. So let me try to relate our discussion to something we are all familiar with. The common English phrasing of the Golden Rule is: "Do unto others as you would have them do unto you." Let us simply rewrite it: "Do unto others as *others* would have *you* do unto them." This I did in the first poem I ever wrote, "Rewriting the Golden Rule" (Chapter 1). Thus rewritten, empathic understanding stands out.

David   An illustration from the art of giving and receiving, derived from your own experience, will make the momentous implications of this rewriting clearer.

YF   As a child, I used to collect postage stamps. My mother bought a collection as a gift for me. I pleaded with her not to do so, saying that I wanted to make my own collection and didn't want her to spend money on something I could collect for free. Moreover, at the time my family was poor, barely able to make ends meet, so I thought the money should have been better spent. The next thing I knew was that she bought me another collection. At that point, I was overcome with unhappiness.

What was going on? Did my mother follow the Golden Rule: "Do unto my son as I would have my son do unto me"? Not necessarily, because she might or might not be pleased if I spent money to buy her a gift. Her reaction would depend on many factors, the most important of which was most likely my heart behind the giving. She definitely did not follow "do unto my son as he would have me do undo him," because her son's pleading was ignored. In other words, she was not empathic in her act of giving. As I now ponder further, I have to ask myself: If my mother was lacking in the art of giving, did I do any better in the art of receiving? Empathy on the part of both parties, then, is the hallmark of a truly dialogic relationship.

This discussion on the art of giving and receiving has practical utility. Next time, on Valentine's Day, readers may want to rethink what makes a "perfect" gift. Roses, chocolates, or other common items that spin doctors of consumerism peddle? Or something, which may or may not be a material thing, that your partner deeply desires? A spiritual journey is like opening a box of delicious chocolates in various shapes and tastes from which the traveler can pick and choose. That's playful. So give your partner a box, and she, if seasoned in the art of receiving, will lure you to consume the chocolates together with her.

Break the rules, but not until you have mastered the grammar of life. The Golden Rule, in either the original or the restated version, cannot be followed unthinkingly. A fundamental problem in the original version is that what you want others to do to you may be unwanted by others. As regards the restated version, would you "do unto others as others would have you do unto them," if what others want you to do to them is destructive or self-destructive? The grammar of life cannot be reduced to simplistic rules.

George Bernard Shaw quips, "The golden rule is that there are no golden rules." Of course, he negates his golden rule by his own remark.

Selflessness in Philosophical Daoism and Buddhism

If the Confucian prescription for combating egoism is not radical enough the same cannot be said of other Eastern prescriptions. The concept of selflessness, common to Daoism and Buddhism, holds the key. To be selfless is to be decentered; to be decentered is an effective antidote to egoism, rigidity, cognitive conservatism, and the like. The decentered self attends to not only what others are thinking, but also what others are thinking about what the self itself is thinking. It is thus better prepared to form dialogical relationships, which are reciprocal and bidirectional.

To Zhuangzi, the sage "uses the eye to look at the eye," "has ears and eyes as images he perceives," and takes his stand "at the ultimate eye." The mind of the perfect person is like a mirror. The selfless, by seeing through all dichotomies, including self and other, is able to "mirror things as they are." Through his metaphors, "losing myself" and "forgetting everything," we may glimpse at the empty mind. Zhuangzi says, "Exercise fully what you have received from nature without any subjective viewpoint. In one word, be absolutely vacuous."

I know the more I become empathic, selfless, and empty of mind the better a listener-therapist I would become. To think of others as "I" comes as close to transcending egoism as it is humanly possible; it is the ultimate of empathy. To have "no self" is the ultimate of selflessness. To be "absolutely vacuous" is the ultimate of emptiness. These ultimate states of mind are beyond the normal range of human experience.

During my episodes of madness, however, empathy, selflessness, and emptiness came readily and enabled me to conduct some of the best classes and therapeutic sessions in my career. I now have an experiential grasp of the exotic states of being that Zhuangzi described. He would be pleased to know that his karma continues to have such a positive effect on human activity more than two thousand years after his death.

The discussion above implies that selflessness may manifest itself differently in normal versus extraordinary states of being or consciousness. In a normal state, selflessness is marked mainly by putting the interests of other people above one's own. In an extraordinary state, it is marked by experiencing "no self" (i.e., an absence of self), corresponding to the blurring of the self-other demarcation—in the extreme, to the disappearance of the distinction between self and nonself. I have used various terms such as *selfless self, selfless-oblivion, selfless-forgetfulness* to depict the manifestations of selflessness in extraordinary states.

Daoism as a Counterpoint to Confucianism

Daoism serves as a counterpoint to Confucian preoccupation with impulse control, social propriety, and status hierarchy, at the expense of personal sentiments and aspirations. It offers a path to spontaneity and personal liberation (Ho, 2023). To be decentered is to embark on a royal route toward liberating oneself from egoism, culturocentrism, and prejudices—toward empathic understanding and relating.

As I now look back on the journey of spiritual discoveries I have taken, philosophical Daoism has colored my development in many ways, particularly my relations with coworkers, my role as an educator, and my artistic fulfillment. Daoism fosters individuality and individual freedom. It is the Chinese counterculture. Not surprisingly, I am attracted to it, intellectually and temperamentally. Regrettably, Daoism has not received due attention from therapists or healers of the mind. Spontaneity and selflessness are two of its key concepts.

Daoists disdain the Confucian affinity for social convention, hierarchical organization, and governmental rule by the scholar class. For Daoists, the good life is the simple life, spontaneous, in harmony with nature, unencumbered by societal regulation, and free from the desire to achieve social ascendancy—in short, a life lived in accordance with the Dao. Thus Daoism champions spontaneity, freedom, and empathic understanding. These Daoist ideas play a significant role in developing our conception of relational and ecumenical spirituality. The sage acts without action and the ruler rules without governing. The intelligent person is like a little child.

To "return to my original face," as I wrote in my diary in the midst of Mania 2, expresses a similar thought. All things are relative yet identical because the Dao is unitary. Being and nonbeing produce each other; each derives its meaning from the coexistence of the other. That's dialectical thought.

Daoism disavows a hierarchical view of the self, society, or cosmos. Unlike Confucianism, Daoism does not regard the self as an extension of, and defined by, social relationships. Rather, the self is but one of the countless manifestations of the Dao. It is an extension of the cosmos. Laozi's *Classic of Virtue and the Dao* speaks of knowing others as being wise and of knowing one's self as being enlightened (Ho, 2023). That seems to imply a differentiation between self and others. Yet the sage has no fixed ideas and regards the people's ideas as his own. All my life I have struggled with the problem of getting rid of "fixed ideas." This problem is especially acute and difficult for professors. In madness, however, I find it easier to do.

Regarded as a mystic of unmatched brilliance in China, Zhuangzi explicitly negates the centrality of selfhood: "The perfect man has no self; the spiritual man has no achievement; the sage has no name." The ideal is thus selflessness.

Yet the selfless person is not without attributes: He becomes a sage in tranquility and a king in activity. The selfless person leads a balanced life, in harmony with both nature and society. In sum, Zhuangzi's conception of enlightenment entails conscious self-transformation leading to the embodiment of "sageliness within and kingliness without."

When selflessness is attained, the distinction between "I" and "other" disappears. One may then act with complete selfless spontaneity. The mind becomes

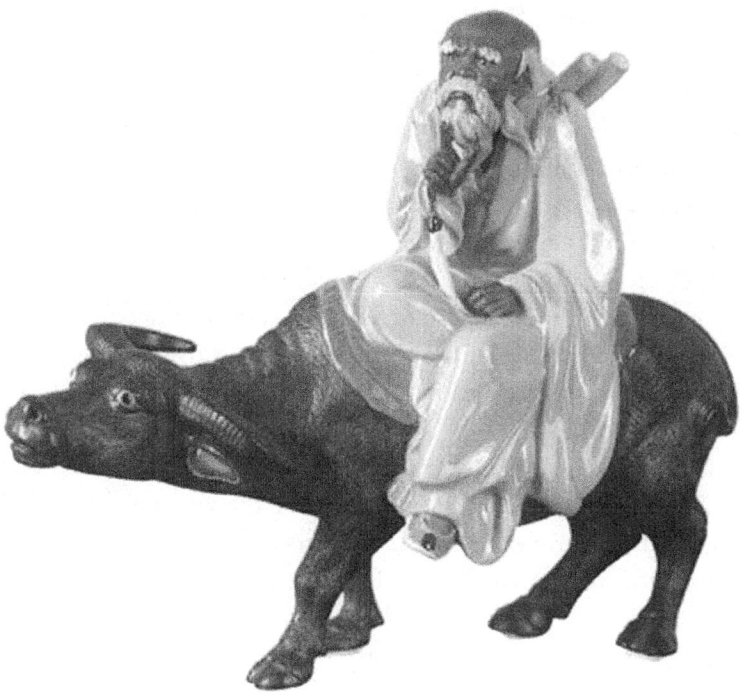

Figure 6.1. Laozi Riding a Buffalo

like a mirror, free from obstinacies and prejudices. Thus, one's thinking is to be liberated from not only external social constrictions but also internal psychological impediments. This idea of thought liberation, transcending one's egoism, occupies a central place in Zhuangzi's writings:

> To be impartial and nonpartisan; to be compliant and selfless; to be free from insistence and prejudice; to take things as they come; to be without worry or care; to accept all and mingle with all—these were some of the aspects of the system of the Dao among the ancients.. . .. Their fundamental idea was the equality of all things. They said: ". . .. The great Dao is all embracing, without making distinctions."

Here is a paradox indeed. Zhuangzi's assault on analysis ("making distinctions") reflects the power of his own analytic faculty. His idea of thought liberation is central to my pilgrimage. Again, in some important ways I am closer to his conception of enlightenment in madness than in normality: more spontaneous, more empathic, and more like a child.

Indigenous to China, Daoism has permeated the Chinese mind, despite the fact that most Chinese have never read the Daoist classics. Laozi's ideas such as *wuwei* (nonaction, not inaction) permeate the language of everyday life. *Wuwei* means avoiding actions that go against the Dao of nature. The Dao of swimming comes to mind as an illustrative example of *wuwei*: Swim *with* the water, not against it; regard it as your partner, not something to be afraid of. I acquire a physical understanding of *wuwei* when I practice Taiji push-hands.

Daoism fosters psychological decentering and egalitarianism. Psychological decentering is implied in the notion of selflessness, the distinction between I and other being absent; it follows naturally from the perspective that the individual is humbled in the cosmic scale of things. Egalitarianism is embodied in the idea of "the equality of all things."

To me, of particular significance is that the relation between women and men is not hierarchical but complementary, like the yin and the yang. Female imagery is used extensively for cosmic and personal creativity. This is especially remarkable in the patriarchal context of Confucian societies.

The Buddhist Path to Enlightenment

The concept of selflessness lies at the core of Daoism. In this regard, Daoism parallels Buddhism. The Buddhist renunciation of selfhood aims to destroy the mother of all illusions. Because the illusion of selfhood is the root of egoism, overcoming it brings forth insight into the true nature of things. Like Zhuangzi, Buddhists use the mirror as a symbol of the mind purified of prejudices.

In Buddhist thought, the state of enlightenment is nirvana (literally, "blowing out," as of a lamp), achieved through moral-intellectual perfection only after strenuous personal effort. It is a state of absolute, eternal quiescence—a transcendent state of supreme equanimity. It is decidedly a state of being, not a literal place. Nirvana is beyond the comprehension of ordinary persons unawakened from the illusion of phenomenal life. "Only a Buddha knows a Buddha": This would preclude me from knowing what Buddhahood or nirvana is like.

Buddhism provides a prescription for enlightenment: Self-renunciation holds the key to salvation. Because life is viewed as intrinsically futile, the goal is deliverance from the self, not from worldly sufferings that have arisen from social conditions. The ideal to be attained, nirvana, is a state of transcendence devoid of self-reference. Buddhism has worked out an elaborate system of practice to enable one to attain transcendence.

Meditation is an instrumentality central to this system. In a state of transcendent consciousness, the subject-object distinction disappears. Cognition is suspended; the self is absent. As claimed by both Buddhists and Hindus, the transcendent state, being transcognitive and hence free from prejudices, enables one to attain higher, even "perfect" knowledge.

The Buddhist path to salvation prescribes ridding oneself of passions and desires, including in particular one's attachment to life. It is based on a total nonattachment from not only worldly objects but also the ego itself. In the language of psychoanalysis, such decathexis is the antithesis of hypercathexis, the profuse and excessive investment of libidinal energy in objects. I experienced hypercathexis during madness: I erotized myself, other people, and the world. From a psychological perspective, nirvana is the antithesis of mania.

Nirvana differs from the Christian or Islamic concept of heaven in one crucial respect: Heaven opens its door to the faithful; nirvana is beyond the reach of most of us. Buddhas are rare in number, as are prophets and saints. They are the few who are willing and able to renounce worldly pleasures and make the supreme effort toward moral-intellectual perfection—the goal of enlightenment.

Humbly, I feel that nirvana is just beyond my reach. However, I find the idea of karma most relevant and useful to my spiritual journey because of three implications. First, karma places responsibility squarely on me for my actions and their consequences. Second, my karma affects the lives of others and is affected by the karma of others; in a sense then, my spiritual journey is linked to those of others, and other people's journeys are linked to mine. My journey is not an individualistic undertaking! This understanding prepares me for developing the idea of spirituality-in-communion. Third, karmic effects have temporal extensions into the future, beyond my individual life.

The Buddhist view may be explained with an analogy. When nirvana is reached, primal ignorance is extinct, as is the causation for the cycle of births and rebirths. An individual candle, when consumed, ceases to be. Yet the light it produced may be transferred to other candles; its "life" continues. A person dies and is truly gone; there remains only the cumulated result of all his words and actions—the karma that will continue to work out its effects on the lives of other sentient beings. Thus, transmigration is really a transfer of karma, not of any individual soul. Reincarnation is really metamorphosis, not metempsychosis: Birth is new birth, not rebirth.

In all, the implications of psychological decentering for spiritual development are enormous. The treasures embodied in the intellectual traditions of the East, particularly Daoism and Buddhism, have pivotal significance for a contemporary understanding of one's place in the world and one's journey through life. They have given me insights on how to develop the Multidimensional Assessment of Spirituality (see Appendix A)

Ambivalence Toward Christianity

I now turn to examine the role that religion plays in my journey of spiritual discoveries. For two millennia, discourse in the philosophy of religion has been dominated by the theocentric traditions of the West: There is one and only one God, omnipotent, omniscient, omnipresent, and everlasting.

The best-known anti-theistic philosophers in the nineteenth century are Karl Marx and Friedrich Nietzsche. To Marx, religion is the sigh of the oppressed creature, the heart of a heartless world, and the soul of soulless conditions. It is the opium of the people, living under the conditions of class exploitation. Nietzsche proclaimed that the last Christian died on the cross. "God is dead" is a truly revolutionary utterance, for a created being to proclaim that his creator is dead.

But it is not until the 20th century that Western philosophers commonly write philosophy without so much as raising questions about God. The more I learn about comparative religion, the more I become aware of the gulf of difference between the monotheistic religions of the West (Judaism, Christianity, and Islam) and the religious traditions of the East.

Brought up as a Christian, I have, however, strong ambivalence toward Christianity. On theological grounds, I doubt the doctrines of original sin, Trinity, Immaculate Conception, Resurrection, Ascension; I have antipathies toward the conception of Hell as everlasting punishment, the negation of the flesh, the Catholic dogma of Papal Infallibility, and so forth. On social grounds, I object to a good many of Christian teachings, such as the opposition to birth control by the Catholic Church, which has dire consequences for the quality of life in many countries, especially the poor.

That's one reason why my journey is not a religious but a spiritual one. But is religion irrelevant to my journey? No. None of the negatives I mentioned seem to have extinguished my strange attraction toward Christianity. It has become an inextricable part of my being. I sense that deep down I am attracted to religion like the earth is to the sun. This strange attraction, which survives countless intellectual questioning, informs me that I must look deeper into the role that religion plays in my journey.

An excursion into my religious history is both necessary and informative. Like other Christian children, I went to Sunday school. The status-conscious behavior of adults in the church put me off; I felt they were hypocrites. To a child, the triangular Methodist church building was huge. Decades later, the building still stands in the same location in Hong Kong; however, to the same child now grown into an adult, it has shrunken in size. Symbolically, as an institution, the church has diminished too.

In the Jesuit school I attended in Hong Kong, religious education consisted mostly of reciting catechisms. That set the stage for my anti-Catholic stance for years. One of my favorite intellectual pastimes was to fire an array of salvos to attack Catholic tenets and push their defenders up against the wall. I would catalog historical embarrassments of the church: the Inquisition, the persecution of Galileo, the compilation of the *Index Librorum Prohibitorum* (Index of Forbidden Books, which includes works of almost every Western philosopher).

Once, at the age of 18, I engaged a priest in conversation while traveling by bus from Ottawa to Montreal in Canada. Before arrival, the priest said something to this effect: "I've held Catholic beliefs all my life. They are basic to my priesthood. My world would collapse if these beliefs are not founded." Sensing the gravity of the situation, I then kept quiet.

When I was a graduate student, I met a priest studying for his PhD in theoretical physics at the University of Chicago. He was obviously an intellect to be reckoned with. One day we engaged in a dialogue on sexuality and sin.

David	According to the Catholic Church, masturbation is a cardinal sin. Why?
Priest	Because in general deriving sexual pleasure outside the context of procreation is sinful.
David	This would include deriving pleasurable sensations from the body, if the act is unconnected with procreation.
Priest	Yes.
David	I have an itch. I scratch it. It relieves me of the itch, and thereby gives me a pleasurable sensation. Is the scratching a sinful act?
Priest	That's a difficult question to answer.

Why the focus on masturbation? While attending a Jesuit school, drummed into my mind was that it is a cardinal (as distinct from a venial) sin, the punishment for which is everlasting hellfire. Because of this, I suffered greatly from conflicts over masturbation during my teenage years, as recounted in Chapter 1.

In actuality, the priest respected the question. I waited in vain for an answer. He was thoroughly imbued with the antisex theology of St. Paul, St. Jerome, and

St. Augustine. The body is as low, filthy, inferior as the soul is high, pure, superior. The lusts of the flesh, prompted by the temptations of the Devil, are locked in eternal battle with the ways of the spirit, supported by the grace of God, within the divided self.

The idea that the body is a hindrance to spirituality is antithetical to holism. In my conception, interconnectedness of the body-mind-spirit as a holistic unit is the ideal, not the triumph of the spirit over the body. In Hypomania 6, it was a physical breakthrough (achieving upright posture after years of hunch back) that led to developments in the psychological and spiritual realms (artistic self-expression and heightened esthetic sensibilities).

Nonetheless, Catholicism has a strong appeal deep inside my psyche, I confess. Such is the allure of religious certainty. My visits to the Basilica of Saint Peter in the Vatican invariably arouse religious sentiments. Upon seeing the *Pietà* by Michelangelo or listening to J.S. Bach, strong emotions of pathos would ensue. Great art and music intertwined with religion. But are those religious sentiments purely religious?

Having received my PhD, I went for my very first interview for a full-time job in a Baptist college in the United States. The interview with the dean of the college went something like this.

Dean   Dr. Ho, you want to teach psychology. Our college has certain fundamental Christian beliefs, which may conflict with those of psychology. For example, Skinner says that man is not much more than a dog. Would you have trouble with this?

Dr. Ho   Man is much more than a dog. He has the capacity to alter the environment and, in doing so, shapes his own behavior. This capacity is human. Dogs don't have it.

Dean   Dr. Ho, you are well qualified. However, there are morals, more important than qualifications.

Dr. Ho   Of course. Would you please enlighten me on what morals you are referring to?

Dean   We had a faculty member, very well qualified academically. But you know what he did? He ran away with the wife of one of our faculty members. Now, Dr. Ho, would you have any difficulty in this realm?

Dr. Ho   Honestly, I can't answer your question. I haven't seen the wives yet.

The interview terminated at that point. Needless to say, I didn't get a chance to lay eyes on any of the wives. Did I really have the guts to say that? Sorry, the reader will have to make his own judgment.

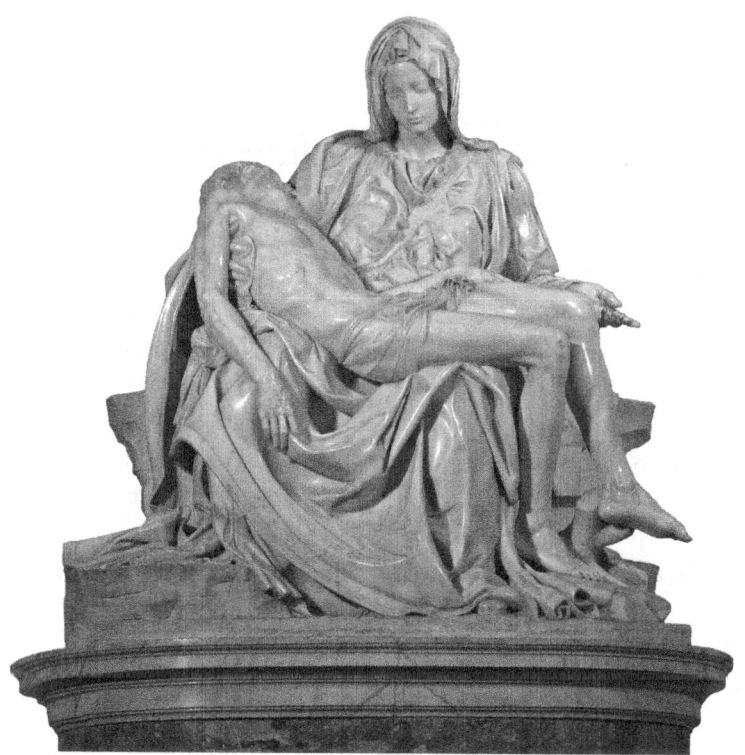

Figure 6.2. Michelangelo's *Pietà*

In Mania 1, I experienced the near-despair of trying to fathom the infinite with a finite mind; the more I knew, the more I became aware of my profound ignorance. I was simply repeating what countless pioneers of spirituality, much wiser than I, have gone through. Reason alone leads to a dead end in a spiritual journey. However, relying on faith *before* reason has exhausted itself is blind faith, which can be outright perilous.

It is the lazy man's cop-out. Ultimately, questions about faith and reason have no answer. Love, beyond faith and reason, is all I know. Why is this beyond the comprehension of so many who profess Christian love?

It was also in Mania 1 that I had hallucinatory visions of seeing myself being nailed on a cross and having intense feelings of pathos for the sufferings of humankind. I felt what Jesus must have felt. Christianity runs deep in my psyche. Am I perhaps more Christian than I dare to admit? I feel real ambivalence. This just about sums up what my religiosity is: I am a Catholic when I enter Saint

Peter's Basilica, an agnostic when I reason, and a Buddhist when I don't think about anything at all.

Spirituality-in-Communion or Spirituality-in-Isolation?

The East and the West appear to resonate in current conceptions of understanding and relating with others. In the East, conceptions grounded in a worldview that stresses the relational character of human existence have always been dominant. In the West, there is growing awareness of the tension between two conceptions of selfhood in terms of self-other relationships: The first, rooted in individualism, is primacy of the autonomous self, through which the world is perceived and understanding is achieved; the second is the dialogic self, to which engagement in self-other dialogues is fundamental. Long eclipsed by the individualistic, the relational conception is now demanding to be heard.

The individualistic and the relational conceptions parallel two fundamental modalities of being, agency and communion. Agency is an autonomous modality, wherein the will to mastery is supreme; it is manifest in actions such as self-protection, self-assertion, self-expansion, self-control, and self-direction: "I am in charge of my own life."

Communion is a relational modality, wherein the sense of being at one with others defines meaning; it is manifest in communal actions like participation, cooperation, attachment, and engagement in dialogues. Agency is accompanied by separation, isolation, aloneness, and alienation; communion by togetherness and union.

Balance between agency and communion is the hallmark of a healthy life. Freedom is achieved through agency; security is obtained through communion. In unison, agency and communion promise a life both free and secure. However, agency without communion is solitary individualism; the life it offers is that of the polar bear, free to roam alone in the desolate cold. Communion without agency has no character; it offers a plain life of security anchored in boring conformity, the extreme of which is like a swarm of bees in a hive.

Agency and communion do not merely coexist; rather, each relies on the other to thrive. Agency may be achieved through communion, as when the agent chooses to surrender aspects of personal freedom for the collective good, and to become more selfless in maintaining solidarity with others. Communion may be realized via agency, in an open and tolerant society that encourages plurality.

Ah, my life has been imbalanced, hence unhealthy, according to what I have just written down: too much agency, not enough communion. My journey of spiritual discoveries has been primarily "personal." It makes a mockery of my claim of being a world citizen: Devoid of fellowship or communion, being a world citizen would be hollow isolation wherever you go, across national, ethnic, or cultural boundaries.

This realization prompts me to take communal actions. But it is difficult. Groups that offer communion are mostly religious and institutional, and I have always kept distance from religious institutions on intellectual grounds. I have religious sentiments, but I find it difficult to accept the fundamental beliefs of theistic religions. But is religion irrelevant to my spiritual journey? This is a pointed question that demands an answer. There is simply no way to escape it.

I have a secret envy of religious folks who have communion. The life of a lonely soul in search of spirituality is heavy. Like fighting a lonely battle, it requires great stamina. There are times when I simply feel tired, emotionally if not intellectually, lacking the strength to go on. Could I not derive more strength in the company of religious folks? That is a comforting thought. But I cannot pretend to be what I am not.

Quakers and Unitarian Universalists

To find a spiritual home, I searched the Internet for the Religious Society of Friends, the Quakers. (Both names appeal to me. The word *Friends* resonates with the second character *Yau*, which means friend, of my Chinese name, Ho Yau Fai; Quakers conjure up imageries of self-expression with abandon, like dancing in a state of Dynamic Relaxation and Meditation. So, there is a predestined affinity.)

Why Quakers? To me, Quakers hold a mysterious attraction: They are deliciously odd. My first encounter with Quakerism took place in Hyde Park in Chicago, back in my student days. I participated in protests against the war in Vietnam, resulting in my being arrested and thrown in jail on one occasion (as recounted in Chapter 1). Quakers are pacifists. So, a natural alliance is formed out of our common antiwar stance.

I attended a Quaker meeting and was initiated into an unusual experience of religious communion. People sat around in a room, quiet, meditative, contemplative. Then a few stood up and spoke, one by one. The words they uttered came from deep within, enlightened and enlightening. No sermon, sacrament, or scripture reading. The meeting engraved an indelible impression into my mind. (As I learned later, this form of worship is "unprogrammed." Another form is programmed or semi-programmed, which resembles the worship practices of other Protestants.) So, my attendance at Quaker meetings in Southern California is a broken continuation of the one I attended in Chicago decades ago. Evidence of predestined affinity?

The core belief of Quakerism is a statement of ecumenicity: There is an indwelling Light within *all* persons. God is directly accessible to all persons without the need of an intermediary priest or ritual. Quakerism rejects, therefore, ecclesiastical authority and "empty forms" of worship (e.g., set prayers, words, rituals).

Going to a Quaker meeting is an inspirational experience in organization behavior, in which I have great interest as a psychologist. Immediately noticeable is a total absence of hierarchical authority. For instance, there are no chairpersons, but "clerks." The gathering appears to be a leaderless group. Nobody issues edicts. Everybody has a place and a voice, to be heard and respected.

The Quaker way of conducting a business meeting is "notorious" for the length of time that may be required for decisions to be reached. Decisions are not made by majority rule. The presiding clerk, guided by the Light, helps the meeting to search for truth and unity. Strongly opposing views are often reconciled through suggestion of a Third Way (dialectics?); quietly resolved in a period of silent worship; or deferred to a later meeting. No vote is taken. When unity is reached, the clerk states "the sense of the meeting"; approval is voiced or apparent, and the minute is recorded.

My past experience with leaderless groups is that they often degenerate into perennial chaos. Not so with the Quaker communion. Things seem to get done! Individual members share a common purpose, manifest in their personal conduct and performance of tasks. They are not externally driven but internally guided. The common purpose they share is not common at all, but a higher purpose imbued with spirituality. This is communion indeed. If Quakerism is so attractive, why don't I become one? I have two reservations.

The first is that I have difficulty accepting some of the fundamentals of Christianity (e.g., the divinity of Jesus), even though I embrace the Christian idea of love. The second concerns Quaker pacifism. I have long been antiwar. During the Cuban crisis in 1962, I wrote to a friend, "I am both nervous and depressed about the present [crisis]. . . when the threat of total extinction by self-destruction is so imminent. Therefore, I have decided, after years of consideration, to dedicate my life to peace." But I am not a pacifist totally, because I hold that there are conditions under which armed struggle (e.g., against tyrannical oppression, ethnic cleansing, genocide) is justified.

Can I still be a Quaker, despite the two reservations? This was the question I put to one of the Quaker "elders." His answer was a definite yes. It put my mind at ease. So I am still treading the Quaker path, learning humbly as I go along. At a Quaker meeting, I was asked to participate in a talent show. I obliged and gave a report on the following imaginary dialogue.

When a Buddhist Meets a Quaker

The lack of talent is no sin, and sin is not a word that Quakers use. So, here I am. This afternoon, I heard a "privileged" conversation between a Buddhist and a Quaker, which I would like to share with you.

Buddhist You meditate. You love to make peace. You want to conserve the gifts of mother earth. You stress the unity of words and deeds. You respect the views and beliefs of others. You are maximally inclusive, not exclusive. You affirm the intrinsic worth of each person. Above all, you believe that Buddha nature lies within each and, therefore, interpersonal encounters are an avenue to enlightenment. Now, a creature that waddles like a duck, thinks like a duck, and talks like a duck is a duck—according to Leibniz's Law of Identity of Indiscernibles. So, I say to you, "You are a Buddhist reincarnate in the guise of a Quaker."
Quaker Quack, quack, quack. But I don't sit cross-legged.
Buddhist I don't quake. That doesn't make me a lesser Quaker than you are.

Buddhism and Quakerism share much in common, such as pacifism, compassion, and universal acceptance of all human beings. Unitarian Universalists neither quake nor sit cross-legged. Yet they shine no less brightly. One visit to Tapestry, a Unitarian Universalist congregation, was enough to convince me that I had found a communion of kindred souls. I can't think of a better name than Tapestry. Here are the seven principles that members of Unitarian Universalist Association of Congregations affirm and promote.

1. The inherent worth and dignity of every person.
2. Justice, equity, and compassion in human relations.
3. Acceptance of one another and encouragement to spiritual growth in our congregations.
4. A free and responsible search for truth and meaning.

5. The right of conscience and the use of democratic process within our congregations and in society at large.
6. The goal of world community with peace, liberty, and justice for all.
7. Respect for the interdependent web of all existence of which we are a part.

When I read these for the first time, I was hit by a sense of amazement. I agree with all the principles completely! They are ecumenical, humanistic, and action-oriented. They encompass timeless, transcultural values, and no dogma. Spirituality-in-communion leaps out from the principles. Words like *religion*, *bible*, and *God* do not even appear. Yet going to the congregation is like attending a Christian church, complete with a sermon, singing of hymns, blessing, and "exchange of gifts" (donation).

Again, the theme of being different emerges in my consciousness. Like Quakers, Unitarian Universalists are small in numbers. Small is beautiful; so is atypicality. Why am I not only atypical but also attracted to the atypical? This is a question I ask myself countless times. Jean-Paul Sartre says that man is condemned to be free. In my case, I am condemned to being different in addition. So be it. As I learned to turn my marginal status into strength a long time ago, so will I learn to truly accept my being different.

Besides, being in the company of the different removes the discomfort of being different. Already, I feel less lonely. I feel I have found, for the first time, a spiritual home. I am no longer a religious refugee. Such is the strength of communion. Like a field of forces, it magnifies the *qi* (energy) within and between persons, resulting in a greater *qi* in the whole of the communion than in the sum of its parts.

A Religious Experience

Toward the end of Chapter 2, I mentioned a transformative religious experience I had in the midst of Hypomania 8. In March 2010, I sent "The Meaning of Easter" to the minister at Tapestry, hoping that it would be shared with members of the congregation. He asked me to read the piece during the service on Easter Sunday.

The Meaning of Easter

Good Friday commemorates the crucifixion of Jesus; Easter commemorates his resurrection. That much we all know. But, in a broader sense, Easter is a time to celebrate the creative power of women. The egg is symbolic of new life.

The Easter egg, in particular, is a symbol of the resurrection of Jesus. It has pagan roots in celebrations of spring, in which the egg represents rebirth of the land. Isn't the creative power of women, then, the secret meaning behind the Easter egg? Easter evokes the eternal pathos of motherhood. Mary gave birth to Jesus, suckled him, rocked him to sleep, and cradled him in her arms; she witnessed her son's scourging, humiliation, and excruciating pain of dying slowly on the cross—while his male disciples have fled in fear. She was a universal Mater Dolorosa.

Resurrection and Ascension are beyond the range of human experience. They are of abstract theological significance: Only when captured in art and music is their triumphant spirit given concrete expression. But Crucifixion is no stranger to human experience. Even thinking about it evokes physical reactions in us. It represents man's inhumanity to man. Easter is time, therefore, to commiserate with the suffering of humankind caused by the actions of humankind. Good Friday is good for a cause.

Before his last breath, Jesus said, "Father, forgive them; for they know not what they do." Friedrich Nietzsche proclaimed that the last Christian died on the cross. He contradicted himself, for he was Christian when he said, "In forgiving and forgetting, things that have happened can be undone." In truth, however, what has been done cannot be undone. Forgetting is neither necessary nor even desirable for magnanimous acts of forgiving. It makes us oblivious to the lessons of history. And, as George Santayana said, "Those who ignore history are condemned to repeat it."

Not even in my wildest dreams had I thought I would be so honored in a religious-spiritual assembly. I complied. But I was still not well enough to drive, so someone from the congregation drove me there. I did the reading, loud and bold. Unexpectedly, I was overwhelmed with emotion. Halfway through, tears began to flow uncontrollably (probably invisible to most of the people present). I might not have been able to complete the reading had there been another paragraph.

The reading was well received. What was remarkable was that, perhaps for the first time in my life, I felt total liberation from egoism. I was concerned not with how well I performed, but with how effectively my message was delivered; attention was focused on the audience, not on me. I felt an inner peace. I experienced authenticity: Emotion and intellect were synergized; I meant every word I uttered. I had the courage to be myself, sensitive, thoughtful, good-natured—displayed in public, unabashedly.

I have rediscovered myself, my original nature that had been buried deep in mundane life. If so, is there a further point to the search for spirituality? Or for enlightenment? Perhaps whatever I have been searching for is not something out there, faraway. Rather, at least a part of it is already here, within my being. I now have a deeper understanding of what it means to "return to my original face."

Later, I described my experience to the minister. He immediately remarked that it was like a religious experience. Courage is central to spirituality, and this is no time to hide my true self, he said. How I wish I could hear such words of affirmation and encouragement more often. The question now is if and how my courage-to-be will be sustained, infused into my life as a world citizen, and expressed through ethical-prosocial actions in the years ahead.

In a sense, all of my adult life has been a preparation for the occasion. At home with being both Chinese and American, creative synthesis, hopefulness, generativity, and a host of other ideas exude from my mind. These are ideas that have given me encouragement and guidance in my spiritual journey. Now I am a witness to their concrete expressions.

7 | Epilogue. I'm Getting There

Let my karma continue to work out its effects on the reader.

The Dao is simplicity itself: to delight in the ordinary things of everyday life, interacting with people, just being alive.

At this point, the reader may wonder, "More opportunities to stride forward to approach enlightenment? That means that you are going to have more episodes." Right on. In what follows, I describe the continuation of my spiritual journey. In Chapter 2, I raised the question, "Since 2005, at least one episode has occurred each year. How long will this last?"

I have now more information to answer your question: My madness has extended into 2021. If the past is a guide, my madness may last indefinitely. So, my episodic madness has become not just predictable, but predictably predictable.

But the reader may sense that, for two reasons, I have a strange calmness in the face of this predicament. First, I have long accepted madness as a part of my life. Second, I see madness as an opportunity for approaching enlightenment, not as something to be feared.

Back to the Original Question

Finally, I am reminded of a central question concerning my quest for spirituality: Has madness led me to enlightenment? By now, the reader should have his answer. And I have my own, not a simple one: Madness has energized my spiritual quest; in this sense, madness has enlightened me.

But I don't have the audacity to claim, and I haven't claimed, to have *reached* enlightenment. Stopping for a moment to survey my present condition, I am humbled by how much I fall short of spiritual fulfillment. Enlightenment, I feel, may be beyond my reach, at least when I am normal.

Have I failed? This question is problematic, and is not a productive way to frame what a spiritual journey is about. A spiritual journey is an ongoing process of development and growth; it has value in itself, regardless of outcomes. Viewed in this light, the idea of a final destination is in itself misleading. After all, the Dao is simplicity itself: to delight in the ordinary things of everyday life, interacting with people, just being alive. Positive forces simply overwhelm negative emotions by their sheer attractiveness.

The word is *delight*. I now know the direction to go. Without the benefit of firsthand experiences, I wouldn't have been able to say all these things about the interaction between spiritual forces and madness. I have good reasons, therefore, to see my encounters with madness as a blessing. A different question is, if given a choice, would I rather be free of madness for a life of greater comfort? Again, the reader should know the answer.

I sense heavy responsibility as I write. I aspire to inform, entertain, and inspire the reader. I assume authorial responsibility to be accurate on factual and historical matters. I adhere to the first principle of healthcare professionals, "Do no harm."

Why? Because spirituality is potentially a dangerous idea that can be abused and mislead people into wayward paths or to evil cults. I thus caution myself not to mislead, and to treat spirituality with the dignity it demands. I shudder when I hear people say with a nonchalant air, "Sex is a spiritual experience." Spirituality is indeed an overused and much-abused word.

Cognizant of the many disparaging remarks I have made about psychiatry, I must also expunge from the mind of the reader any possible misunderstanding that it is of no use whatsoever. Being inadequate or incomplete is not the same as being useless. So seeking psychiatric help may be warranted, even necessary, if and when you have a mental disorder.

To bridge different domains of learning, East-West and psychology-spirituality, is demanding; to relate personal and universal experiences is doubly so; to bridge and relate in a way that makes the whole story relevant and meaningful to the reader is even more so. No wonder I find writing this book a challenging journey within a journey, humbling yet fulfilling.

One particular issue in serving as a bridge in East-West learning stands out. The Western tendency is to conceive of spirituality in terms of personal development and growth. The individual self is affirmed, leading to greater autonomy, self-esteem, and self-mastery. These ideas I accept.

Yet, informed by Eastern ideas of the selfless self, more and more I see my spiritual journey as a movement away from the individual self to a self-in-relations (with others, nature, and the cosmos). In particular, I see liberation from egoism as central to this journey.

Is there a contradiction between the Eastern and the Western approaches to spirituality? No. Again, creative synthesis works best. We can embrace both the Western affirmation of the self and the Eastern ideas of the selfless self.

I would go as far as to say that achieving the selfless self requires a healthy, integrated individual self to begin with; and that selflessness enhances the health of the individual self. Further, a healthy self is one that is necessarily engaged with others, being in the world. Therefore, embark not on a journey of spirituality-in-isolation, but of spirituality-in-communion.

Sharing My Karma with Fellow Travelers

The thought that this book is ultimate self-disclosure is unsettling, especially to an author who is not inclined to self-disclose. For a while, I struggled with whether writing this book was a good idea. In the end, the decision to proceed won the day, motivated by the purpose to share my karma with fellow spiritual travelers. Nothing is more gratifying to an author than to find his work useful to readers.

Karma is an abstract idea that comes to life in the concrete. Most recently, I found one such concrete expression of karma in a chance encounter with a young woman who came from Hong Kong to Southern California, where I am now living, to attend a wedding. After a brief mutual introduction, I discovered that she is now working in the center at the University of Hong Kong, where I worked during my golden age. Whereupon, she blurted out, "Are you that legendary professor?"

Central to the purpose of being useful is to normalize abnormality as an integral part of human experience, something not to be ashamed of. Abnormality or madness may be kept under control, rendered harmless, and even harnessed to add color to life.

1. Madness is not that horrible and not all bad: You may learn to master it, even to harness its creative energy to advance your spiritual development.
2. The self-creative self: You have the potential to transform, even create your own self.
3. Spirituality-in-communion: Your journey in search of spirituality does not have to be lonely; look for kindred souls as fellow travelers.
4. Enlightenment is the acme of attraction (unavoidably, an understatement): Like a magnet, it draws you toward it, even if it is beyond the reach of most of us. Don't feel you have failed if your journey has not brought you there. The search for spiritual fulfillment is rewarding in itself. It can be a playful, joyous process in which you find delight in daily living.
5. Beware of the perils of spiritual emptiness resulting from inaction, from being lukewarm or noncommittal: estrangement, meaninglessness, and burnout.

If an author says, "I don't want to brag about my own work, because bragging goes against the spirit of humility in which I try to lead my life," is he nonetheless bragging? I will, therefore, neither brag nor self-efface. What I can say is that, speaking from personal experience, I have derived much comfort from the ideas I have written about. Among these are the powerful ideas of love and hope that can draw people out of despondency and energize them to proceed with their journey.

The Art of Loving for All Seasons

For all seasons? In all cultures? Grandiose, isn't it? Nevertheless, my message about love reaffirms the universality of humankind, and counters the excesses of "multiculturalism" now in vogue in the Western world. Some truths about the art of loving are eternal and culture-transcendent. But who has the audacity to proclaim what they are? At the risk of going beyond myself, I offer a distillate of some insights.

1. Only when the self forgets itself can total communion with another be achieved.
2. Do you have someone around whom you feel free to hit or scold (lovingly, that is), and who feels no less free to return in kind? You are blessed if you do.
3. Love presupposes the need to forbear devastating disappointments as part of life. It comes naturally when you are no longer obsessed with pursuing it.
4. Blessed is the person who finds the greatest joy in making others happy.
5. Blessed is the couple for both of whom the inner and the outer selves are one.

Love is indeed quintessential to any spiritual journey. Now, if only you and I put into practice the art of loving that has just been articulated. . ... Here, an additional word of encouragement is fitting.

Blessed are fellow travelers in our spiritual journey. You may not feel loved, but you will love others, so they may love more.

You may be near exhaustion, but you will not give up. You may be defeated for now, but you hold your heads high with dignity. You may be in turmoil, but you will continue to search for direction. You don't yet see your destination, but you are about to see the light of dawn.

My personal journey is incomplete. I can't help feeling a deep sense of humility, in the face of my many failures and the difficulties ahead. I have a long way to go. In fact, the longer the better, for the end of the journey is also the end of life *as we know it*.

Gone, but not gone.
I will be here,
Here with you.
My karma will continue
To work out its effects,
Through this book,
On sentient beings,
Of which you are one.

If that be the case, then this book will have served its intended purpose.

Part II
Transcending the Clash of Opposites

Embodied within the sickness of each individual is a microcosm of the sickness of his society and culture.

Thematic Grouping of Chapters

The chapters in Part II are categorized into four thematic groups: Normality versus Abnormality, Individual versus Collective Madness, Eastern versus Western Culture, and Spirituality versus Spiritual Emptiness. Here, I must make clear that the use of the word *versus* may be misleading from a dialectical standpoint. In terms of logic, each of the pairs of opposites may be construed as inclusive disjuncts (X or Y, or both X and Y), not as exclusive disjuncts (X or Y, but not both X and Y). This implies that the four opposite pairs may coexist. Thinking further, the use of the word *clash* implies coexistence, for there would be no clash between X and Y if they do not coexist. The application of dialectical thinking confronts the clash of opposites, leading to a resolution of contradictions.

From a dialectical stance, change and development result from contradictions between events occurring in various biological, psychological, and sociocultural progressions or crises, the resolution of which leads to further development.

Ho and Yin (2016) state that "spiritual fulfillment goes above and beyond ordinary existence that is conditioned by biological and sociocultural givens in which a person is situated" (p. 281). In other words, discontent with the ordinary is the mother of spiritual development. Ho and Wang (2009) stress that metacognitive reflectiveness grounded in dialectical thinking plays a vital role in therapeutic movement.

Dialectical thinking protects us from pseudodichotomies because it provides us with the analytic power to reveal the basis of their faulty reasoning (Ho, in press-a). Pseudodichotomies pervade our daily lives. People, psychologists included, speak of *emotions versus reason*, for instance. In actuality, both feelings and thinking are invariably involved in any action. A dialectical conception sees no contradiction between emotionality and rationality. It promotes the unity of emotion (pathos) and intellect (logos) in actions. What has to be added, however, is that to relinquish the control of reason over feelings safely presupposes a mature mind that has gained mastery of impulse control, so that unbridled feelings will not go rampant. Break the rules, but not before you have mastered the grammar of life.

Rejecting the Pseudodichotomy Between Nomothetic and Ideographic Studies

Dialectics reject the pseudodichotomy between nomothetic (derived from the Greek word *nomos*, meaning law) and idiographic (from *idios*, one's own) methods. Nomothetic methods (exemplified in Part II) are procedures and methods designed to discover general laws or principles; they tend to rely heavily on the use of quantitative or statistical techniques. Idiographic methods (exemplified in Part I) aim to understand a particular individual or phenomenon; they tend to rely on intensive case studies over a prolonged period of time.

There is no reason to exclude data obtained from intensive case studies in the discovery or formulation of general laws. In particular, atypical or exceptional cases that do not conform to prevailing scientific beliefs must not be ignored. To be done well, idiographic studies have to be guided by established general principles, without which the investigator would be groping in the dark. The interplay between nomothetic and idiographic methods promises greater achievements that neither one may obtain alone.

The unity of nomothetic and idiographic methods parallels the dialectics between the general and the particular: successive cycles from the general to the particular, and from the particular back to the general. We apply general principles to the study of a particular phenomenon, in the process of which we may discover that the phenomenon cannot be fully accounted for by the principles. We would then modify the principles successively until the phenomenon is accounted for satisfactorily—leading to a new body of knowledge.

Dialectical psychology takes a fundamental stand in rejecting any contention that the psychopathology of an individual may be adequately understood without reference to the whole of which the individual is a part. In particular, it rejects the investigation of individual psychopathology without reference to interpersonal, individual-group, and individual-society relations. Therefore, the analysis of mental disorders necessitates recognition of at least three components: processes internal to the individual (inner dialectics, e.g., psychopathological processes), processes external to the individual (outer dialectics, e.g., societal pathologies), and interactions between internal and external processes. Dialectical psychology demands attention to the interdependence, as well as tensions and contradictions, among all three components.

Stated in another way, the microcosm of an individual's disorder reflects the macrocosm of societal disorder within which it is embedded. In particular, intrapsychic conflicts reflect contradictions found in external reality; and the condition of each individual reflects societal health and pathologies.

The reader may also notice that dialectical thinking provides guidance on how to resolve apparent contradictions throughout this book, such as those between normality and abnormality, individualism and collectivism, and Eastern and Western values. Resolving contradictions involves the process of dialectical synthesis that leads to an advancement of understanding. Cultivation in the art of dialectics will facilitate problem solving in *all* domains of human activity—including the diagnosis and treatment of the mentally ill with which we are chiefly concerned in this book.

Thematic Group 1

Normality Versus Abnormality

Thematic Group 1 concerns diagnosis and psychopathology in the psychiatric literature; I have drawn on legends and literary works as well. Its aim is to confront the pseudodichotomy between normality and abnormality. This pseudodichotomy leads people to think that a person is either normal or abnormal categorically. In truth, normality may coexist and clash with abnormality. A person's mental condition may change across time, situations, and especially interpersonal relationships. It is specious to construe psychopathology as static or unchanging.

Religious luminaries, such as George Fox the founder of Quakerism (later named the Religious Society of Friends), deserve special attention. They force us to face the coexistence of madness and religiosity that looms large throughout history in diverse geographical locations.

What are the complications and consequences involved when a person is pronounced abnormal? According to what standards? By whom? To which audience? Turning to the *Diagnostic and Statistical Manual of Mental Disorders* (DSM) is of little help. Modeled after medical diagnosis, the DSM is based on a rather narrow view of mental disorders.

Suppose you have been diagnosed as suffering from a mental disorder. That can be scary. But relax! In the bible of psychiatric diagnosis (i.e., DSM), the term *mental disorder* encompasses a wide range of human misery indeed, ranging from mild, common disorders (e.g., adjustment or anxiety disorders) to the severe (e.g., schizophrenia). Having taught and practiced clinical psychology for decades, I venture to say that very few of us would escape from falling into one or more of the DSM mental disorders at some time in our lives. In other words, the abnormal outnumber the normal; or, it is "abnormal" to be normal.

The set of three chapters in Thematic Group 1 comprises Madness as Creative Energy: Self-Observations; Psychiatric Diagnosis and Its Pitfalls; and Psychopathology of Religious Luminaries. Together, they illustrate that value judgments of good versus bad (or evil) cannot be fully separated from psychiatric diagnosis.

8

Madness as Creative Energy: Self-Observations

This chapter begins with acknowledging that my account of the workings of the mind during episodes of unipolar mood elevation is based on only one case. However, it is a self-study of an exceptional case by a mental health professional, based on his firsthand experiences. Being a self-study raises questions of objectivity. To address this issue, I rely on a rereading of my diaries, which is replete with cautionary remarks about my inflated self-confidence. I also engage in extensive correspondence with friends and colleagues about my condition, which has helped to guard against bias.

Prior to the age of 58, I had no history of severe psychiatric disturbance. Then something happened that profoundly changed my life, unexpectedly and inexplicably. From 1997 to 2021, I have had altogether 22 episodes of elevated mood disorder, 20 hypomanic and 2 arguably severe enough to be considered manic. From these episodes, I have gained invaluable firsthand experiences that inform on the workings of the mind driven by the creative energy of madness.

My firsthand experiences raise significant issues concerning diagnosis, the nature of mood disorders, as well as the failure of mental professionals to recognize the positive aspects of abnormality (see "On Being Strange in Normality as in Madness" in Chapter 3). In what follows, first I present a self-diagnostic exercise based on diverse sources of information. Next, I discuss diagnostic issues and the place of madness in creativity in cultural context.

Atypicality is the most salient feature that emerges from the self-diagnosis. This atypicality is manifest in enhanced health, physical, mental, and spiritual; creativity; and literary-artistic-esthetic sensibilities. I rely on a dialectical conception to discuss the place of madness in creativity: Each transforms, and is transformed by, the other. In a nutshell, the objective of this self-study is to shed light on how and the conditions under which madness may be viewed as creative energy.

A Self-Diagnosis

The primary data consist of (a) a thorough self-study completed when I was a graduate student in clinical psychology, (b) diaries written during or around episodes, (c) a free association done in the midst of a manic episode, and (d) correspondence with friends and colleagues about perceptions of my behavior during episodes. (See Appendix C for details; also Ho, 2014a, 2014b, 2016.)

The following is an excerpt from my diaries written in the midst of a hypomanic episode (with ellipses and added materials in square brackets). I have deliberately kept the reproduction exactly as it was written (excepting spacing between paragraphs) to reflect my thought process.

> physical fatigue, but tremendous energy, mentally active, auto racing, voice recovered, very alert, but the body needs rest and sleep [...]
>
> takes 20 minutes to find my underwear, distractible, how annoying [...]
>
> I have a theory about intelligence the brain is the same but after removal of repression the whole bloody unconscious is available the raw emotions [...] no repression = greater intelligence, creativity = intelligence infinite association of ideas all at once [...]
>
> in just a split of a second, it's gone, can't recall, and lost memory, forever [like] Korsakoff syndrome? Keep trying to reconstruct the past when immediate memory cannot be transferred to long term memory like a funnel, can't hold water
>
> Use [delete use] logic, make distinctions, fear, now I know what ob-compulsive is!? (joy and delight) save this file before it's lost, but I dare not!!!
>
> No longer able to process thoughts, recollect, obsessive, like the brain is no longer able to function properly [...]

Stupid, can do only one thing at a time, keep on forgetting what I had been doing a minute ago, start looking the things ("I spend most of my life looking for things", in the past, previously, no, in the past, previously, ... compulsive!!!!!) keep on forgetting thoughts I had just a while ago [...]

not the same ob-compulsive in youth, excitation beyond the ability of the central nervous system to cope with that memory, creative associations
nothing to do with forbidden/sexual [thinking Freud doesn't apply]
same brain → self-reprocessing → different brain [→] self-creation potential!
"It's nonsense, from a science point of view; uninspiring from a literary point of view"

These passages, input into my computer as fast as I could, read like an outpouring of a stream of consciousness. They illustrate my intense struggle with brain fatigue, disturbances of memory and executive functioning. Flight of ideas and distractibility, two classic symptoms of mania, were clearly present. The thought that my memory was "like a funnel, can't hold water" was scary. There were also lucid moments of reflectiveness, during which I brought my inflated self-confidence down to size. Of my thinking output, I wrote: "It's nonsense, from a science point of view; uninspiring from a literary point of view." I mused that "I spend most of my life looking for things."

Also salient was the obsessive-compulsivity I struggled to rid myself of. I experienced "joy and delight" when I felt freed from its grip. However, obsessive-compulsivity and creativity can "coexist." I theorized that the obsessive-compulsivity was due to "excitation beyond the ability of the central nervous system to cope... nothing to do with forbidden/sexual (Freud doesn't apply)." I thought of the potential of brain alteration through self-reprocessing: "same brain → self-reprocessing → different brain [→] self-creation potential!" The most interesting idea was that I had "no repression anymore." The consequences must be profound: Truly "no repression = greater intelligence, creativity = ... infinite association of ideas all at once."

Here is another excerpt from my diary, also written in the midst of a hypomanic episode, about my physical and psychological condition.

My physical condition was one of great imbalance. The body was near exhaustion. The mind remains active, running on fast time. I felt thirsty all the time. I felt hot, where others may feel cold. Aware that my energy reserve might be depleted, I moved around slowly to conserve energy.

Recollections of remembrances may throw fresh insights informative on brain functioning. The positive side was the creativity. Like boundaries between the conscious and the unconscious had vanished. The unconscious became accessible. Retrieval of information was superefficient. In addition, association of ideas was facilitated, fast, but I also felt overwhelmed by these endless associations.

Similarly, I had to try to focus on one thought. While staying focused, a myriad associations. The next moment, the memory of what I had just been thinking about was gone. Attempts to recall were usually futile. I became obsessive about keeping memories from being lost. So I tried to record my thoughts on paper or in a computer file. Thus, brain fatigue may well be the mechanism for obsessive symptoms. I have also experienced this when the air con is turned off. Mild cerebral anoxia. I don't want to say that this applies to all forms of obsessive phenomena. These obsessive phenomena I have described are qualitatively different from the psychoneurotic varieties described in the psychiatric literature.

This diary recapitulates the theme of brain fatigue expressed in the preceding episode. However, the contrast in the quality of writing between the two episodes cannot be more striking. This reflects the fact that dramatic changes in cognitive functioning can occur as a function of fluctuations in energy level. And here is an abridged version of my diary written around the end of my first manic episode.

Clearly, my manic period was marked by extraordinary creativity, heightened aesthetic sensitivity, depth of feelings, and deep humility. These positive, delightful features are significant: They define the nature of my mania. Definitely, racing thoughts, faster than usual, appeared. Sometimes I was obsessed with losing these thoughts, which I couldn't utter fast enough, let alone put down in writing. Speed was also manifest in an extraordinary sensitivity to cues in social interaction. Watching films or TV shows provided delightful occasions for predicting the next scene, what the actors would say and do. My predictions showed uncanny accuracy, as if I had overtaken the role of the director. That was empathy: I and the director became one. Probably I conducted some of my best psychotherapy sessions or workshops, during which my empathy joined forces with the courage to be myself.

I glimpsed into the mystical-transcendental. But one concern I had was that the combined forces of heightened sensibility and intensified emotionality can be hazardous. I might be too easily fired up by ephemeral ideals and thus act impulsively. Or I might be overly attached to, and hence enslaved by, objects of pleasure or beauty. However, I thought that the Buddhist attitude of nonattachment may keep overattachment at bay: engaged and involved with worldly objects, without being possessive; letting go of fixations. It differs from detachment, which refers to emotional noninvolvement with and disengagement from the world....

Retrieval of information and association of ideas were superefficient, so much so that I was overwhelmed by my own outpouring of creativity. I became obsessively attached to ideas and objects, including the self. I had no physically aggressive or destructive tendencies, although direct expressions of verbal aggressiveness sometimes exceeded my normal level.

I have not been able to duplicate the feats achieved during my first manic episode, at least not as dramatically: self-healing, the completeness of the no-mind state of emptiness, and the willful visual hallucinations. The depth into which I had gone was proportional to the extent to which my social relations suffered. Finally, here is a diary written around the time of one of my late episodes.

> I enter into a state of selfless-oblivion, like a trance. I experience disinhibition like I had never experienced before. I become spontaneous, liberated. My mind explodes. Creative thoughts and flashes of insight rain down fast. I see beauty everywhere, in people's faces, in living things, and in the cosmos. Simply, I am enjoying life.

The positive tone is characteristic of the later episodes I have had, which tend to be mild. Increasingly, I welcome them with open arms and, more significantly, feel that I am gaining mastery in control of their place in my life.

To summarize, the psychiatric symptoms, as well as a composite of psychophysical, affective, cognitive, perceptual, and social functioning across all 22 episodes are presented in Table 1. A perusal of this table reveals no depression of clinical severity. Among the plethora of symptoms, some can hardly be characterized as pathological (e.g., enhanced creativity, literary-artistic-esthetic sensibilities, and capacity to enjoy life); some pertain to gains in health, physical, mental, and spiritual (e.g., liberation from obsessive-compulsivity and self-condemnation by a punitive superego). This is not to deny that psychiatric symptoms have indeed incurred occupational and social costs. It should also be noted that psychophysical and cognitive-perceptual features figure more prominently than affect features, contrary to the typical pattern described in psychiatric texts.

The overall picture is characterized by imbalances: ecstasy intermingling with anguish; maintaining a sense of psychophysical well-being while suffering from inability to fall asleep, physical exhaustion, and depletion of reserves; hyperactivity coexisting with mental or physical fatigue; alterations between bursts of creative output and cognitive disturbances (e.g., extreme forgetfulness or mental confusion). More so than mood elevation, depth of feelings (in both positive and negative directions), it may be argued, describes my condition accurately.

Diagnostic Issues

The question of whether or not unipolar mania constitutes a distinct disorder remains controversial (Nurnberger, Roose, Dunner, & Fieve, 1979; Perugi, Passino, Toni, Maremmani, & Angst, 2007; Yazici et al., 2002). However, reported prevalence rates of mania without major depression from two large-scale epidemiological studies of adolescents and young adults (Beesdo-Baum et al., 2009; Merikangas et al., 2014) fall in the range of 1.7%–1.8%. As Angst (2015) has noted, these rates are higher than even those of schizophrenia. Furthermore, recent reviews (Angst & Grobler, 2015; see also Mehta, 2014) reveal considerable evidence (derived from epidemiological, clinical, treatment, cardiovascular, and genetic studies) pointing to the existence of mania as a distinct disorder. Obviously, the phenomenon of unipolar disorder with only hypomanic and/or manic episodes refuses to be unheard.

My firsthand experiences counter much of the psychiatric literature on mood disorders. The presumption of a shift in polarity between mania and depression is inherent in the use of the term *bipolar*. Having had 22 episodes of euphoria and none of depression, I cannot be said to have suffered from a bipolar disorder at all. If so, attempts to accommodate cases such as that of mine within a bipolar category would lead only to a linguistic-conceptual conundrum.

There are also other atypical features of diagnostic significance: age of onset; absence of identifiable precipitating factors; salience of psychophysical and cognitive-perceptual features; and enhanced literary-artistic-esthetic sensibilities. Most importantly, there is no impairment serious enough to incapacitate occupational or daily functioning. Self-reflection and self-monitoring, both indicative of metacognitive functioning, play a crucial role in maintaining my capacity to function. Even in the depth of madness, I would frequently ask myself, "Am I mad or enlightened?" This has helped me greatly to deflate my supreme self-confidence, keep in touch with reality, and avoid causing more harm to myself or others. All these clinical features summate to a most atypical case that casts doubt on the deficit model according to which mental disorders are viewed solely or primarily in pathological terms.

We need to clarify a diagnostic issue in the cultural context of the East. The evidence suggests that pure or unipolar mania is more common in non-Western cultures (Angst & Grobler, 2015). Significantly, the third edition of the *Chinese Classification of Mental Disorders* continues to list, as in the second edition, "recurrent mania" (without depression, bipolar disorders, or cyclothymia) as a subtype of mood disorder.

Given the combined forces of heightened sensibility and intensified emotionality, I was self-enchanted during madness. Fortunately, self-reflectiveness saved me from being captured by the allure of virtual pleasures. My self-enchantment did not result in psychotic-like or bizarre behaviors, a culture-bound syndrome commonly known in China as *zouhuorumo*, which translates as "catching fire, entering demon." It is listed as a mental disorder "due to qigong" in the Chinese Classification of Mental Disorders (Chinese Society of Psychiatry, 2001) under the category of culture-related disorders. *Zouhuorumo* is thought of as a transient psychotic state found among qigong practitioners thought to have gone astray due to excessive or improper practice (literally, qigong means "breath work," and may be translated as "vital energy work").

One essential feature is a loss of control and reality testing; the practitioner cannot disengage himself from qigong and return to the nonqigong state. *Zouhuorumo* shares common features with the physiokundalin syndrome described by Greyson (2000). It should be distinguished from the demon possession syndrome, in which the patient believes he is "possessed" by an exogenous demonic agent. It may also be interpreted as a type of reactive psychosis or as the precipitation of an underlying mental illness. An estimate from human rights groups of about 600 people, or 0.01% of the 60 million qigong practitioners in China, have received psychiatric treatment (Lee & Kleinman, 2002). Not being an advanced qigong practitioner, I am certain I did not suffer from *zouhuorumo*. However, it is important to be cognizant that bizarre behaviors manifest in *zouhuorumo* may also appear in hypomania or mania and confound diagnosis.

In Buddhist thought, the ideal to be attained, nirvana (literally, "blowing out," as of a lamp), is a state of absolute, eternal quiescence, achieved through ridding oneself of passions and desires, including one's attachment to life. It is a state of enlightenment achieved through moral-intellectual perfection only after strenuous personal effort—a transcendent state of supreme equanimity (Ho, 1995).

In the language of psychoanalysis, nirvana may be described as an infantile state of precathexis, before libido has been invested in objects. Purposeful ridding of passions and desires may be described as decathexis, which should not be confused with anticathexis, the opposition to cathexis by the ego or superego (Ho, 1995, 2014a). Decathexis should be further distinguished from withdrawal, a maladaptive defense mechanism. It is the antithesis of hypercathexis, the profuse and excessive investment of libidinal energy in objects. From this perspective, mania may be conceived as the antithesis of nirvana.

In my case, especially during the two manic episodes, I did enter into states of transcendent consciousness devoid of self-reference, such that the subject-object distinction appeared to have vanished. In such a state, cognition was suspended; the self was absent. Furthermore, I experienced self-enchantment: I erotized myself, other people, and the world. The underlying mechanism, I would argue, is hypercathexis.

The Place of Madness in Creativity

Since ancient times, a common perception is that genius and madness are closely associated. There is good reason for genius to be associated especially with bipolar disorders, among the great variety of mental disorders. Hyperactive mental activity and grandiosity are conducive to creative productivity.

Socrates declares, "If man comes to the door of poetry untouched by the madness of the Muses, believing that technique alone will make him a good poet, he and his sane compositions never reach perfection, but are utterly eclipsed by the performances of the inspired madman."

Aristotle asks, "Why is it that all men who are outstanding in philosophy, poetry or the arts are melancholic?" The answer, I venture to suggest, is that feelings of anguish, self-rejection, and hopelessness in the depths of depression provide the raw materials for creative production. Melancholia, therefore, bars no creativity.

Kierkegäärd writes, "A poet is an unhappy being whose heart is torn by secret sufferings, but whose lips are so strangely formed that when the sighs and cries escape them, they sound like beautiful music" (Thomte, 1948/2009, p. 27).

There is empirical support for linking creativity to psychopathology, especially mood disorders (Andreasen, 1987, 2008, 2011; Jamison, 1993; Kyaga et al., 2011). My firsthand experiences lend further support to this linkage. During madness, I was inspired; creative ideas rained down faster than I could cope. I had supreme confidence, with a touch of "megalomania," enabling me to write without inhibition or self-doubt. I could become self-enchanted, captured by the allure of my own runaway thoughts, resulting in a blurring between the virtual and the real, *as if* I had entered into *zouhuorumo*. I erotized myself, other people, and the world. I yearned to share my creative insights with others. These were favorable conditions for productions of inspirational creativity (Ho, 2016).

From a psychoanalytic viewpoint, with repression vanished, the unconscious became accessible; my mind functioned with holistic oneness, interconnected. Superefficiency in memory retrieval and ideational association may then result from undoing or bypassing repression with ease, thus enabling me to gain unhindered, direct access to the unconscious, a condition for creativity as postulated in psychoanalytic theory.

Such superefficiency has the effect of enhancing my aesthetic, empathic, and cognitive capabilities. This conception may augment or even modify the psychoanalytic theory of creativity. It receives support from a recent study of highly creative individuals by Andreasen (2011): (a) Introspective accounts suggest that unconscious processes play an important role in achieving creative insights, and (b) neuroimaging studies indicate that the association cortices are the primary areas activated during the state of "REST" (random episodic silent thought). Of special relevance to the notion of cognitive superefficiency is the finding that highly creative individuals have more intense activity in the association cortices when performing tasks that challenge them to "make associations."

The High Costs of Cognitive Superefficiency

There is a heavy cost to be paid for the superefficient retrieval of past memories: I may be endlessly haunted by embarrassments over faux pas, failures to meet personal standards, disappointments over betrayals of trust, and other unpleasantries. I may still harbor resentment toward people who caused me great pain. To cleanse my mind, I practice self-healing harder. Success is only occasional, when I find the resentment subsided, gone perhaps.

Additionally, a price has to be paid for creativity in madness due to cognitive superefficiency: Mental fatigue is a prominent symptom that often prevents me from doing work requiring concentration for days. Another observation is that mental fatigue becomes increasingly severe in later episodes. As I age, a decline in cognitive abilities, particularly short-term memory, is unmistakable in my normal daily life. Remarkably, this decline has no effect on superefficiency in memory retrieval or fluency in articulation during abnormal states. Oftentimes, everything seemed to have speeded up, in my thinking, talking, writing, responding to social cues, and so forth.

In the midst of Hypomanic 13, which incredibly occurred while I was in the process of writing an academic article, mental fatigue prevented me from serious writing for several weeks. So I indulged myself in playing the game of *Weiqi* (*Go* in Japanese, *Baduk* in Korean), without question the most complex board game ever invented, via an Internet website. Despite dedicated practice, I was never strong enough to attain the status of an advanced player. Though mentally tired, I was able to play *Weiqi* because the game requires focus on only one thing, namely, how to plan one's moves to win.

One night, in a state of near mental exhaustion, I suddenly found myself able to recall what I had studied and seen the strategies of grand masters decades earlier. Then my skill improved by leaps and bounds, enabling me to compete with advanced players. There were many other similar, though less dramatic, experiences in memory recall (e.g., of events long past, what people had said or done but had forgotten themselves). All these constitute a convincing demonstration that superefficient retrieval of past learning and memories may occur during episodes (Ho, 2016).

Two more important points deserve attention. First, clearly fatigue is distinct from sleepiness. Fatigue, both physical and mental, was intensely felt. But I did not feel sleepy. Second, mania is characterized by unusually high levels of energy and activity. In my case, I fluctuated between high and low levels of activity. I felt that my energy reserves were depleted after sustaining a period of high levels of activity. I was running on a "low battery," and I had to conserve what little energy I had.

In all, both mental fatigue and remembering too much of the painful past, which I regard as the costs to be paid for cognitive superefficiency, stand out as prominent features in my case. Cognitive superefficiency may be the mechanism underlying a host of my firsthand experiences: physical symptoms such as fatigue and shaking chills; psychiatric symptoms such as talkativeness and flight of ideas (which I experienced as an "infinite association of ideas all at once"); cognitive symptoms such as heightened sensitivities and bursts of creativity.

A reading of *Fatigue as a Window to the Brain* (DeLuca, 2007) suggests a new avenue for understanding conditions such as those I have experienced. High energy consumption by the brain may result from hyperactive neural activity, involving probably the sympathetic autonomic nervous system. This hyperactivity may lead to superefficiency in memory retrieval and in forming remote semantic or conceptual associations, but at the cost of mental fatigue.

My conjecture that mental fatigue may result from increased energy consumption by the brain during manic or hypomanic states has received empirical support: Proton magnetic resonance spectroscopy shows that acute manic patients have elevated glutamate/glutamine levels within the left dorsolateral prefrontal cortex (Michael et al., 2003). Yüksel and Öngür (2010) have reviewed the growing evidence for glutamatergic abnormalities in mood disorders from magnetic resonance spectroscopy studies. More generally, Kaidanovich-Beilin, Cha, and McIntyre (2012) claim that there exists an intimate link between the brain and sugar metabolism. Thus, the connection between metabolic disturbances and neuropsychiatric disorders has been strengthened by recent clinical studies.

Conclusion

The psychiatric literature is replete with studies showing cognitive deficits in patients suffering from mania or hypomania (e.g., Martínez-Arán et al., 2004). My intention is not to dispute the results of these studies, but rather to draw our attention to the limitations of research based on the deficit model.

First, we need to guard against overgeneralization, for there may well be a subset consisting of exceptional or atypical patients who show little or no deficits. More importantly, albeit relatively small in numbers, they are often among the more creative members of humanity.

Second, alternative interpretations of findings concerning cognitive deficits should be entertained. A parsimonious interpretation is that the deficits result from the lack of sleep, rather than from mood elevation per se. A more plausible interpretation is that they result from not only sleep disturbance but also mental fatigue due to high energy consumption by the brain associated with hyperactive neural activity.

Third, as in my case, the presence of cognitive disturbances does not necessarily preclude outpourings of creativity. My self-observations have provided some evidence in support of the contention that superefficiency in memory retrieval and ideational associations is a mechanism underlying creativity in euphoric states and, more generally, of viewing madness as creative energy.

Table 1. Psychiatric, Psychophysical, Affective, Cognitive, Perceptual, and Social Features

Area of functioning	Manifestation
Psychiatric features	
Unusual mood elevation	Euphoria. Inflated self-confidence. Irritability not a significant feature. No grandiosity or psychotic features.
Flight of ideas	Rapid succession of ideas or verbalizations with abrupt shifting from one idea or topic to another. Especially pronounced during manic episodes.
Talkativeness	Under pressure to keep talking. Usually kept under control, especially in later episodes.
Impulse control	Usually able to exercise adequate impulse control. Absence of high-risk activities, except in manic episodes.
Psychophysical functioning	
Inability to sleep	A major symptom in all episodes, except the last two, which accentuated fatigue. No decreased need to sleep but did not feel sleepy.
Extreme fatigue	Experienced depletion of energy after engaging in demanding physical or mental activities. Had to conserve energy with extreme measures, such as half shutting my eyes (a Yoga technique), avoiding all unnecessary talking or movements.
Shaking chills	Present in episodes beginning from the 7th, even in hot weather. Progressively worsened.
Strong libidinal drive	Increased sexual thoughts and activities.
Engagement in physical activities	Driven to physical activities such as martial arts (mostly Taiji) and dancing to music, no matter how tired. Ushered into a self-rewarding state of selfless-oblivion.
Infused with *qi* (energy)	Experienced an energy flow throughout my body, feeling strong. Occasionally, though briefly, after practicing Taiji.
Posture	Rid of hunchback posture that had existed for years, maintaining upright posture during episodes.

Table 1. Continued

Area of functioning	Manifestation
Motility	Enhanced kinesthetic sense in dancing, practicing martial arts, and so forth when entering into a state of selfless-forgetfulness.
Blood pressure	Sometimes lowered to the point where medication is no longer needed, for periods lasting up to over 1 year.
Hiccups and gastrointestinal imbalances	Occasional hiccups that lasted on and off for some 5 hours in the middle of the night. (Perplexed, I consulted a Taiji master, who said, "It's a good thing.") End result indeed beneficial to my health, felt a sense of extraordinary well-being, rid of gastrointestinal imbalances or disturbances I have had for years.
Self-healing and bodily relaxation	Self-healing of an injured knee and ridding it of pain in a transcendent state. Sharpened proprioceptive perception enabled me to be sensitive to tightness or weakness, even past mild injuries. Total body relaxation achieved extends into normal states.
Affective and emotional functioning	
Depth of feelings	Experienced ecstasy; serenity and inner peace intermingling with anguish.
Uninhibited expressiveness	More expressive than usual. Usually kept within the bounds of social acceptability, except in the two manic episodes.
Liberation from self-doubts	Feeling at home in the cosmos. Saying to myself, "Life is wonderful." Liberation from self-condemnation by a punitive superego.
Humility	Humbled by the collective achievements of humankind, the vastness of the cosmos.
Magnanimity	Strong feelings of pathos, compassion, and *da'ai* ("big love" in Buddhism). Predominance of love over hatred.
Cognitive functioning	
Mental confusion	Unable to perform simple tasks, such as arithmetic calculations. At worst, disoriented, unable to parse whole sentences.

(*Continued*)

Table 1. Continued

Area of functioning	Manifestation
Distractibility	Secondary to fatigue. May be highly goal-directed when energy level permitted.
Metacognition	Maintained self-reflectiveness and self-monitoring throughout all episodes. Aware of my extraordinary condition at all times.
Superefficiency in memory retrieval	Able to retrieve memories rapidly, even those of past decades or of infancy.
Creativity	Able to make remote association of ideas. Often flooded with novel ideas, some of which have lasting value. The mind seemed to be working continually at full speed, even during sleep.
Articulation	Enhanced verbal fluency, articulation, to-the-point expressions.
Empathy	Enhanced capability to feel the feelings of others and to anticipate what people will say or do accurately.
Freedom from compulsivity	Became spontaneous, less inhibited. Totally relieved from obsessive-compulsiveness.
Perceptual functioning	
Alteration in time perception	Cease to be obsessive about living by the clock. Occasionally hours would pass without my awareness, surprised when I looked at my watch.
Alteration in auditory perception	Occasionally, while listening to music, my tolerance for volume diminished dramatically; somehow the music did not sound right.
Supersensitivity in olfactory perception	On one occasion, able to smell unpleasant odors from a swamp more than a hundred feet away, even though there was a steady breeze blowing.
Willful hallucinations	Dramatic willful hallucinations in the first manic episode: seeing myself nailed on a cross and feeling pathos for humankind, *as if* I were Jesus; transgender experiencing.

Table 1. Continued

Area of functioning	Manifestation
Social functioning	
Occupational functioning	Not compromised, except in one manic episode.
Social relationships	Caused considerable anxiety in my family and among my friends and colleagues.
Humor	More humorous, colorful, and entertaining during social gatherings.
Generosity	More generous in helping others in need, both in terms of time and money. Engaged in philanthropic activities.
Literary-artistic-esthetic sensibilities	
Enhanced esthetic sensitivity	Seeing beauty everywhere, in people's faces, in ordinary objects, in nature (e.g., the roots of a tree, the droning sound of cicadas). Enhanced capacity for art appreciation.
Music appreciation	Magnified emotional responsiveness to music stood out in all episodes. Listened and danced to music for hours daily.
Literary output	Wrote poems. Sent literary messages to friends and colleagues.
Appreciation of life	Delight in "just being alive." Enjoying the simple activities of daily life, including those normally resisted (e.g., brushing my teeth).

9

Psychiatric Diagnosis and Its Pitfalls

The bible of psychiatric diagnosis, Diagnostic and Statistical Manual of Mental Disorders, is responsible for the closing of minds in psychiatry.

Done correctly, a psychiatric diagnosis serves to clarify the nature and extent of the mental disorder a person may have. That's useful information for taking preventive or curative measures. Trouble comes, however, when a psychiatric diagnosis is taken to be the alpha and omega of understanding. In this chapter, I discuss the limitations of the *Diagnostic and Statistical Manual of Mental Disorders*, cultural relativism and the definition of abnormality, and the dialectical tension between the particular and the universal. This discussion informs us on the pitfalls of psychiatric diagnosis, with special reference to a question that concerns many parents: Is our child suffering from any of the Attention-Deficit and Disruptive Behavior Disorders?

Liberation from the *Diagnostic and Statistical Manual of Mental Disorders*

To expand our horizons, consider the different ways or criteria by which a mental disorder, or its absence, may be judged (see Table 1).

A person may be diagnosed by a qualified professional as suffering from a mental disorder on the basis of some identified defect or pathological process. He may (or may not) subjectively feel unwell, with complaints such as "I'm going to have a nervous breakdown." He may be "abnormal" in either a positive or negative direction according to some statistical norm (e.g., scoring unusually high, or low, on a psychological test of intelligence). He may be deemed as deviant by acting in ways that are considered outside the bounds of social or cultural acceptability. He may have failed to maintain interpersonal relationships or meet the demands of adaptation (e.g., holding onto a job). He may fall short of some ideal of psychological health such as self-realization, selflessness, nobility or integrity of character.

Finally, diagnostic judgments may be made at different points in his life-span development. As a child, he may have fallen significantly below the maturational norms of his age group and be diagnosed as having a developmental disorder. As an adult, he may interpret his mental disorder in a larger religious or spiritual context (see Chapter 10, Chapter 18). This is not unusual, but ironically the bible of psychiatric diagnosis has given virtually no attention to the religious-spiritual dimension of abnormality.

These criteria do not necessarily and probably do not yield the same judgment. A person may be judged to be mentally ill by one criterion (e.g., diagnosis by a professional) but not so by another (e.g., his own subjective feeling). Diagnosis is no simple matter. To add more complication to the life of a diagnostician, consider the case of a person who wants to lead others to think he is mentally ill (a form of manipulation), does not think he is mentally ill himself but is judged to be mentally ill by professionals. I have, in fact, come across such cases.

Serious consequences follow if you have been pronounced to be abnormal. First, the diagnosis itself is likely to cause or to exacerbate anxiety. It may lead to a labeling effect: The psychiatric label is a stigma. Consequently, it may intensify the tension between how you view yourself and how you are viewed by others. An awareness of such tension may help you to negotiate the path back to health.

Cultural Relativism and the Definition of Abnormality

Clearly, value judgments are implicit in psychiatric diagnosis. The need to consider value judgments becomes even more critical when the diagnosis of a person

Table 1. Conceptions and Criteria of Normality and Abnormality

Conception of normality/abnormality	Criterion
Psychopathology	Internal defects and/or pathological processes
Subjective feelings	Self-report, complaints
Statistical reference	Population norms
Deviance	Social, cultural, religious norms
Adaptation	Meeting demands for interpersonal, social, and occupational functioning
Health (not the same as absence of illness)	Ideals such as self-actualization, selflessness, nobility or integrity of character
Life-span development	Maturational norms for children; psychological maturity, spiritual growth for adults

from a different cultural background is made. This brings us to confront the issue of how norms, beliefs, and values differ across cultures.

Cultural relativism presents a challenge to psychiatry: It views abnormality as a *deviation from cultural norms*, not in terms of psychopathology. Most of us would consider cannibalism gruesome and abnormal. Now suppose we relocate to a different time and place, to a cannibalistic bribe. Would cannibal behavior be considered abnormal? No, if cannibalism is the only behavior in question—in accordance with the thesis of cultural relativism. But yes, if his cannibal and other forms of behavior deviate from the norms of his tribe. Violating the taboos of his tribe, by far the most serious, is the significant factor to consider, rather than cannibal behavior per se. This point is important. The person in question is not just cannibalistic: Questions of impulse control, understanding of and ability to abide by cultural norms, and so forth—and hence psychopathology—have to be raised. In short, defining abnormality solely in terms of deviation from cultural norms may grossly oversimplify the issues involved.

Given an extreme form of cultural relativism, the task of defining abnormality would be grossly simplified: Behavior is abnormal if, and only if, the culture in which it occurs labels it as such. In effect, psychiatric diagnosis has been reduced to a matter of conformity-deviance on the part of the person in question and of acceptance-rejection by culture.

A grave implication follows. Cultural acceptance renders abnormal behavior (as judged by mental professionals) normal. Nonacceptance regards deviant individuals as being abnormal—particularly visionaries ahead of their times. If this were so, the task of the therapist would be reduced to helping clients to "adjust" (i.e., conform) to their cultural norms. Of course, we don't have to embrace such extreme relativism; and rejecting it does not mean negating the importance of considering cultural factors in psychiatric diagnosis.

Dialectical Tension Between the Particular and the Universal

A closely related question, which is is as old as the social sciences, concerns the tension between the particular and the universal. Norms, beliefs, and values supposedly shared by virtually all known cultural groups, albeit not necessarily in the same manner, are *cultural universals*. Those shared by only a cultural group or related groups (e.g., the ethic of filial piety in Confucian cultures) are *culture specific*.

The thesis of *universality* presupposes the existence of core values shared by the majority of cultural traditions, although their concrete expression may take different forms. It entails the identification and extraction of commonalities across cultures. Values such as love, courage, justice, and wisdom may be identified as plausible universals because they are rooted in the world's great philosophical-religious teachings and are upheld in virtually all cultural traditions (Ho & Ho, 2007). Conceived at a high level of abstraction or generality, universals allow for cultural variation in interpretation and expression. Nonetheless, universals imply that there are irreducible standards for human conduct.

To a universalist "objectionable" practices abound. Foot binding in China, practiced for centuries to make women more "attractive," is one. Chastity belts designed for the wives of Crusaders, Medieval knights gone off to fight Moslems (the "usefulness" of which may be left to our imagination), are largely a myth that nonetheless reflects on the Medieval mind about how much violations of female chastity threatened the knights' manhood.

Female genital mutilation is still practiced widely in Middle Eastern countries. Often referred to as female circumcision, it comprises all procedures involving partial or total removal of the external female genitalia or other injuries to the female genital organ, whether for cultural, religious, or other nontherapeutic reasons. Another example should be added, if only to avoid the impression that different norms exist only between ethnic or cultural groups: abortion as murder, a position held vehemently by the pro-life camp in opposition to the pro-choice camp in the United States. We should also take note that all examples cited entail the female body and sexuality. Is this purely coincidental? Can we avoid taking a stand on the ethical issues they bring?

Social scientists who adhere to *cultural relativism* refute this implication. Standards, they claim, are subject to temporal and geographical variations; what is right or wrong, normal or abnormal, is relative to the cultural group in question at a specific period in history. Moreover, to pass judgment on the cultural practices of another group is to commit ethnocentrism or, more precisely, culturocentrism, considered as a cardinal sin. Cultural relativists prefer to rely on the concept of *deviance*: What is deviant in one cultural group may be accepted even as standard practice in another, and vice versa. Viewed in this light, madness is a manifestation of deviance, not of mental derangement.

Before deciding on whether we agree with relativism or universality, let us witness an imaginary debate between relativist Dr. R and universalist Dr. U. At the end, we will be better informed on where we stand on the issues. Here, we need to make explicit a distinction between two related, but distinct, issues of this debate, the cultural and the ethical. At stake is the question: Is human dignity universal or culture specific?

An Imaginary Debate

Dr. U Misguided cultural or religious pluralism can corrupt into moral relativism, a curious and dangerous position denying that there are irreducible standards for human conduct. Moral relativism poses a threat to ecumenicity, which affirms universalistic values and principles. Thus, tension exists between the embracement of diversity and the threat that this embracement may pose. Indiscriminate admittance of cultural or religious beliefs and practices may be as deadly as embracing the Medusa.

Dr. R Universalistic doctrines of morality disregard cultural diversity. In contrast, ethical relativism allows any culture to define what it regards as right or wrong. As a cultural relativist, I reject the idea of universal norms, simply because there are no norms accepted in or common to all cultures. As an ethical relativist, I refute the idea that cultural values may be ranked on primitive-to-advanced or bad-to-good dimensions. In particular, I reject the notion of a pathogenic culture or subculture in which its social pathologies or mental disorders are rooted in some of its cultural norms. Cultural relativism leads to ethical relativism: There is no way to reach consensus across cultures; or to decide if one set of norms or values is better, or worse than another.

Dr. U We may stand our argument on its head, and affirm general, culturally invariant principles by challenging ethical relativists to negate them: Can you name a single culture that rejects appropriate behavior, and affirms deviant behavior, defined according to its own norms? Alternatively, can you think of a single exception to the universal principle that all cultures affirm appropriate behavior, and negate deviant behavior, according to its own definition of what is appropriate and what is deviant? Similarly, it is both possible and necessary to formulate general, higher order ethical principles according to which lower order principles may be judged.

Dr. R You are treading toward the issue of *ethical relativism*. Universalistic doctrines of morality disregard cultural diversity; in contrast, ethical relativism allows any culture to define what it regards as right or wrong. Throughout history, universalism has sometimes assumed the form of absolutistic doctrines, which have not served humanity well. The rise of relativism parallels the decline of the absolute. Knowledge is power; absolutistic knowledge is tyrannical power. The institutionalization of absolutistic knowledge confers upon its possessor absolutistic authority and control over others. Absolutism should prod us to become aware that knowledge can indeed be a dangerous thing.

Dr. U To say that absolutistic doctrines have not served humanity well sounds like a universalistic, not relativist, statement!

You imply that any set of values is as good as another for humankind when you reject the idea that some cultural norms may be pathological and hence pathogenic. In so doing, you remove the motivation for cultural change for the better. But cultures do change and benefit from intercultural fertilization. Take foot binding, for instance. Chinese people now look back on it as a backward practice that oppressed women. The world is moving toward the idea that there are fundamental values, such as human rights, even if consensus on defining those values has not been achieved.

Are cultural relativists simply amoral or immoral as well? Cannibalism is repugnant, but not evil or pathological. But female genital mutilation, which violates the rights of women to health and sexual fulfillment, flies in the face of the idea of progress. Violation of human rights, ethnic cleansing, genocide, and other forms of terrorism are plainly heinous. To deny that some cultural norms may be unethical or pathological opens the door to condone all these practices. Beware that ethical relativism may be used inadvertently to silence critics and paralyze action in defense of human dignity.

Dr. R By documenting cultural variation, cultural relativism provides ammunition for ethical relativism, which promotes toleration, if not acceptance, of cultural values that diverge from one's own. Tolerance of diversity is what the world needs more of.

Dr. U Extreme cultural relativism can amount to *incommensurability*, the absence of common conceptions and perspectives. Incommensurability means that there is no common ground, and hence no possibility, for communication or

Dr. R   mutual understanding between divergent cultures, leading to misunderstanding, even mistrust. Not an appetizing position to take at all.

Dr. R   Not all cultural relativists take such an extreme position. Ethical relativism champions diversity and counters uniformity. It has a rightful place particularly in this age of globalization when the identities of many cultures are under threat. In 2008, the Australian government made a historic apology to the Aboriginal people for a six-decade policy of forced resettlement. In the early 1900s, thousands of mixed-race children were taken from their families and sent to live in orphanages, mission homes, or Caucasian households. Now, this is truly the mark of a civilized nation. Will the Government of the United States apologize to African and Native Americans?

Dr. U   I'm for it. But note that you have raised ethical relativism to universal status: Acceptance of cultural diversity is a universal principle. This contradicts relativism, which disallows universal principles!

Dr. R   I have no problem with accepting ethical relativism as a universal principle. Each culture is free to define for and by itself what is good and what is bad, *except* to disallow other cultures the same privilege.

Dr. U   Embodied within your refined version of cultural relativism is a universal principle: All cultures are equal. There is simply no way to escape from universality. Consider now the logic of self-application in the case of ethical relativism. You assert that there is no way to decide if one set of values is better or worse than another. Ethical relativism is a set of values, and so is universalism. Then, on what grounds can you negate universalism and affirm ethical relativism?

Dialectical Synthesis

The ideal is diversity within unity: That would be the end result of continuing the dialogue in which Dr. R and Dr. U are engaged. Universalism in keeping with pluralism allows for, even welcomes, culturally diverse understandings of human dignity.

Closely allied with universalism is equifinality, which entails the idea that the same ultimate goal may be reached from different paths. Anyone is at liberty to define his own chosen path for leading a dignified life, *except* to disallow others the same privilege. In principle, there may be as many developmental paths as there are individuals.

In conclusion, I affirm the dialectical synthesis between unity and diversity. Intercultural fertilization enriches our understanding of human dignity as an ecumenical ideal. This ideal, diversity within unity, is both principled and tolerant: Ecumenicity without tolerance succumbs to absolutism; unprincipled ecumenicity absorbs unwanted elements and risks becoming tainted. The tension between principled discernment and tolerance drives its further development. A major task lies ahead of us: to identify and catalog commonalities as well as differences in conceptions of human dignity among the world's philosophical, religious, and cultural traditions (see Chapter 17).

Is Your Child Suffering from ADHD?

Cultural factors figure prominently in the conception, identification, and treatment of abnormality (see Chapter 16). For the purpose of illustration, I choose to focus on the assessment of Attention-Deficit/Hyperactivity Disorder (ADHD) and of aggressiveness in children. Cultural expectations and tolerance are particularly relevant to the diagnosis of conditions like ADHD, which are familiar to parents and teachers as a source of great irritation and headaches. Hyperactivity, for instance, is by definition activity beyond the normal limits of tolerance. Many parents have been compelled to ask, "Is our child really beset by ADHD and to what extent?"

Cultural Differences in Patterns of Socialization

Psychological research has shown that early Chinese and Japanese socialization patterns are in line with the demands of Confucian-heritage cultures, in which overriding importance is attached to impulse control (Ho, 1994, 1996, in press-b; Ho et al., 2012). The disposition toward impulse inhibition manifest early in life is a precursor of the same disposition to be found in adulthood. This disposition is adaptive in the Confucian cultural context, characterized by its great demands of social control, intolerance of deviance, and pressure toward conformity. The mother is the chief agent of impulse control in the earliest period of the child's life. A cross-cultural study shows that Japanese mothers expect early mastery of emotional maturity, self-control, and social courtesy.

In comparison, mothers in the United States expect their children to achieve early mastery of verbal assertiveness and social skills in interaction with peers. It would thus appear that early maternal expectations and behavior are strategically adaptive for preparing children to meet the demands of the culture in which they mature.

Research on traditional Chinese values (Ho, in press-b; Ho et al., 2012) shows that parental education is *negatively* correlated with both folk and ideal values. Additionally, father's education surpasses mother's education in the absolute size of the correlation with folk values; in contrast, mother's education surpasses father's education in the case of ideal values.

A significant implication follows. Traditionally, parental roles are sharply differentiated in Chinese societies. The paternal role is that of an educator-disciplinarian, in addition to that of a provider; the maternal role is primarily that of a protective, nurturant caretaker. The data obtained suggest, however, that mothers with high levels of education have an eroding effect on Chinese traditionalism, particularly in terms of its ideal values. Increasingly, women appear to be playing a major role in cultural changes, in view of their marked increase in educational level in recent decades.

Cultural Expectations and Tolerance

The failure to meet cultural demands is one of the most important standards by which judgments of abnormality are made. However, complications in judgment arise because demands may vary considerably in different cultures. Hence, clinicians in different cultures may vary in their readiness to assign various diagnostic categories to the child. This variation arises because often diagnostic labeling depends less on the seriousness of the behavior in question than on social expectations and level of tolerance toward the behavior.

Furthermore, whether or not the child is brought to the attention of the clinician in the first place is a function of the tolerance level of adults around the child in question. The boisterous, disobedient, or delinquent child is much more likely to arouse concern in his parents and teachers than his sullen, socially withdrawn peers—not because he is necessarily more disturbed psychologically, but because his disruption to the orderly patterns of everyday life is more apparent.

Dramatic differences in expectations and tolerance exist between Chinese and Western (especially American) cultures. In Chinese culture, great importance is attached to the exercise of control over impulses that may disrupt societal order (Ho et al., 2012). Thus, Chinese parents are highly concerned with the training of impulse control, beginning early in the child's life. In contrast, American parents are inclined to be worried that their children may not be socially well-adjusted unless they are outgoing, active, and, for boys, assertive, perhaps even aggressive.

Also to be considered are differences in the uniformity and pervasiveness of expectations. Traditionally, Chinese expectations toward children are extremely stable and uniform, as if it were inconceivable that children could behave differently from what is expected of them. It is the weight of this uniformity—of the whole culture—that bears down upon the child to exercise self-control. In contrast, American expectations tend to be characterized more by heterogeneity than by homogeneity. Questions concerning how children should be treated occasion lively debate and controversy.

Aggressive Behavior

A closely related topic to be discussed concerns the lack of aggressive behavior observed in Asian children, in comparison with American children. I have often been pressed by Western psychologists for an explanation, but I really cannot offer one. Rather, I would turn the question around and ask how the high frequency of aggressive behavior in American children can be explained. This is because I do not wish to be committed to the theoretical position that aggression, as distinct from the capacity for aggression, is a necessary component of the biological nature of humans. It may be argued that what needs to be explained is the presence rather than the absence of aggression.

Again, the difference in cultural expectations between China and America is striking. In China, the child's aggressive behavior is regarded as antisocial and consequently suppressed. In America, a certain amount of aggression is to be expected; an absence of aggressive behavior, especially in boys, might even arouse suspicion of "wimpiness." Chinese parents are typically upset if their children get into a fight. American parents may be worried about their son's "masculinity" if he runs away from a fight. Many years ago, an American psychologist visiting China told me that he felt uneasy because he failed to see any fighting in kindergartens and schools he visited; he felt relieved when he finally observed one incidence of fighting between two boys, who were unaware of his presence. His view of human nature had been reaffirmed!

Many Chinese immigrants to the United States I talk with have expressed the concern that their children need to protect themselves from physical fights in school; some have advocated arming their children with martial arts. Perhaps this explains why *kung fu* has become particularly popular among young Chinese-Americans and why to them Bruce Lee was such a popular folk hero. The fact is that violence is highly visible in America, in the mass media as it is in real life. The violence of the frontier days has permeated and remained alive in the psyche of American society. Could the belief that aggression is inherent in human nature lead to accepting violence as a way of life? And hence to a greater likelihood of its occurrence?

Concluding Remarks

The central point is that psychiatric diagnosis has to be liberated from its bible, the DSM that has been instrumental in the closing of psychiatric minds. Cultural factors figure prominently in the conceptualization, recognition, and assessment of abnormality. In particular cultural expectations and tolerance play an important prominent role in the assessment of ADHD and over aggressiveness in children.

As a parenthetical thought, one wonders if there is a tradeoff between self-control and individuality. Is the suppression of individuality a price to be paid for achieving self-control at an early age? Is hyperactivity or poor impulse control, at least in part, an unfortunate by-product of misinterpreting individuality to mean unlimited freedom?

In answering these questions, it is important to negate a faulty assumption: the incompatibility between self-control and individuality. Dialectical thinking would not allow for such an assumption; rather, self-control is not self-suppression, and individuality does not mean disregard of limits. Therefore, a preferred way to formulate the question is: "How can one achieve self-control, without loss of individuality? Alternatively, how can one preserve one's individuality, while exercising self-control?" My answer is that the unity of self-control and individuality is a step toward the mastery of life. This is a key point in Chapter 3.

As a psychologist who has lived and worked in both the East and the West, I feel deeply that each has much to learn from the other. What is desirable for Western children is to strengthen impulse control and social courtesy; to be less demanding and less aggressive. Among children in the East, to be more assertive, autonomous, and adventuresome; less conforming and impulse inhibited.

10

Psychopathology of Religious Luminaries

Collectively, religious luminaries manifest a museum of psychiatric symptoms.

Psychiatry deals with the diagnostic question of what is normal or abnormal, which is conceptually distinct from the ethical question of what is right or wrong. In actual practice, however, the questions of normality-abnormality and of good-versus-bad are inseparable.

In diagnostic decisions, ethical questions are considered as well, particularly with regard to antisocial or conduct disorders. Similarly, in moral judgments, the question of abnormality would be raised when a person behaves in a way that is pervasively and consistently judged as wrong in his culture.

Nonetheless, to distinguish between abnormality and wrongful behavior is a major achievement of psychiatry. A person suffering from an abnormal condition is mentally ill, not bad; to be treated, not punished. Historically, this has not always been the case. During the Middle Ages in Europe, many of those prosecuted and punished for deviating from the Christian faith would be viewed as mentally ill, not "evil," in the modern age.

Are madness and evil necessarily connected? This is a question that has been reawakened in recent decades. The association of madness and violence has been strengthened by human bombers in the Middle East and elsewhere who blow innocent people and themselves up in the name of God or Allah. This compels us to reassess the connection between madness and evil. At the same time, we must also reexamine the long history of violence committed in the name of religion and, more fundamentally, the duality of good and evil in religious or ideological fanaticism.

The duality of good and evil looms large in religiosity. In this chapter, I attempt to differentiate between the good from the evil directions in which religiosity, coexisting with madness, may take: in other words, between benign and malignant madness. Religiosity and spirituality are distinct, though overlapping, concepts.

A major difference concerns the propensity toward violence. Religiosity may carry with it potential perils of dogmatism, cultism, extremism or, worse, fanaticism. Because religious experiences pertain to the ultimate questions of life, the danger of their occurrence in violent forms rings a grave alarm. The likes of evil cults ending in mass suicide and religious militants who murder in the name of God are magnified consequences of violent tendencies wedded to religious fervor.

In contrast, spirituality has an inherent immunity to guard itself against these perils, because of its propensity toward humility, contemplativeness, and self-reflection. Exemplars of spirituality (e.g., prophets, mystics, Arhats) may be tormented by self-doubt or guilt; they may be given to self-denial—but not to suicide bombing or other forms of wanton outbound aggression.

Religiosity and Madness

Like religiosity and spirituality, religiosity and madness are overlapping concepts. Logically, this implies that neither is a necessary or sufficient condition for the other. It is possible to be religious without being mad or be mad without being religious, be neither, or be both. The last category, being both religious and mad, may comprise only a minority, but an important minority.

Religion may enter into madness in the form of hallucinations or delusions with religious content. In some cases, these psychiatric symptoms are merely byproducts of madness; they disappear with its termination. In other cases, symptoms with religious content constitute the core of madness—that is to say, religion is now wedded to madness, a highly incendiary condition.

In still other cases, and these are the most interesting of all, religiosity takes on a life of its own, coexisting with madness, and transforms the person's life in two possible directions, one toward the good and the other toward evil. When that happens we may witness the arrival of a new prophet or another monster. That is why a study of the psychopathology of religious luminaries throughout the ages may be so illuminating.

An account of great leaders of religious movements, Gautama, Jesus, Muhammad, St. Francis of Assisi, George Fox, and many others, reveals some recurrent patterns. Their career paths are tortured paths, characterized by most, if not all, of these elements: an triggering event leading to intensive religiosity; intense, fierce inner struggle; isolation and solitude; being a voice in the wilderness, figurative or literal; self-denial, to an extreme; temptations of great force, typically of lust for sex or power, that are eventually overcome; experience of enlightenment; preaching to increasingly larger multitudes; rejection by orthodoxy or, worse, being branded as a heretic and persecuted; surviving persecution; and, finally, recognition as a religious leader.

Together, these great religious leaders of the world manifest a museum of psychiatric symptoms (e.g., hallucinations, delusions of grandeur). Whereas genius tends to be associated with manic-depression, religiosity-spirituality tends to be associated with paranoia. Medical authors have long adduced biblical evidence to allege that no less a leader than Jesus suffered from paranoia. Albert Schweitzer (1913/2011), the renowned medical missionary to Africa, wrote his doctoral thesis, entitled *The Psychiatric Study of Jesus: Exposition and Criticism*, to refute this allegation.

In this connection, religious leaders (Jesus and Saint Paul) are among the historical figures who score highly on the Psychopathic Personality Inventory, as reported by Oxford psychologist Kevin Dutton (2016). (The Inventory comprises three factors: Fearless Dominance, Self-Centered Impulsivity, and Coldheartedness.) Of critical importance, however, Jesus and Saint Paul both have low scores on Coldheartedness; Jesus has low scores on Fearless Dominance as well. Mahatma Gandhi has low scores on all three factors.

How do we interpret these results? First, psychopathic dispositions are common historical figures in leadership positions. Second, leaders characterized by fearless dominance enhance their charisma for drawing multitudes of followers; in and by itself, fearless dominance may not lead to disasters. Third, a combination of fearless dominance and self-centered impulsivity, especially when coupled with coldheartedness, portends incendiary tragic consequences.

George Fox and Quakerism: The Tortuous Road of a Religious Movement

No one to my knowledge has come out for a psychiatric defense of George Fox, who founded Quakerism (later called the Religious Society of Friends) in 17th-century England. For this reason, I have chosen Fox as a case study of how religious fervor wedded to madness need not lead to more, but rather to less, violence in the world.

Fox was a troubled and searching youth drawn to religious concerns. He was shocked by what he saw as the failure of the "professors," that is, the professing Christians, to live their beliefs. At age 19, Fox left home on a spiritual quest, during which he challenged religious leaders everywhere to answer his questions. Nowhere did he find satisfaction. In 1647, having "forsaken all the priests" and in despair, he heard a voice, saying "There is one, even Christ Jesus, that can speak to thy condition."

To Fox, this was a direct, immediate, and transforming experience of God. It was to become the heart of his message and ministry, marking the beginning of the Quaker movement. Predictably, Fox was persecuted. He was imprisoned eight times. He suffered cruel beatings and deprivation. But he was an indomitable figure. Nothing would drive him to detract from his dogged persistence to spread his message. His *Journal* and other writings continue to be the basic works of Quakerism.

Anyone who succeeds in leading a religious movement into maturity, surviving untold hardship and persecution, has to be a religious genius. The probability of success, though statistically significantly different from zero, is still near zero. But Fox was also a mad genius. A reading of his *Journal* makes clear that Fox was a deeply disturbed man. Paranoid ideation leaps out from the pages. As a clinical psychologist, I detect one extremely disturbing aspect in Fox's case: his obedience to, and acting out, hallucinatory commands attributed to some external authority. An excerpt from his *Journal* (emphasis added):

> The word of the Lord came to me, that I must to thither [to the city of Lichfield].... Then was I commanded by the Lord to pull off my shoes. I stood still, for it was winter: but the word of the Lord was like a fire in me. So I put off my shoes.... Then I walked on about a mile, and as soon as I got within the city, the word of the Lord came to me again, saying: Cry, "Wo to the bloody city of Lichfield!" So I went up and down the streets, crying with a loud voice, Wo to the bloody city of Lichfield! ... As I went thus crying through the streets,

there *seemed* to me to be a channel of blood running down the streets, and the market-place *appeared* like a pool of blood.... After this a deep consideration came upon me, for what reason I should be sent to cry against that city, and call it the bloody city! ... *afterwards* I came to understand, that in the Emperor Diocletian's time, a thousand Christians were martyr'd in Lichfield. So I was to go, without my shoes, through the channel of their blood, and into the pool of their blood in the market-place, that I might raise up the memorial of the blood of those martyrs.

What if the commands had been of a more violent-destructive sort? The use of the words *seemed* and *appeared* suggests an awareness of the distinction between appearance and the real thing. The "deep consideration" is a clear indication of a self-reflective mind (or metacognition) at work. The word *afterwards* is significant, for it informs us that the crucial historical information about Lichfield comes after Fox's venture into the city. The martyrs' blood then gives Fox's actions perfect rationalization and elevation to the status of religiosity.

His *Journal* also reveals a total commitment to his religious quest; indifference to his physical and, more significantly, social costs that the quest entails. To Fox, how others perceive and react to his actions are irrelevant. Surely, here is a mark of egomania. But is there anything evil in his actions? The answer is no. That is the critical question that may differentiate religiosity from evil. To conclude, Fox is a religious genius, paranoid but not evil. William James (1902/2002) says, in *The Varieties of Religious Experience*:

> A genuine first-hand religious experience like this [of George Fox] is bound to be a heterodoxy to its witnesses, the prophet appearing as a mere lonely madman. If his doctrine prove [sic] contagious enough to spread to any others, it becomes a definite and labeled heresy. But if it then still prove [sic] contagious enough to triumph over persecution, it becomes itself an orthodoxy; and when a religion has become an orthodoxy, its day of inwardness is over: The spring is dry; the faithful live at second hand exclusively and stone the prophets in their turn.

Great religious leaders share some common attributes: They have charisma; they have an unshakable belief in their own righteousness; they have a singularity of purpose, to spread their message or doctrine; their determination is resolute, even ruthless, and no sacrifice is too great a price to pay to reach their goals. Contagiousness comes from the combination of these attributes. Now the same combination is found in the leaders of evil cults, of whom there are few examples more destructive and revolting than James Jones. Moreover, if religiosity is extended to the larger domain of ideology, then we may easily find men of genius who are both mad and evil, of whom Adolf Hitler must lay claim to being the Führer. How can benign madness and malignant madness be differentiated?

Duality of Good and Evil

Judgments of good and evil are made, not on psychiatric or scientific, but on ethical grounds. So the severity of psychiatric disturbance, if any, is irrelevant. The biblical parable "Every tree is known by its fruit" provides a hint on how we may proceed. Suppose we look at two trees, Fox and Hitler, and see how they are known by their fruits, Quakerism and Nazism. Suddenly, the contrasts cannot be sharper at every turn.

Quakerism: The Indwelling Light Is Within All Persons

Nazism is too well-known to require an introduction. For now, a brief introduction to Quakerism will suffice. Early Quakers were so named because they were said to tremble or quake with religious zeal. The nickname Quaker stuck, now devoid of its original derisiveness. Quakers are also known as Friends, belonging to the Religious Society of Friends. Quakerism was a radical movement against hollow formalism, for a return to the original gospel truth, in the aftermath of the Protestant Reformation.

George Fox, the leader, believed that the Scriptures must be read in the same Spirit that inspired those who wrote them. He and his followers rejected the ecclesiastical authority of their day. Their movement represented a call to return to the original, primitive Christianity. Predictably, Quakers were branded as heretics and persecuted. Quakerism has survived but has shown resilience in preserving its original intentions, not to become itself orthodoxy. Today, the friendly Quakers, no longer quaking, may be seen doing their work for peace and the betterment of humankind everywhere.

The central beliefs of Quakerism are at once simple and deceptively simple. Simple, because they are stated in simple words, accessible to most people. Deceptively simple, because deeper meanings rooted in Quaker traditions and the "testimonies" of exemplary Quakers cannot be understood in words alone. They have to be lived, witnessed in the deeds of daily life.

Without getting too deeply into Quaker theology, I find this core belief to be the most illuminating: There is an indwelling Seed, Christ, or Light (which may be interpreted as metaphors) within all persons that, if heeded, will guide them and shape their lives. From this simple idea springs a wealth of spiritual implications.

The core belief is a statement of ecumenicity: The Light is within *all* persons, that is, everywhere. It erases, therefore, the artificial divide between the secular and the religious, so that all of life may be lived in the Light. Each person I meet is potentially inspired and inspirational. When I shun or reject one, I deprive myself of an inspirational channel to spirituality; when I embrace one, I enrich myself spiritually.

What a creative and powerful idea! God is directly accessible to all persons without the need of an intermediary priest or ritual. Quakerism rejects, therefore, ecclesiastical authority and "empty forms" of worship (e.g., set prayers, words, and rituals). All persons are to be equally valued. No wonder the Quaker organization is an ultimate democracy.

Buddhism and Quakerism share much in common. Of the world's major religions, Buddhism stands out in its appeals: nonviolence, compassion, and respect for life in all its forms. Through supreme effort, a person has the potential to reach enlightenment (Ho, 1995). This idea is truly radical, for it implies the possibility of altering the cosmic flow of events, namely, breaking the cycle of births and rebirths, through conscious self-direction. In sum, both Buddhism and Quakerism are champions of human dignity.

Judge by the Fruits of Two Trees

With this brief introduction to Quakerism, we are now better positioned to make a judgment. The fruits of Fox may be found in Quakers' humanitarian mission of service outreach, programs of education and social action; the fruits of Hitler are death by the millions, unprecedented destruction, and the Holocaust.

Quakers were victims of persecution; Nazis persecuted innocent victims. Quakers are led by love; Nazis are consumed by hate. Quakers do not have a creed, but "testimonies" expressed in individual lives and collective actions; Nazis have *Mein Kampf* as their bible. Quakerism is inclusionary, tolerant of diversity; Nazism is exclusionary, obdurate in its insistence on purity.

Quakers believe that each person has the divine potential to be guided by an indwelling Light or Truth, without the need for intermediary priests; Nazis demand absolute obedience to the Führer. Quakers believe in self-direction and self-determination; Nazis excel in mind control.

Quakers are pacifists; Nazis are warmongers. Quakers value the individual man, woman, and child equally, without distinction; Nazis believe in Aryan superiority. The Quaker Way of decision making and governance is not the rule of the majority, but a deliberate process of resolving differences, in which the opinion of every single person is respected and heard; Nazi governance is the embodiment of totalitarianism, where the voice of the Führer drowns out all others.

Concluding Thoughts

Religiosity is not always benign; when it is based on absolutism or wedded to fanaticism, it can be outright dangerous. However, there is no necessary or predestined connection between madness and evil. Benign and malignant madness can be differentiated on the basis of directional actions toward good or evil taken by a mad person. Yes, we may identify mad geniuses who have acted as champions of human dignity throughout history. Again, madness may be linked to good rather than to evil, to peace rather than to violence, and to human dignity rather than to degradation. We may reflect on this hypothetical chain of possibilities: Devoid of madness, religious leaders would lose much of their charisma, singularity of purpose, and resolute determination; consequently, the world might be deprived of its great religious traditions. Is this a good or a bad thing? I'm not sure. The reader has to answer for himself.

Thematic Group 2

Individual Versus Collective Madness

Most of us, professionals or laypersons, are conditioned to think of mental illness as an individual phenomenon. Psychopathology is indeed located within the individual. But the collective manifestations of psychopathology by a group of people become sociopathology.

Extraordinary social pathologies have appeared in many guises throughout history. Mass madness emerged during the last half of the Middle Ages in Europe, involving the widespread occurrence of collective disorders such as group hysteria. Dancing manias (epidemics of raving, jumping, dancing, and convulsions), commonly known as St. Vitus' dance, appeared in Europe. In the marketplace, the town's people would dance wildly, tear off their clothes, beat one another, roll on the ground, drink, sing, or talk incessantly. Such frenzied excitement may be viewed as a transient sociopathological phenomenon in which fears and tensions might be collectively released.

In the United States, the rise in homicides, suicides, cases of opioid addiction, and the like are certainly not individual phenomena, but are rooted in the current sociopolitical climate characterized by loss of civility and societal order, political polarization, increasing disparity between the rich and the poor. The reader may come up with more examples of collective madness in the modern world. She may also decide on the extent to which the Trump phenomenon (described in Chapter 13) falls into the category of collective madness.

Even the *Diagnostic and Statistical Manual of Mental Disorders* acknowledges the existence of nonindividual mental disorders, such as Shared Psychotic Disorder (Folie à deux). However, its lack of attention to interpersonal, individual-family, individual-community relations in which the individual functions constitutes a major flaw. From a theoretical viewpoint, system theory and particularly family and marital therapy are based on an analysis of these relations, not on the single person alone.

The ethical, societal, and political contexts of mental health and disorder are examined in this thematic group of chapters. The ethical concerns values underlying mental health practice; the societal provides a framework for a better understanding of the mental health crises in America and China; finally, the political puts the focus on the alliance between Trump and evangelical Christians.

11

Societal Mental Health Crises in America and China

> *Your birth was a crisis, for you and your mother, to which you owe your life outside her womb.*

> *The record of accomplishment of the American mental health establishment can only be depicted as collective impotence.*

The Chinese term for crisis *weiji* consists of two characters, *wei* (peril) and *ji* (opportunity). Embedded in this term is the message that the perils of life provide opportunities to overcome them and consequently to grow.

This message echoes the problem of evil that bedevils Christianity: Why should there be human pain and suffering if God is omnipotent, omniscient, and perfectly good? (For a discussion on the birth of evil, see Ho, 2019b, Chapter 4.8 "Descent into Hell: A Dialogue Between Jesus and Lucifer.") The Christian answer is that allowing evil may make possible greater goods: Evil affords humans opportunities to demonstrate their forbearance, fortitude, and moral stamina. It tests and strengthens their faith in God. Those who have suffered will be eventually compensated. Salvation lies in acceptance, not in questioning God's purpose.

But what exactly is a crisis in the first place? Crises follow us like a shadow throughout our lives. Birth is a crisis, for you and your mother, to which you owe your life outside her womb. The causes of a crisis are many, some natural, some unnatural: being laid off, going through a divorce, losing a significant other, or facing a life-threatening event (e.g., diagnosed with a severe disease).

I am now going to make a bold statement: There is no *necessary* connection between a crisis and personal trauma. A crisis may be defined objectively, in terms of how it is rated on a scale of severity by a representative group of people. It may also be defined subjectively, in terms of how it is perceived personally and how it affects the person concerned. The crucial question is how you react to the crisis. It is also entirely possible that a person does not construe as a crisis what other people do in the first place. In that case, there is no trauma to speak of.

Here is another bold statement to make: There is no *necessary* connection between the severity of the initial trauma and the outcome after a time period. A person may be traumatized by, surviving and recovering from, and even thriving through a crisis (Ho, 2019b, Chapter 5.6 "Crisis Intervention: From Traumatization to Psychological Growth"; Chapter 5.7 "Coping with Life's Misfortunes: Forbearance and Meaning Reconstruction").

Also, note that I am introducing the term *societal mental health* in the title to underscore my thesis that it makes no sense to conceive of the mental health of individuals without reference to the collective mental health of communities and of societies as a whole.

The Mental Health Crisis in America

What Do These Figures Tell Us?

According to the National Institutes of Health, "Nearly one in five U.S. adults live with a mental illness (46.6 million in 2017)." Suicide mortality rates per 100,000 people have risen consistently from 1999 to 2016. The corresponding rise in the number of drug overdose deaths is more dramatic: In 2017, 47,000 Americans died by suicide in comparison with 70,000 from drug overdoses.

Researchers Anne Case and Angus Deaton (2020) have grouped together deaths caused by suicide, drug overdose, and alcoholic liver disease as "deaths of despair." The effect of these deaths is so large in the United States that life spans have decreased since 2015. For many people, daily life lacks the structure, status, and meaning it had before, as the researchers explained. People feel less connected to an employer, a labor union, a church or community groups; they are less likely to be married, and more likely to report being unhappy.

On May 11, 2022, the American Medical Association released a statement on overdose deaths:

> We know the overdose epidemic is ravaging this country, and the National Center for Health Statistics tally of about 107,000 deaths in the past year confirms the problem is getting worse. Behind the numbers is thousands of grieving families. We need to help patients and their families with medically proven approaches to addiction.
>
> Among the actions we recommend . . . hold insurers accountable for repeated, willful violations of state and federal mental health . . . and substance use disorder parity laws.
>
> At this time next year, we hope that the treatment landscape has changed, and we again will not be shaking our heads about the damage caused by this epidemic.

The most noteworthy point in the statement is to "hold insurers accountable for repeated, willful violations" of laws. That is a clear admission that the epidemic of overdose deaths is driven by socioeconomic forces over which the medical profession is powerless to control. My prediction is less optimistic: We will continue to be shaking our heads in the foreseeable future.

The figures I have reported are alarming. They are telling us that the overall mental health status of Americans is poor in comparison with most other rich countries. Furthermore, socioeconomic status is a major determinant of health and life expectancy: an unmistakable reflection of the underlying socioeconomic pathology associated with increasing disparity between the rich and the poor in American society.

When the figures are gauged against the enormousness of the American mental health establishment, a great irony stares us in the face. According to the United States Department of Labor's Bureau of Labor Statistics (2017), there were over 577,000 mental health professionals practicing in the U.S. whose main focus is the treatment and/or diagnosis of mental health or substance abuse concerns. Numbering 166,000, clinical and counseling psychologists continue to make up the largest segment of mental health professionals. In all, the U.S. mental health establishment, particularly the psychological, dwarfs those in other countries. The record of accomplishment, however, can only be depicted as collective impotence.

As a professor of clinical psychology, I have pointed to this great irony in *Rewriting Psychology: An Abysmal Science?* (Ho, 2019b; see also "The Limitations of Psychologism" in Chapter 12). Of what use is clinical psychology if it does not solve the pressing mental health problems of the day? A thorough professional self-examination is long overdue.

Mass Shootings in America Is Preventable Evil

Witness the deadly shooting in Las Vegas on October 11, 2017, one of the worst in a seemingly unending repetition of senseless mass slaughters in American society. One noteworthy and perverse reaction was the rise in stock prices of firearm companies following the shooting, which means that more people will die from mass shootings in the future. In contrast, gun-control laws enacted in Australia have resulted in a dramatic decline in firearm-related deaths, especially suicide.

Confronted with such psychosocial pathologies, psychologists have no effective answer. Here again is a paradox: A society that has an army of psychologists appears nowhere near to solving its psychosocial problems. In particular, a country that has more therapists (and other mental health professionals) than the rest of the world combined is also unable to solve its mental health problems.

Meanwhile, an industry of health promotion has emerged on an unprecedented scale. Transcendental meditation, yoga, and mindfulness-based stress reduction, and the like, all originating from Asia, appear to have gained more popularity in the United States than in Asia itself. Repackaged, they are promoted in an organized business fashion, but devoid of their religious-philosophical roots.

Why does psychology have such a poor record of solving societal and mental health problems? Partly because psychologists, preoccupied with micro phenomena, tend to neglect macro problems relevant to the human condition. Misguided by psychologism, they expend their energies on curative measures (e.g., psychotherapy) rather than on preventive actions (e.g., community-based programs aimed at enhancing the health of individuals and communities, strategies for conflict resolution and tension reduction).

Treating the Mentally Ill as Criminals

In January 2021, the police in Rochester, NY, released body-camera footage showing how multiple officers, while responding to a "family trouble" call, ill-treated a 9-year-old girl while in obvious distress. In one video, she was shown sobbing and struggling against the cuffs as officers tried to force her into a patrol car. The officers chided her; one told her she was "acting like a child." She responded: "I am a child" and pleaded with them to stop forcing her into the car. The video shows, minutes later, an officer pepper-spraying the girl, leaving her crying in the back seat.

Obviously, the police officers were not just using excessive force; they were behaving in the most uncaring, unprofessional manner toward a child. There is, however, another aspect of this case that deserves no less attention. The police officer who responded to the call for help was told that the girl was "suicidal." If so, why didn't he refer the case to a social service agency with personnel trained to deal with such family troubles or mental disturbances?

Not long ago, Pete Earley wrote for the Washington post: "Americans with mental illnesses make up nearly a quarter of those killed by police officers." He has highlighted mental illness as a specific issue that many experts believe is crucial to reducing police-related violence. One major reason is that very often police officers, rather than mental health professionals, are the first to respond to mentally ill individuals displaying socially disruptive or violent behavior.

To understand why we have come to such an abnormal situation, I recommend reading *Insane: America's Criminal Treatment of Mental Illness*. The author Alisa Roth (2018) states: "There's an epidemic of police shootings of people with mental illness." The book is an exposé of the mental health crisis in our courts, jails, and prisons. America has made mental illness a crime: Jails in New York, Los Angeles, and Chicago each house more people with mental illnesses than any hospital; as many as half of all inmates in America's jails and prisons have a psychiatric disorder. Perlin and Lynch (2018) have forced upon public consciousness the shaming and shameful arrest policies of urban police departments in the United States in their treatment of persons with mental disturbances.

To gain a historical perspective, let me draw on my experiences as a clinical psychologist working with state mental hospitals (see Ho, 1965). Back in the 1960s, these hospitals were places of hopelessness, where inmates were commonly locked up in smelly wards and given no effective treatment. The one I worked in was a monstrosity with more than 5,000 inmates, passive, resigned, and in despair.

More than half a century later, prisons have in large measure become our mental asylums: The Bureau of Justice Statistics estimates that some 365,000 American adults with serious mental illness are behind bars and an additional 770,000 are on probation or parole. Mentally ill Americans are behind bars because, too often, they have nowhere else to go. Two generations of policy have led to the mass closing of state mental hospitals (such as the one I worked in) without providing adequately for community backup mental health services.

Back in the nineteenth century, Dorothea Dix, influenced by Quaker reformers, fought a heroic battle for "lunacy reform" to obligate the government to provide humane care for the mentally ill in large-scale asylums. Today, some thoughtful mental health professionals are calling for a return of the asylum or, to use a much better term, "therapeutic community." What irony! We really haven't made any progress in almost two centuries; meanwhile, the mentally ill have suffered more indignities.

Stopping the Police from Killing the Mentally Ill

Finally, how may we reduce police-related violence? The problem with police brutality will not go away unless we confront its root causes: racism, inequality, the pervasive breakdown of the family among minority groups (too many adult men locked up in prison), too many guns around (thanks to the NRA), and relying on "superior fire power" to solve what are basically social problems.

Police in the United States are already the most militarized among democratic countries. The so-called nonlethal weapons (rubber bullets, flash-bangs and beanbag rounds) regularly used by law enforcement officials can cause serious, and even fatal, injuries. One analysis found that 15 percent of people injured by rubber bullets and similar objects were left with permanent disabilities. Also, research suggests that tear gas could amplify the spread of the coronavirus.

Equipping the police with nonlethal weapons is very costly. So, one reasonable way of stopping the police from killing the mentally ill suggests itself: Reallocate at least a part of the resources for procuring more and more nonlethal weapons used by police officers to enhance the capability of mental health agencies. Correspondingly, procedural-structural changes have to be made such that mental health professionals, rather than police officers, would be the frontline workers to respond to mentally ill individuals displaying socially disruptive or violent behavior. Instead of dialing 911, another hotline should be provided for the mentally ill and their families, relatives, or friends to ask for help from mental health professionals.

Would police departments object to such a reallocation of resources? Reason would suggest that the answer is no: Police officers are trained to prevent crime, not to deal with madness. Wouldn't they gain pride by ridding themselves of the stigma of being killers of mentally ill people? In any case, political leaders in a democracy have an obligation to ensure that police departments operate to protect all citizens, not to kill illegally or unnecessarily.

Psychology and Psychiatry in China

The status of Chinese social sciences pales in comparison with that of the physical sciences, which lead the world in some specific areas such as quantum computation and space exploration. In particular, my overall assessment is that social psychology has always been the least developed among the social sciences. The system discriminates against publications in Chinese. Academics scramble to publish in English-language journals or books because publications in Chinese count much less in promotional evaluations.

A Note on the Historical Development of Psychiatry

Mental disorders have long been recognized and described since ancient times. Here is a quotation from the *Yellow Emperor's Classic of Internal Medicine* composed during the Han dynasty (206 BCE–220 CE) or later:

> The person suffering from excited insanity initially feels sad, eating and sleeping less; he then becomes grandiose, feeling that he is very smart and noble, talking and scolding day and night, singing, behaving strangely, seeing strange things, hearing strange voices, believing he can see the devil or gods.

Today, practitioners of traditional Chinese medicine (TCM) work closely with physicians trained in Western medicine. TCM is holistic in nature, devoid of the body-mind dichotomy conceptualization of the West. Disorder is thought to be resulting from the loss of balance between forces or energies that are both antagonistic and complementary to each other. It therefore follows that treatment is a matter of restoring balance, through changes in lifestyle and diet, acupuncture, therapeutic massage, taking herbal medicine, or other techniques.

TCM is based on systemic-dialectical thinking. Interactions between yin-yang and the five elements (or five phases) are of paramount importance. These interactions include those between physiological subsystems within an individual and between an individual and his social or natural environment. The philosophical basis of TCM is grounded in empiricism (clinical observations); the causes of mental disorders are believed to be natural rather than supernatural; the goal of treatment is health and longevity, not just the curing of disease.

Psychiatry as a medical specialty is a modern achievement. Its development in the People's Republic of China (PRC) provides a stark contrast to that in America, particularly with respect to its lack of resources, manpower, and scientific research. As Ho (1974) reported:

> Pre-1949 China had only a handful of trained psychiatrists and almost negligible facilities for treatment relative to the needs of this populous country.... There were only a few psychiatric hospitals located in major cities and only about 50 to 60 psychiatrists in the whole country; large numbers of mental patients were roaming the streets, left unattended. (pp. 620–622)

The development of psychiatry in the PRC represented a progression in shifting the focus of attention from individual patients to the entire social milieu in which they live and work. A trend in the approach to treatment may be discerned: decreasing reliance on physical techniques (excluding acupuncture) and especially the use of drugs, accompanied by increasing attention to the therapeutic potential of social interaction.

Several salient features deserve attention: belief in the educability of patients and hence in their curability; stressing patients' self-reliance and acceptance of responsibility; using a variety of treatments, including techniques based on TCM; emphasizing "collective help" and downgrading "professionalism"; and, most important, putting prevention first.

It should be noted that Ho's report covers developments up to 1974. Nonetheless, what is worthy of attention is that the Chinese were able to put their ideas into practice on a massive scale within a relatively short period of time. Furthermore, these ideas were not imported, but have emerged from experience gained through practice within the framework of Chinese sociopolitical culture. Mental health workers elsewhere are challenged to the extent that the Chinese experience has provided a viable alternative to existing approaches: It demonstrates what can be done when the whole society is mobilized and when limited resources are utilized effectively.

Clinical Death During the Great Cultural Revolution

Ironically, in the early days of the People's Republic, Marxist critiques of psychological testing held sway. Now, development is largely instrument driven, rather than concept driven. Clinical psychologists seem to rely on instruments to define their identity and maintain their respectability. Without their tests, would they know what to do? Do they "serve the people" (a slogan in China)?

During the Great Cultural Revolution, psychology was banned as an academic discipline for ideological reasons—in a way that outperformed Lysenko's suppression of genetics, supported by Stalin, in the Soviet Union during the 20th century. The decisive blow to psychology came from the propaganda chief of the Communist Party, Yao Wenyuan (one of the "gang of four" during the Great Cultural Revolution), who denounced psychology as bourgeois metaphysics, not only useless but also dangerous in undermining communist ideology.

Bizarre as it may now occur to us, he began his denunciation with the choice of an unlikely target: a psychological study of color and form preferences! This led to a complete shutdown of all psychological activities in academic and research institutions. I have to admit that Yao's "creative use of language" as a weapon has few equals in terms of perversity and destructiveness.

Why is psychology such a dangerous thing? Because it is privileged to make pronouncements on human nature. To Mao Zedong, bourgeois pronouncements on human nature serve to nullify class antagonism and blunt class struggle (Ho, 1978). The so-called theory of human nature is an ideological product of the ruling classes enshrined as a universal truth. Mao insisted that people's thoughts and feelings, even love, are invariably stamped with their class character, without exception. He stated in 1942:

> There is only human nature in the concrete, no human nature in the abstract. *In class society* [italics added for emphasis], there is only human nature of a class character. . . . The human nature boosted by certain petty-bourgeois intellectuals . . . is in essence nothing but bourgeois individualism. (p. 394)

The statement leaves open the question of what human nature would be like in a classless or communist society. Individual variation is a given in Mao Zedong Thought, as it is in Marxism. Marx's statement, "From each according to his ability; to each according to his needs," clearly implies a recognition of individuality.

Thus, what Mao repudiated was bourgeois individualism (indiscipline, selfishness), not creativity or individuality; what he upheld was the solidarity of the working class, not total uniformity. Unfortunately, this important point has not been grasped by his dogmatic, doctrinaire followers. During my visit to mainland China in 1971, when psychology was in a state of clinical death, the cadres I talked with negated individuality: Uniformity in following Mao Zedong Thought was paramount; individual differences were of no consequence.

Translated from Chinese, Mao Zedong Thought is a noun phrase in which *Thought* is capitalized and grammatically singular to underscore its established status as an integral body of knowledge. It results from the collective efforts of learning from the summation of experience and is characterized by dialectical thinking (see Ho, 2019b, Chapter 2.2 "Dialectics of Thought and Action: A General Method for Problem Solving"; in press-a). I am not amused when Mao's followers, infected with a syndrome commonly known in China as "cognitive ossification," follow Mao Zedong Thought as if Mao thought only once!

The demolishment of psychology during the Great Cultural Revolution is surely the darkest chapter in the history of psychology. Mental health practice did not merely undergo a crisis; it sank into a state of clinical death. What can we learn from it? Never forget that psychology or any other social science does not exist in a vacuum: It is always under the influence, even control, of the sociopolitical system within which it operates.

Catching Every Imaginable Disease in Western Clinical Psychology

My perusal of psychology journals in China reveals many of the same "malpractices" that I have found in Western journals. In addition, copycat research borrowed from the West is common. There is an overabundance of technical, soulless research aimed at the development of measuring instruments; but a dearth of needed research devoted to addressing pressing societal problems. It pains to see scarce resources diverted to socially irrelevant activities (e.g., constructing yet more self-report questionnaires and administering them to students). We may know more about psychology, but less about people (similarly, more about sociology, and less about society)—as in the West.

As regards mental health, there is the same bias as in the West for treatment over prevention and for intervention at the individual level over the group or collective levels. I question the direction into which clinical psychology in China is going. Look at the *Chinese Journal of Clinical Psychology*, the first Chinese language journal in clinical psychology. It is clear that clinical psychology (as elsewhere) is heading for scientism, overspecialization, and narrow professionalism—That is to say, the Chinese have caught every disease imaginable in Western clinical psychology.

Environmental and population psychology, both urgently needed, are still only at an embryonic stage of development (see Chapter 15).

Concluding Thoughts

Statistics is anything but boring. The statistical figures I have reported tell us that individual mental health is intertwined with societal mental health, and that there is no hope of addressing the mental health crisis in America until we confront the root cause of the country's societal pathologies arising largely from its structural socioeconomic inequalities. The reader may have noticed the sense of urgency with which the author writes about the mental health crisis in America. Please then accept this author's invitation to participate intellectually in the subsequent search for solutions. As to mental health practice in China, my strongest wish is that its future development will embrace the systemic-dialectical thinking inherent in traditional Chinese medicine, and not catch the "disease" now afflicting American clinical psychology and psychiatry.

12

Values Underlying Mental Health Practice

The superior physician treats the country, the middle physician treats the person, the inferior physician treats the disease...The superior physician treats the disease before it arises, the middle physician treats the disease as it is developing, the inferior physician treats the disease after it has already developed.
—Sun Simiao, renowned Chinese physician, circa 541–682 CE

American society is in dire need of psychological prophets to preserve lifestyles and social institutions that serve our profound needs for intimacy and community.

Let us examine the application of psychology to mental health. Psychologists are fond of talking about self-actualization. But what is the point of unleashing the individual's creative potentialities, only to witness that they cannot be fulfilled because of degrading social conditions? How honest is it to say that the individual has unlimited choice, when in fact most people in this world are locked in their situation and are severely limited in what they can choose? Self-actualization is escapism unless it entails active participation in social change.

The Limitations of Psychologism

Why does psychology have such a poor record of solving societal and mental problems? Partly because psychologists, preoccupied with micro phenomena, tend to neglect macro problems relevant to the human condition. Misguided by psychologism, they expend their energies on curative measures (e.g., psychotherapy) rather than on preventive actions (e.g., community-based programs aimed at enhancing the health of individuals and of communities, strategies for tension reduction and peace).

Psychology has yet to make its mark at the macro level, in dealing with societal problems such as crime, mass shootings, social injustice, the increasing disparity between the haves and have-nots; or with survival problems confronting humankind as a whole, such as environmental degradation, mass migrations born of despair, interethnic strifes, and outbreaks of war (civil, regional, or global).

Thus, attention should be drawn to the fallacy of pan-psychological approaches to solving recalcitrant problems that have their roots in the pathology of sociopolitical systems. That is why we must redefine psychology's boundaries and priorities. We need a clearer delineation of problems that may be dealt with psychologically (e.g., through psychotherapy) versus those to which psychological approaches are irrelevant or nonapplicable.

I contend that the potent determinants of mental health and, more generally, the quality of life are located externally in the sociopolitical system, not internally within the individual. Mental health professionals are handmaidens of those with the power to make decisions which have serious bearings on mental health, or caretakers of a society that has failed to meet the mental needs of its members. They promise little more than some emotional release or consolation—transitory, illusory escapes into "mental health"—while social conditions which dictate the quality of life remain unchanged. The idea of mental health then turns into an opiate of the mind—as Marx says of religion. In the face of ugly social reality, we make a travesty of enhancing the individual's potentialities.

According to the present conception, the realization of human potentiality differs from self-actualization, which humanistic psychologists have long extolled. Rather, it takes a dialectical form (Ho, in press-a): the collective actualization of individuals-in-community and, simultaneously, the reflection of this actualization within the individual self. This conception is far removed from Friedrich Nietzsche's Last Man in *Thus spoke Zarathustra*, the human condition of mass stagnant mediocrity.

The imperative need for an examination of the value assumptions underlying psychological practice becomes all the more apparent when we reflect on the paradoxical situation in America: A society which has more clinical psychologists (and other mental health professionals) than the rest of the world combined appears nowhere near to solving its mental health problems. Clearly, the answer to these problems does not lie in escalating manpower and other resources alone. I submit that there are deeply entrenched value orientations in American society which impede mental health efforts and which, more fundamentally, lie at the root of many of its psychosocial pathologies.

Self-Reliance Rooted in Individualism

Presently, I confine myself to the discussion of one of the most salient of these entrenched values, namely, self-reliance rooted in individualism. Applied to the mentally disturbed, self-reliance is a major determinant of how they will be viewed and treated by society. Two broad classes may be distinguished: first-class patients who remain self-reliant and are in a position to secure professional help on a private basis, and second-class patients who have to rely on publicly funded institutions or drop out of the societal system altogether. Among mental health professionals, too, the same class distinction may be discerned, in most cases depending on whether the professional is engaged in private practice (or in a privately funded institution) or employed in a publicly funded institution (Ho, 1965).

The ideological basis for this class distinction may be traced to the Protestant ethic, in particular, the Calvinist doctrine of predestination. Psychologist Rotenberg (1974) argues that the underlying beliefs of Protestantism and of people-changing systems are inherently contradictory. According to the doctrine of predestination, all people-changing systems are futile in the final analysis. Further, the same doctrine classifies people into two dichotomized groups, on the basis of their success or failure (mainly material) here on earth: the "good-elect" and the "wicked-damned." In psychopathology, this dichotomy translates into classifying people into the "treatable-elect" (neurotics) and the "untreatable-damned" (psychopaths, psychotics) groups. Psychotherapists have shown a traditional preference for treating the former while shunning the latter.

I would argue that the same underlying ideology has been a major factor which impedes the community mental health movement in the United States. Despite the early enthusiasm for community mental health centers, their promises have remained largely unfulfilled. Worse, prisons have in large measure become our modern mental asylums.

Deeply ingrained in the American psyche is a stubborn resistance, even hostility, to the idea of using public resources to help people who are unable to take care of themselves and have failed to meet the primary requirement of social adequacy, that is, self-reliance. If salvation is a matter of individual responsibility, then it is up to the individual to make the necessary efforts for change. If you live in a slum, then it is up to you, and you alone, to try to move out of the slum, improve your lot, and be counted among the "successful-elect." Of course, the slum remains, and countless others remain the "wicked-damned."

There is clearly an ideological bias underlying traditional approaches to intervention (e.g., counseling and psychotherapy) that define the individual, not the individual-in-community, as the object of treatment. At rock bottom, individualism is alien to the notion of community; and the doctrine of predestination, in particular, is antithetical to values embodied in the concept of community mental health.

As a therapist, I cannot accept the Calvinist doctrine of predestination. My conception of salvation is ecumenical, hence inclusionary. Salvation extends to all humanity; no one is excluded. Furthermore, personal salvation is linked to the salvation of others. This conception clashes with Christian fundamentalism head on (see Chapter 13).

Crisis in Values

In recent years, perceptive observers have voiced their concern over the deterioration of traditional values in American society. Individualism vulgarized and reinforced by misguided moral relativism leads to the absurd and dangerous position that there are no standards of conduct whatsoever.

Bizarre behavior is sanctioned in the name of originality; antisocial behavior is rationalized on the ground that society, not the individual, is sick; even psychotic-like behavior may be somehow regarded as "normal" if it "fits" into some subcultural or countercultural context. Ironically, individuality degenerates into conformity, under the social pressure that one has to display one's "uniqueness"—being apart and different from, and hence superior to, the crowd. Freedom degenerates into rampant irresponsibility, disregard for others, or just plain selfishness. The symptoms of a crisis in values can be read.

The late George Albee (1977), a champion of primary prevention, attributes the deterioration of traditional values to the decline of the Protestant ethic, which

Weber has identified as the spirit of capitalism. Albee states: "The ethic underlying the survival of capitalism is disappearing as the system struggles to create an impulse-indulgent society of consumers, and psychotherapists have become the new gurus explaining life's elusive purpose."

Edward Sampson (1988) has characterized the self-contained individual as one "needing or wanting no one, avoiding interdependence and contact with others so as to secure one's own satisfaction." He argues that "in an era in which collective problem solving is necessary, the perpetuation of self-contained, individualistic conceptions can stifle psychology's efforts to contribute to resolving contemporary social issues."

I submit that clinical psychologists, especially those enthusiastic about the encounter movement (sensitivity training, T-groups, encounter groups) in America, have been instrumental in promoting self-contained individualism, wittingly or unwittingly. Psychologist Sigmund Koch has denounced the movement as providing "a convenient psychic whorehouse for the purchase of a gamut of well-advertised existential 'goodies': authenticity, freedom, wholeness, flexibility, community, love, joy. One enters for such liberating consummations but settles for psychic striptease." The late Professor of Clinical Psychology S. J. Korchin (1976) has a more forgiving, balanced assessment:

> The encounter movement started ... as a protest against the growing loss of a sense of psychological community in contemporary America. At its best, it is a groping toward new social institutions and new life styles to replace those which no longer serve our profound needs for intimacy and community. At its worst, it perverts and cheapens those needs. . . .. In a time of deteriorating social values, it may also represent a frenzied quest for individual pleasure and indulgence which serves as an escape from confronting the true problems.

Korchin is accurate in his diagnosis. It would then make better sense to identify, preserve, and enhance those social institutions and lifestyles rooted in the culture that serve "our profound needs for intimacy and community," rather than to rely on the artificiality of creating new ones. If humanistic psychologists like Maslow and Rogers are the modern prophets of individualism, then Albee, Korchin, and Sampson are among the counterprophets who insist that we must search for alternatives to confront "the true problems."

In contrast to self-contained individualism, collectivism affirms that to preserve and enhance the well-being of the group is the supreme guiding principle for social action. As such, collectivism is exemplified by the traditional Chinese ethos. Individuality is negated to the extent that pressure toward conformity is exerted on members of the group. In return, the members are assured of collective economic and psychological security inaccessible to the individualist. Built-in group mechanisms would ensure that their basic needs are met. Each member of the group is related to other members in a network of interlocking responsibilities and obligations. The spontaneity in the readiness to give and to accept aid is an element lacking in formalized public aid institutions.

I would add that a cardinal symptom of the deterioration of traditional values is the manifestation of individualism in the mass culture under new guises, variously described as the "new narcissism" and "self-contained individualism." Peter Marin describes the new narcissism as a "trend toward deification of the isolated self" and "lifeboat ethics." A classic statement of the new narcissism is the so-called Gestalt prayer written by Fritz Perls in 1969.

> I do my thing and you do your thing.
> I am not in this world to live up to your expectations,
> And you are not in this world to live up to mine.
> You are you, and I am I, and if by chance we find each other, it's beautiful.
> If not, it can't be helped.

In *Culture of Narcissism*, Christopher Lasch considers narcissism to be both a cause and an effect of rampant individualism. His widely popular jeremiad published in 1978 put narcissism on the cultural map of America, prompting intellectuals to become concerned with the purported rise of narcissism as well as to engage in endless debates about America's self-image as a nation of narcissistic individuals. A notable example is Elizabeth Lunbeck's *The Americanization of Narcissism*, a scholarly book published in 2014.

Loneliness Is Lethal

In Chapter 6, I have already raised the question of spirituality-in-communion versus spirituality-in-isolation. Loneliness and social isolation are among the true problems in the age of narcissism and self-contained individualism. In the United States, a survey by the American Association for Retired Persons in 2018 found 1 in 3 adults older than 45 is lonely. Loneliness and social isolation constitute one of the important factors contributing to suicide.

There is also substantial evidence that being socially connected reduces the risk for premature mortality; conversely, lacking social connectedness increases the risk (see the *Public Policy and Aging Report* published in January 2018). Moreover, the risk estimates exceed those associated with obesity, air pollution, smoking, and physical inactivity. Additionally, an American Cancer Society study of 580,000 people found that the most isolated White Americans were up to 84% more likely to die from all causes than the least isolated.

Clearly, in light of such evidence, loneliness and social isolation have yet to receive due attention from public health institutions. Everywhere, I see single individuals doing their own thing, without a partnership or family. In public places, it is quite a sight to see a line of individuals all looking at their cell phones, without paying the slightest attention to the people around them. The rise of Facebook, Twitter, and the like is both a symptom and a cause of loneliness: a symptom because they meet a need of the lonely; a cause because obviously the more time you spend on such media the less time you have for face-to-face social interactions. American society, as elsewhere, is in dire need of psychological prophets to preserve lifestyles and social institutions that serve our profound needs for intimacy and community.

In the United States, prescriptions for anti-anxiety medications rose and sleep-aides have increased significantly during the pandemic; and psychiatrists prescribed 86% more for psychotropic drugs, primarily antidepressants. Prescriptions such as these can lead to a sort of addiction or pathological dependency on medication. What is profitable for pharmaceutical companies is abhorrible for a nation already having too many over-medicated individuals.

Actually, Americans have been "social distancing" long before the pandemic. The Joint Economic Committee reported that, between 1974 and 2016, the number of adults who said they spent an evening with a neighbor at least several times a week dropped from 30% to 19%. Not surprisingly, a survey by the American Association for Retired Persons in 2018 found 1 in 3 adults older than 45 is lonely.

Unfortunately, such is the preexisting condition under which the coronavirus contagion arrives in America: The deaths of despair (caused by suicide, drug overdose, and alcoholic liver disease) are already alarmingly high. More suicides and other mental health problems will add to the lethal consequences of the pandemic as people practice necessary, even compulsory, social distancing—locked up as "prisoners" in their homes. There is no excuse to regard such a tragic outcome as unforeseen.

Reallocate Resources: Put Prevention First

Many lessons may be learned in the light of negative aspects of the American experience. In particular, what are the strategies to be adopted that may abate tragic outcomes such as an increase in deaths of despair? In this connection, first it is noteworthy to see a Minister of Loneliness appointed in 2018 for the more than 9 million adults who are "often or always lonely" in the UK.

I would argue strongly that we should allocate more resources to prevention rather than cure: Create, sustain, and vitalize participatory communitarian programs aimed at enhancing the health of individuals-in-relations and of communities. The rationale is that it makes better sense to identify, preserve, and enhance those social institutions (e.g., the family) and lifestyles rooted in the culture that serve our profound needs for intimacy and community, rather than to rely on the artificiality of creating new ones (e.g., sensitivity training, T-groups, encounter groups).

These cutting remarks, please note, are coming from a clinical psychologist who has spent decades of his professional life teaching and training therapists. When will mental professionals wake up to the fact that relying on curative measures (e.g., counseling or therapy) alone will not fulfill their collective responsibility? People are fundamentally social creatures that do not thrive in loneliness, lack of security, or violence.

A strategy for prevention and intervention suggests itself: Support systems rooted in the culture may be mobilized to help people in difficulties. In this way, cultural forces are enlisted to serve psychology. Unfortunately, again, too many psychologists in China (and, more generally, in Asia), having been captivated by the values of Western individualism, fail to appreciate and capitalize on this strategy. This would contribute to their sense of alienation, which is rarely articulated. A moment of reflection, too, suggests that there is no reason why the same argument presently advanced cannot be applied in Western contexts as well. Collectivist values offer an antidote to the excesses and misdirection of self-contained individualism.

In Maoist dialectics (Ho, 1978, 2019b, Chapter 2.2 "Dialectics of Thought and Action: A General Method of Problem Solving"; in press-a), individualism and collectivism are not mutually exclusive categories. Rather, they represent an instance of the identity of opposites, according to his philosophy of contradiction. The implication is that it is possible to create a form of social organization in which the best elements of both are preserved: individuality, freedom, democracy, human rights, and the intrinsic worth of the individual from individualism; selflessness, discipline, the unity of purpose and action, and collective creativity from collectivism. To be extirpated are indiscipline and selfishness from Western individualism; pseudoharmony, complete uniformity, paternalism, and hierarchical social ordering from Chinese collectivism.

Likewise, the individual and the group are not to be seen as antagonistic entities. To begin with, each depends on the other for its existence: Without individuals, there is no group to speak of; without the group, the very notion of individual identity loses meaning. With individual variation, there will be no contradictions to impel change, and the group would come to a standstill. Without a functional group, there would be no security for the individual. Hence, the individual must assume responsibility and participate in the betterment of society, in the process of which he may transform himself to be a better person. The importance that Mao accords to individuality counters the collectivist inhibition of individuation; his conviction in the inherently unlimited human potentiality for self-transformation adds a new, profound dimension to our conception of human development.

Concluding Thoughts

In an American community for "active seniors" where I now live, I see elderly folks taking a walk with their dogs, but rarely with young children. The community seems intent on discouraging young people from being present, enforced by its many regulations. In large measure, dogs have replaced humans for companionship. I think to myself, "Dogs show unconditional positive regard toward people unconditionally. In this respect, they excel over people. But they don't talk back! I still miss the people I knew who talked back to me." Meanwhile, an industry has sprung into existence—psychotherapy for dogs, which is probably more successful than psychotherapy for humans. You can guess why. In contrast, going into a Chinese restaurant, I see many of the tables are occupied by families of three generations. Eating a meal is time for the grandpas and the grandmas to enjoy the company of their grandchildren.

We are now prepared to provide an answer to the question: What is the optimal role of psychologists, individually and collectively, to address the emerging challenges of the 21st century? The first point to be acknowledged is that the challenges are grave, exemplified by the menace of what I call the Trump phenomenon (described in Chapter 1), with symptoms such as social divisiveness, moral degeneration among politicians, resistance to COVID-19 vaccination based on scientific illiteracy—Please do not think that authoritarianism wedded to immorality is unique to the United States.

The second is the need to formulate strategies for social action that are rational, effective, and possible within the constraints of our limited powers. I must also ask if we are ready to take a stand on moral issues and assume responsibility for collective actions to meet the grave challenges facing humankind.

How can psychology be reinvented to serve the people? My answer: Why can we not retain our life rooted in the security of family and communitarian institutions that meet our profound needs for intimacy—without losing our freedom, individuality, and respect for human dignity? Changing our conception from individuals-in-isolation to individuals-in-community marks a starting point. A creative synthesis of collectivism and individualism, in which the best elements of both are preserved, points to a hopeful direction for the future of psychology in the East as well as in the West. On the other hand, a society in which the worst elements of both are present is not one people would want to live in.

Actually, I myself find it odd that, as a psychologist, I have to attack psychologism. In particular, I have "poured cold water" on the overreliance on individual therapy among mental health practices—even though I have devoted a bulk of my professional life teaching and training therapists. In the eyes of some of my colleagues, I may be viewed as a "traitor" to their cause. So be it.

The reader may find that my assessment of psychology is too harsh and may disagree with some of my viewpoints. If so, this might be the beginning of a fruitful dialogue. As Confucius says, "The gentleman is conciliatory but remains distinctive vis-a-vis others." And nothing would please me more than to see the day when a reinvented psychology sheds its abysmal symptoms. But why have I talked about Maoist dialectics? (Refer to the introduction to Part II again, if necessary.)

13

The Trump Phenomenon and the Politics of an Unholy Alliance

Knowledge is power; absolutistic knowledge is tyrannical power.

Extreme fundamentalist Christians and Islamic militant jihadists are mirror images of each other.

This chapter presents two related main topics. The first is a psychiatric case study of Donald Trump, a past president of the most powerful nation on earth; going beyond this case study is what I call the Trump phenomenon as a manifestation of socioeconomic pathologies that run deep in America. The second is the political alliance between Trump and powerful evangelical leaders. Together, these two topics reveal the workings of religious and political forces that shape the formation of collective psychosocial pathologies.

Trump and the Trump Phenomenon

History is replete with psychopaths in leadership roles invested with great powers who have caused untold miseries to peoples under their rule or in countries they invade: the likes of Tomás de Torquemada, Heinrich Himmler, Pol Pot, and of late Putin. This lends itself to a question that concerns all of humankind: Is Donald Trump mentally deranged, immoral, or both?

Trump makes an extraordinary case study. He spends a lot of time tweeting, instead of governing. His tweets show impoverished ideation, not to mention subpar literacy. His compulsive use of "trust me" and "believe me" betrays a lack of inner conviction. His habitual denials of lying, publicly seen as lying, are ludicrous. They would qualify him as a pathological liar if he does lack the ability to know that he is lying when he is in fact lying; if he does not lack that ability, he would be a doubly dishonest man denying that he is lying when he knows he is.

Trump is the personification of narcissism. More than that, American Senator Bernie Sanders has said repeatedly that Trump is a pathological liar and is the most dangerous president in American history. Pathological lying is a manifestation of paranoia, a serious mental disorder.

I would like to clarify some relevant clinical points of interest. Different types of liars (e.g., occasional, habitual, and pathological) should be distinguished. Pathological liars are among the most interesting to study; having succeeded in deceiving themselves, they are quite unable to distinguish between fact and fantasy. Also, the presence or absence of an intention to falsify information is a critical factor to consider. The presence of such an intention implies that in the mind of the liar is a distinction between two versions of reality: a "false" version for deceiving others, and a "true" version to be concealed from others. So, is Trump immoral, mentally deranged, or both?

Case Studies

Case studies of Trump by psychiatrists, psychologists, journalists, and even members of his extended family are readily available. Trump's mental impairment is dangerous because he also shows strong psychopathic traits. According to a study by Oxford psychologist Kevin Dutton (2016), Donald Trump has more psychopathic traits than Adolf Hitler.

So, not surprisingly there is consensus among psychiatrists that Trump is mentally deranged. Bandy X. Lee (2019) has edited a book entitled *The Dangerous Case of Donald Trump: 27 Psychiatrists and Mental Health Experts Assess a President*. Dr. Lee invokes the "Duty to Warn" rationale: "Public trust is violated if the profession fails in its duty to alert the public when a person who holds the power of life and death over us all shows signs of clear, dangerous mental impairment."

Americans who voted for Donald Trump should not be surprised that White supremacists and neo-Nazis, emboldened by *their* President, have inflamed ethnic tensions. Contrary to what many have said about him, Trump is highly consistent, hence predictable, in terms of his words and deeds "on many sides," such as bigotry, get-even mentality, chauvinism, narcissism, dishonesty, shamelessness, total lack of self-reflection, and other qualities too numerous to catalog. The trouble, however, is that he is also impulsive, erratic, oblivious to his own inconsistencies; that makes him dangerously unpredictable.

Trump caused great distress to other people worldwide. But according to Allen Frances, also a psychiatrist, Trump "shows no signs himself of experiencing great distress." Really? Just look at his body language, his defensiveness, his increasing tendency for throwing temper tantrums, and so forth. Trump's psychopathology would be far more serious if indeed he is incapable of experiencing distress—the mark of a psychopath devoid of conscience. Nonetheless, I agree with the second part of Frances' statement: "Trump isn't crazy, but our society is."

The Trump Phenomenon

Even more alarming is what I call the Trump phenomenon, one that portends unprecedented perils facing humankind far more than Trump as a person per se. The frightening concentration of power in a handful of political leaders, on whose decisions our survival depends, means that their idiosyncratic dispositions or actions can have magnified, even fateful, consequences for all of us.

The Trump phenomenon is a reflection of the underlying fear of losing supremacy among Americans. Angry about dysfunctional politicians at various levels of government, Americans have chosen a president who is more of the problem than the solution: The cure is worse than the disease, as in medicine. Even now, well after his incompetence and evil intentions are there for all to see, Trump still has a large following, especially among older, less educated, blue-collar Whites.

How does the Trump phenomenon manifest itself? Simmons (2018) has documented how increasing systemic humiliation is associated with the rise of Donald Trump. Just see too the shameless, cowardly Republican politicians who dare not offend Trump and sell their souls for political gain; Fox News as well as conservative, hawkish ideologues that breed political illiteracy; large segments of fundamentalist Christians who speak and act in non-Christian ways. Readers interested in learning more about the Trump phenomenon may read *The Room Where It Happened: A White House Memoir*, authored by a man who was part and parcel of that phenomenon, namely, John Bolton.

The Trump phenomenon is also a manifestation of socioeconomic pathologies that run deep in America: political polarization, societal divisiveness, loss of civility, plutocracy leading to increasing sociopolitical polarization, domination by the military-industrial complex, racism and prejudice, loss of civility and sense of direction. Collectively, these pathologies forebode an irreversible decline in American leadership on the world stage.

Americans have become fed up with their government and insecure about their future. Trump's followers, in particular, are desperate enough to "drink venom to quench their thirst," as a Chinese saying puts it. Finally, the consequences of failing to confront the menace of the Trump phenomenon are too horrible for contemplation.

Trump's "America First" betrays the underlying insecurity that America is losing its leadership in the world. It smacks of "Deutschland über Alles" (Germany above all), a phrase from the German National Anthem, which Nazis reinterpreted as a rallying cry for hegemony and territorial expansion. But the original intention of the Anthem was to place unified nationhood above regional differences. The lesson is that a divided, polarized America cannot be first among equals.

The Unholy Alliance

The politics of societal pathology has not received the attention it deserves, particularly when the roots of the pathology is intimately linked to religion. For this reason, I have decided to delve into the politics of the spectacular rise of evangelicalism and its linkage with the Trump phenomenon.

In June 2020, Trump was honored by the Gateway Church in Dallas, one of the largest megachurches in the world, during a Roundtable on Transition to Greatness: Restoring, Rebuilding, and Renewing. Here is a sample of what he said, followed by enthusiastic applause: "I think the concept of chokeholds sounds so innocent and so perfect"; sending the National Guard to go in Minneapolis to do their work (e.g., tear gassing) was "like a miracle," "a beautiful scene," and "like a knife cutting butter." Observe the mutual admiration in the following excerpt of exchanges between Trump and evangelical leaders.

Trump	So I want to thank Pastors Robert Morris and Steve Dulin. They're great people. (Applause.) Great people with a great reputation. . . .
Pastor Morris	Lord, we need you. We need you at this time in our country. And I thank you for our President. I thank you, Lord, for our leaders. . . . I know in the Bible that, when something was emphasized, it was repeated: "holy, holy, holy". . . . And I thank you for this

	administration. And, Lord, we pray [sic] your blessings and your guidance today on this meeting, in Jesus name.
Bishop Jackson	Father, we thank you so much for what you're doing today. You have revealed so many things that are untoward, even evil. But we ask, according to Isaiah 50, verse 4, that you would give us the tongue of the learned that we should know how to speak to the heart of this nation. . . .. We have a great, courageous President who's a problem solver. And let him speak as your mouthpiece and act as your instrument. . . .. Amen.

This assemblage of evangelicals serves to show strongly they have bonded with Trump, ready to invoke Divine Providence to support him. This bonding may be seen also from survey data. Researchers estimate that around 25% of Americans consider themselves to be evangelical. In 2016, 80% White evangelicals supported Trump over Hillary Clinton. And in May 2020, the Pew Research Center reported that 59% of White evangelical Protestants say the Trump administration has helped evangelicals; most other religious groups tend to be as divided as the U.S. adult population as a whole.

Why does Trump appeal to so many evangelicals? Are they all nincompoops? Astounding, inasmuch as he has persistently violated virtually all basic Christian values: committing the deadly sins of pride (speaking like an egomaniac), covetousness (exploiting his privileged position for personal gains), envy (of Obama), lechery (having sex with a pornstar and other women), and wrath (inciting mob violence).

Actually, however, Trump's appeal to evangelicals is highly predictable, deeply rooted in the psychology of closed mindedness and how it relates to dealing with fear and insecurity. No less predictable is the alliance between the Trump administration and White evangelicals forged by religious, cultural, and political forces running deep in the American psyche. Viewed in this light, the alliance between Trump and evangelicals is an instance of collective psychosocial pathology; it also points to the significance of the political context in which such pathology is manifest.

Explanations for the Alliance

Some obvious explanations for this alliance come to mind. First, evangelicals receive tremendous support to their religious agendas, beliefs, and sentiments (e.g., anti-abortion, abhorrence toward LGBTQ, fear of Muslims) from the Trump administration, particularly powerful officials who are self-identified as evangelicals (Pence and Pompeo). Of course, Trump the consummate opportunist gets what he wants in return: much needed votes from a numerous, reliable religious group. To him, the means justify the ends, no matter how immoral and destructive to democracy.

A second explanation is based on ethnic-cultural considerations, specific to the White folks among evangelicals, who feel increasingly threatened of becoming a minority: It has everything to do with numbers. Trump's hostility toward welcomed immigrants (such as those from the "shit-hole" countries from Latin America) resonates with White evangelical sentiments of being God's favorite among all the peoples on earth.

A third explanation is that salvation reigns supreme to an evangelical. It is highly personal, individualistic; social-collective interests are of a secondary concern. The cardinal aim is to ensure entrance into Heaven and the avoidance of eternal damnation in Hell through embracing Jesus Christ as your personal savior. Everything else is irrelevant or at best secondary in importance. This single mindedness relegates everything else (e.g., social actions for the collective good, social programs aimed to alleviate poverty, affirmative action) to a lower order of priority. Viewed in this light, evangelicalism breeds political illiteracy, which Trump exploits to advance his political agenda.

A fourth explanation is that evangelicals and Trump share common visions in various domains. Some are based on anti-intellectualism and distrust of science (e.g., upholding creationism, rejecting evolution among evangelicals, rejecting scientific evidence on climate change by Trump). Trump's tilted foreign policies in favor of Israel (e.g., moving the American embassy to Jerusalem the Holy City), in sharp contrast to the demonization of and aggressiveness toward Iran, bring great joy to evangelicals.

Thus, the Trump-evangelical alliance solidifies through mutual benefits to be gained. After solidification, rationalization of incongruent convictions sets in: Advancing evangelical privileges overrides concerns over Trump's grave personal flaws, chaotic leadership at home or abroad, and indifference to the sufferings of underprivileged and minority groups.

Delving Deeper into the Human Psyche

Even seasoned commentators, however, have not paid due attention to a more fundamental reason for the Trump appeal to evangelicals deeply rooted in the human psyche: the psychology of closed mindedness and how it relates to dealing with fear and insecurity. To fill this lacuna, I draw from three books that help to answer the puzzling question: Why do so many evangelicals support Trump?

The first book is *The Power Worshippers: Inside the Dangerous Rise of Religious Nationalism* by Katherine Steward (2020). For too long the Religious Right has masqueraded as a sociocultural movement preoccupied with a number of cultural issues, such as abortion and same-sex marriage. Steward's investigative research reveals a disturbing truth: The Religious Right is a political movement that seeks to gain power and to impose its vision on all of society; America's religious nationalists are not just fighting a culture war, but are waging a political war on the norms and institutions of American democracy.

The second is *The Closing of the Western Mind: The Rise of Faith and the Fall of Reason* by Charles Freeman (2005). Freeman traces the closing of the Western mind to the early days of Christianity, when Emperor Constantine declared it the official religion of the Roman Empire. This first alliance of church and state led to the abandonment of the Greek intellectual tradition. Christian leaders stifled debate and dissent to establish an orthodoxy and solidify their position within the state. This development thrust the Western world into the Dark Ages.

The third is *Rewriting Psychology: An Abysmal Science* (Ho, 2019b), which contains extensive discussions of the dialectical tension between reason and religious faiths.

Reportage: Personal Encounters with Evangelicals

I have learned much from direct encounters with evangelicals. A conversation with an evangelical took place soon after the storming of Capitol Hill on January 6 this year. This is the gist of her account of what happened: "The police deliberately let the protestors go inside to set a trap, which resulted in one protester being killed." She remained oblivious to the fact that there were few arrests, in stark contrast to previous massive suppressions of peaceful protests against police brutality all over the country. She made no mention of the violent nature of the storming and its destructive consequences to the democratic institutions of America.

This evangelical dislikes Biden because he is "weak." She is not by nature a violent person herself. But she has demonstrated an amazing ability to distort, rearrange, or simply turn a blind eye to facts that run counter to her political leanings. Other extensive conversations with her reveal an extreme bias in selecting her information news, and her lack of ability to discern facts from rumors, lies, or fake news—a living demonstration that lies or conspiracy theories reiterated ad nauseam may become "facts."

I dwell on this case because she is representative of many other evangelicals. Born into a Christian family, I have had plentiful interactions with evangelical Christians. Once, I said to a group lecturing me on gospel truths, "If Trump goes to Heaven, I don't want to be there!" Thereupon, I was suitably reprimanded. They had failed to grasp the intended facetiousness of my remark.

In another encounter, I was told in no uncertain terms that I would go to Hell. Once I attended a well-established Christian church that was new to me. After the service, I was received as a newcomer. A designated host was assigned to introduce to me the basic teachings of the church. Here is the gist of the introduction.

Host   [Going straight to the point] Mr. Ho, are you a Christian?
Mr. Ho   I was baptized when I was a child.
Host   That doesn't mean you will go to Heaven, unless you make a commitment to accept Jesus Christ as your personal savior. [At this point, my host took out a copy of the Bible and proceeded to give me a lecture on who will go to Heaven and who will go to Hell.]
Mr. Ho   I get it. That means countless Christians will go to Hell, and so will I.
Host   That's right. Many Christians don't know it.
Mr. Ho   What about the masses of humanity who are not Christian? Hell will really get crowded.
Host   That's why we must bring the Bible to them. Now, Mr. Ho, are you ready to make a commitment?
Mr. Ho   [politely but firmly] I will think about it.
Host   Are you ready to accept Jesus Christ as your personal Savior?

It was the most direct, face-to-face encounter I have had with fundamentalist evangelicalism. I visualized a match burning my finger and then everlasting hellfire engulfing my whole body. What warped mind, human or divine, could conceive of such sadism? I was not angry because there was nothing personal about the encounter, though marked as it was by utter insensitivity. But I was dejected, because there are so many fundamentalist Christians who think and act with such certainty, with such a sense of mission. Like my host, they act as reincarnates of the Crusaders.

Viewed in this light, the encounter reaffirms my observation that in many ways extreme fundamentalist Christians and Muslim militants are mirror images of each other. That's why the acrimony is bidirectional. I feel an inner chill. I fear for the future of peace. I tremble at the thought that the voices of reason, which pale in insignificance against the loud trumpets of extremism, can be drowned out of existence.

I cannot help thinking that fundamentalism, chafing under the term fundamentalists applied to themselves in the 1920s in North America, puts both believers and nonbelievers in an impossible moral position. Fundamentalism assigns the nonbeliever to eternal condemnation, if he refuses to be "born again"; or makes him a liar if, out of fearing Hell alone, he surrenders to his "personal savior." It would give no comfort to believers in the knowledge that a majority portion of humanity will not share with them the joys of their salvation; it would cause them great pain, if that portion includes their significant others.

This is not just an abstract theological issue. Coming from a Christian family, I have many relatives who are Christian. Some are fundamentalists. What pains me greatly is to witness the progressive closing of the mind stemming from their religious beliefs. How should they feel if they really believe they would find me not in Heaven, but in Hell?

Absolutism and the Closing of the Mind

Knowledge is power; absolutistic knowledge is tyrannical power. This observation applies most suitably to evangelicals, for whom the grounds for belief rest on appeal to testimony (e.g., a public recounting of a religious conversion or experience) and to dogmatic authority (e.g., gospel truths and revelations). Rational analysis and scientific evidence are regarded as anathemas.

In short, the mentality of evangelicals typifies those of closed mind individuals. Are closed minded individuals likely to be drawn to evangelicalism in the first place? Or do evangelicals become progressively solidified in their closed mindedness after they have been immersed in the ideological baptism of evangelicalism? I think that both statements have merit. Closed mindedness and evangelicalism are mutually reinforcing. In the extreme, evangelicalism leads to ossification of the mind; groupthink has taken over, leaving no room for doubt, independent thinking, or creativity.

Once the mind is closed, psychological defense mechanisms come readily into play, such as compartmentalization (e.g., total separation of Trump's leadership from his defects of character), denial (e.g., "Trump hasn't lost the election"), rationalization (e.g., "Trump isn't responsible for the storming of the capital by violent mobs because . . . ."), and projection (e.g., "I am not violent, they are").

As a clinical psychologist, I have studied the speaking and writing patterns of evangelicals in both face-to-face interactions and social media such as Facebook. These patterns are characterized by the frequent use of preachy monologues;

superlatives, extreme qualifiers or quantifiers (e.g., always, never, everyone, nobody, absolutely).

Evangelicals are at home with absolute certainties; correspondingly, they have difficulty with conceptualizing in terms of probabilities. Their thinking pattern is characterized by a dichotomous right-versus-wrong or true-versus-false mentality that precludes meaningful dialogues (e.g., pro-life versus pro-choice) with groups who do not subscribe to their beliefs.

They are likely to have difficulty in dealing with contrafactual statements such as, "If the moon were made of green cheese, then . . .." Their likely response would be to cut the utterer short: "Impossible, the moon is not made of green cheese!" From this, it would not be difficult to predict how the evangelical mind is likely to respond to a conditional statement beginning with "if God did not exist, then . . .." These patterns, of course, may be easily found in Trump's speeches and writings: repetitive, simplistic, absolutistic, absent of self-reflection, and so forth.

The closing of the mind provides the fertile soil for biased selections of information sources, rearrangements or distortions of facts to conform to a preordained narrative, lack of discernment between facts and rumors or fake news, and so forth.

What drives this process? I submit that fear and insecurity underlie the closing of the mind. The emotional gains here on earth may be seen: a quick-and-easy reduction of fear and insecurity, plus comfort and support in a company of other people who believe in exactly the same faith as you do.

My mother, born into a Christian family, was a fearful and insecure person. As a child, I bore witness to her numberless recitations (in Chinese), "The Lord is my shepherd. . .." Years later, it dawned on me that her recitations imply total submission, as that of a flock of sheep to their shepherd and his shepherd dogs. An insecure mind addicted to absolutistic beliefs is vulnerable to self-deception. And a collectivity of such minds provides the fertile soil for conspiracy theories; in the extreme, for national paranoia. In sum, there is an emotional basis for trading freedom for security.

The Price to Be Paid: A Surrender of Self-Ownership

Faust trades his soul for worldly knowledge and pleasure; Dorian Gray exchanges his soul for eternal youth; and evangelicals forfeit their freedom of thought for a ticket to Heaven. In all cases, a terrible price has to be paid. For evangelicals, that price is the closing of the mind that entails submission to or, even worse, domination by a "strong" authority figure—a surrender of self-ownership. Thus, Trump is invited into their lives.

Total submission is the antithesis of the American spirit of confidence and overcoming challenges. Nonetheless, it does offer a great "benefit": You do not have to think; just follow the leaders, such as your pastor regarding your religious life and Trump regarding your political views. And when your pastor and Trump become buddies, it's a godsend. The trouble is that opinion leaders, religious and political, tend to be power hungry, greedy in gaining more followers. History is replete with absolutistic opinion leaders (e.g., self-proclaimed prophets, popes) who want to monopolize the platform for pronouncing what is right or wrong, thus denying other leaders the same privilege.

Many Catholics in the modern age may feel embarrassed about the inglorious histories of the Inquisition against alleged heretics (e.g., Galileo) and the *Index of Librorum Prohibitorum* (*Index of Forbidden Books*) listing the works of almost every Western philosopher in its day. In many respects, Pope Francis has emerged as a prominent figure of progressivism and a spokesman for the underprivileged, the marginalized, and the dispossessed segments of humanity.

In contrast, evangelicals have regressed to the Dark Ages. They excel in their aggressive stance to claim theological authority. They have appropriated the Bible, interpreted literally, to advance their version of Christian fundamentalism. Meanwhile, liberal or progressive theologians look in awe at the evangelical assault on reason, without being able to hold it in check. They are losing the cultural war on the religious front to the superstars of televangelism.

Will America Become a Theocracy?

The rise of evangelical political power sets the stage for absolutism. As Katherine Steward and others have shown, America's religious nationalists, the power worshippers, are waging a political war, highly organized and well-funded by the rich and powerful, on the norms and institutions of American democracy. The evangelical "generals" of this war are turning religion into an instrument for domination. They rely on a dense network of think tanks, advocacy groups, and pastoral organizations embedded in a community of international alliances, united not by any central command but by a common antidemocratic vision and will to power. Following the money that fuels this development, Steward traces much of it to a cadre of superrich, ultraconservative donors and family foundations. I see this as another indication of growing plutocracy in the United States.

Christian nationalism is the fruit of the closing of the Western mind described by Charles Freeman (2005). It forms the common cause of a global movement that seeks to destroy liberal democracy and replace it with nationalist, theocratic, and autocratic forms of government. In particular, its militaristic forms of expression constitute a continuation of America's long history of violence (e.g., massacre of Native Americans, slavery) that Jill Lepore (2018), a Harvard history professor, has documented in *These Truths: A History of the United States*.

From a long-term perspective, the most worrying is an organized attempt to imprint the legality of hard-line Christian values in American society. Since Trump became president, the religious right has unleashed a wave of legislation across the United States. The Congressional Prayer Caucus Foundation was established by a former Republican congressman aimed to "protect religious freedom, preserve America's Judeo-Christian heritage and promote prayer." Developed by a collection of Christian groups, a playbook known as Project Blitz, has provided state politicians with a set of off-the-shelf pro-Christian "model bills," which may be used verbatim to facilitate the introduction of new legislation. This would undo the separation of church and state and thus tilt America toward theocracy.

Concluding Thoughts

The Trump phenomenon continues after the Trump presidency. Emboldened by Trump, evangelical fanaticism and far-right ideologies are amalgamated into a most sinister political machinery not seen since the end of the civil war. The successes of this machinery have been stunning, affecting virtually every aspect of American life.

Democracy can best defend itself against the onslaught of its many enemies only when there are enough informed citizens who have the ability to discern truths from falsehoods and to engage in dialogues for the common good. Viewed in this light, this critical essay is an indictment of the massive failure of American education to cultivate politically literate citizens.

And what about the issue of loss of freedom versus insecurity deep in the human psyche? That is the perennial dilemma that confronts all of us. But we can escape from the horns of the dilemma by proclaiming that freedom and security are not mutually exclusive; they may even be interdependent. And remember that the rise of democracy correlates with the decline of absolutism.

Thematic Group 3
Eastern Versus Western Culture

Kindred souls countenance no cultural barriers to communication.

With two cultural parents, One Chinese and one Western, I write with the passion of a person who has been transformed into a thoroughly bilingual-bicultural person, empowered to build intercultural bridges.

> East is East, and West is West.
> Excesses in one mirror deficiencies in the other, and vice versa.
> Each has something from which the other needs to learn,
> And something that the other should reject.
> East is West, and West is East:
> The world will be a better place.

This thematic group introduces readers to the contrasting sociocultural contexts between the East and the West that give rise to different patterns of living, normal or abnormal. In Chapter 14, I caution readers on the limitations of viewing Chinese as collectivists and Americans as individualists, an oversimplified view that has been reinforced by the works of cross-cultural psychologists.

In Chapter 15, I make the point that the country's socialist ideology may be overwhelmed by exposure to Western influences following the open-door policy.

The population policies have a powerful impact on the fabric of Chinese society based on kinship. Imagine a social world in which you don't have siblings, aunts or uncles; as a child, six adults (four grandparents and two parents) may well be constantly competing for your attention and affection. Chinese society has been transformed from old-age centeredness to child centeredness.

Lastly, in Chapter 16, legends and literature provide a rich source of insight into family pathology. A comparative study of Chinese and Western sources points to three directions. The first is to recognize the pathogenic aspects of some cultural demands (e.g., Confucian precepts of filial piety). The second is to acknowledge that filicide is far more common than patricide. The third is a reinterpretation of the Oedipal myth in terms of submission versus challenge to authority figures.

14
Two Ways of Life: Chinese and American

The Christian belief in the person-in-community is easily polarized into two heresies, individualism and collectivism.

—R. L. Shinn

In what ways are Chinese collectivists and Westerners individualists? This is a key question to be answered in this chapter. Individualism and collectivism are exceedingly complex concepts, central to debates over how society is to be organized. In recent decades, cross-cultural psychologists have shown an upsurge of interest in individualism and collectivism, which may be described as nothing short of phenomenal.

This statement should be qualified, however. Collectivism is often not accorded the status of a key construct in its own right; it is treated as a counterpart of individualism. This imbalance reflects an underlying ideological bias toward individualism in the social sciences, psychology in particular. In actual fact, however, collectivism has been by far the more representative mode of human existence found throughout the ages and in diverse parts of the world.

Students of Chinese society are often confronted by a paradox. On the one hand, traditional Chinese ethos is generally regarded as exemplary of collectivism. On the other hand, no less a person than the founder of the Republic of China, Dr. Sun Yat Sen, has depicted Chinese people as "a pile of loose sand." As witnessed by the present author, this accusation is echoed by remarks frequently made by people of various persuasions such as, "Chinese people do not work together well to achieve common goals." How shall we deal with the paradox?

Individualism and Collectivism: A Dialectical Approach

Are Chinese really collectivists and Westerners individualists? Indubitably, you have heard a great deal about individualism versus collectivism among psychologists and business managers who borrow ideas from them indiscriminately. My advice: Don't believe everything they say.

At the outset, it should be realized that the terms of individualism and collectivism in different languages may have different connotations and are thus likely to evoke different cognitive and affective responses. For instance, whereas in English the term *individualism* connotes positive values affirming the individual, in Chinese it connotes selfishness or placing self-interests above those of the group, a lack of concern for others, and aversion to group discipline. *The Modern Chinese Dictionary* published in Beijing in 1981 defines individualism as follows (in my translation).

> The incorrect thoughts of considering everything from the viewpoint of the individual; putting individual interests above those of the group; concerned only with oneself and not with others. Individualism is the product of the system of private ownership of the means of production. It is the basic nucleus of the worldview of the capitalist class. Its expression has many forms, such as individual heroism, libertarianism, departmentalism, factionalism, and so forth.

This, I may add, is a clear demonstration of how lexicographers work under the stricture of doctrinaire ideologies.

In English, *collectivism* connotes a negation of the individual; in Chinese, it has positive connotations affirming the solidarity of the group. This poses a challenge to cross-cultural researchers: to develop conceptually and, more ambitiously, metrically equivalent measures of the two constructs to be used in different linguistic communities.

The connotation of a term, positive or negative, is a reflection of the cultural values it expresses; in turn, these values are instrumental in shaping psychological thought. Traditionally individualism tends to be highly valued in psychology; humanistic psychologists, in particular, have long extolled the autonomous, unique, and self-actualizing individual. Collectivism is regarded as antithetical to individualism. Voices of dissent to such dichotomous conceptualization are, however, being heard. The debate hinges on how the two concepts are defined by various authors. Attention must be turned, therefore, to the diverse conceptions of individualism and collectivism.

Individualism

As it is expressed in the Judeo-Christian tradition, individualism affirms the uniqueness, autonomy, freedom, and intrinsic worth of the individual; at the same time, it insists on each one assuming responsibility for one's own conduct, well-being, and salvation. Individualism eschews uniformity and favors individuation.

Thus, a society organized on the basis of individualistic values tends to maximize opportunities for variation; individuals would tend to be polarized on the continuum of success and failure in life. The idealized successful person, according to the modern spokesmen for individualism, the humanistic psychologists, is the self-actualizing individual.

Alas, to most people, self-actualization is but an unrealized potential; on the other end of the continuum, there remain vast numbers of people in misery or at war with society. The individual must assume responsibility for his failures. For, upon reaching adulthood, all members of society (excepting those with serious physical or mental handicaps) are supposed to be capable of defending their rights, making their own decisions, and in general looking after themselves—in short, self-reliant. Accordingly, a society which puts the premium on individualism would be ill-disposed to those who have failed to achieve self-reliance. In particular, individuals who become a public liability, for example, those on public welfare, invite contempt and rejection.

In contemporary psychological thought, the dominant conception is exemplified by the definition of individualism as believing and behaving as if one's efforts and goal attainments are unrelated to or independent from efforts toward the goal attainment of others. Central to this conception is the notion of the autonomous individual, whose identity, responsibility, and achievements are defined independently of the group.

Alternative Conceptions

An intellectual hurdle is to be overcome, however, is to transcend this dominant conception and to consider alternative viewpoints. Psychologist M. Rotenberg

(1974) makes a distinction between alienating individualism and reciprocal individualism; obviously, the former has negative, and the latter positive connotations. Reciprocal individualism comes closer to Asian conceptions of selfhood.

In a similar vein, Edward Sampson (1988) distinguishes two indigenous psychologies of individualism. One is self-contained individualism, characterized by firm self-nonself boundaries, personal control, and an exclusionary conception of the person or self; this psychology is dominant in U.S. society today. The other is what he terms *ensembled individualism*, characterized by fluid self-nonself boundaries, field control, and a more inclusive conception of the person; this psychology has a greater worldwide presence (see also Ho, 2019a, Chapter 3.3 Selfhood and Identity: East-West Contrasts).

Reflections on American Society

Rotenberg and Sampson have prompted me to reflect on how cultural myths rooted in individualism permeate American society, such as the following.

1. You have freedom of choice concerning your life over which no one else should circumscribe or exercise control. (A fateful example: Millions refuse to be vaccinated, thus endangering lives, their own and those of others.)
2. How you express yourself and fulfill your personal aspirations is your own business: "I do my thing and you do your thing." (Indulgent and socially irresponsible? Individualism misconstrued, banalized?)
3. You can be whatever you want to be, achieve whatever you want to achieve, provided that you believe strongly enough in yourself. (Thus, educators, psychologists, and therapists trumpet "positive thinking" and "self-esteem," rather than hard work and perseverance as the foundation for success. Can self-esteem be obtained without effort and trial? Do outcomes depend on psychological factors such as self-confidence, without regard to external reality, socioeconomic, political, and environmental?)
4. You are OK just the way you are. (Congruence between the real and the ideal self, in the manner of humanistic psychologists, such as Carl Rogers. By this count, psychopaths are the most congruent.)
5. Everyone can be the President of the United States. (I hope not!)
6. The good life is one from which unhappiness is expunged from the individual's psyche (see Ho & Ho, 2007, for an assessment of subjective well-being research).

7. Medical science and technology will one day succeed in turning back the biological clock, conquering diseases and rid humankind (at least the rich) of suffering completely. Commercial interests fuel the wellness industry, with claims that lead Americans to falsehoods about unlimited health and denials of psychophysiological decline as a natural consequence of aging (see Barbara Ehrenreich, 2018, *Natural Causes: An Epidemic of Wellness, the Certainty of Dying, and Killing Ourselves to Live Longer*; Kate Bowler, 2018, *Everything Happens for a Reason, and Other Lies I've Loved*).

These cultural myths amount to what may be called the *illusion of unlimited personal freedom*. This illusion is predicated on the failure to acknowledge, on ethical grounds, social responsibility; and on scientific grounds, reality.

To its credit, America does not conceal its disgraces. So, informed professionals frankly admit that their country with an overwhelming superiority in resources for social science research is also a country visibly beset by more than its share of societal problems. In contrast, professionals in China are often under political pressure to keep silent (see Chapter 15).

Collectivism

Historically, collectivism has appeared in many varied forms: in tribal societies, ancient empires, the communism of early Christians, the communes of the People's Republic of China, the kibbutzim of Israel, and the experiments in communal living in American society. No less varied are the political ideologies that legitimize their existence: Collectivism is no more necessarily wedded to totalitarianism than to democracy. Neither does it necessarily require the negation of the individual. What is asserted, rather, is that individual well-being and security derive from those of the collective. Mutual support and interdependence are hallmarks of collectivism.

Mutual Support and Interdependence

Common to the various forms of collectivism is the emphasis on the interdependent nature of human existence, and the insistence that the interests of the group or collective take priority over those of the individual. Collectivism affirms that to preserve and enhance the well-being of the group is the supreme guiding principle for social action. Accordingly, members of the group are expected to subjugate their own inclinations to group requirements. Furthermore, collectivistic organization rests on the principle of reciprocity, such that each member is related to other members in a network of interlocking responsibilities and obligations.

Collectives are thus organized on the basis of two fundamental principles: One, *the priority of collective interests*, governing the vertical individual-collective relationship; and two, *the reciprocity of responsibilities and obligations*, governing both vertical and horizontal interpersonal relationships within the collective.

Groups and Collectives

In the research literature, the terms *group* and *collective* are most commonly used to refer to collectivistic social units. *Collective* is the preferred term when we refer to a larger, more inclusive unit; a collective may comprise a number of smaller units. The term *group* should be understood to mean a collectivistic group. This is because not all groups are collectivistic; specifically, groups not organized on the basis of the two stated principles are not. For instance, a number of self-contained individuals may constitute a group, if they are not merely a collection of unrelated individuals acting in isolation; but such a group would hardly qualify as a collectivistic social unit.

Collectives are of many kinds. All are, however, invariably defined by their members' common social connections, based on for instance: blood and marriage ties; tribal or ethnic origin; caste; institutional affiliation, formal or informal; and nationality. They may be ranked in terms of their inclusiveness, for example, family, clan, tribe, country, and international or ecumenical organization. The units within a collective may be ordered hierarchically, as in the army.

Organizational Structure

Total collectivism demands that hierarchical structure is maintained: The interests of the lower level unit must be subservient to those of the higher level one. Thus the priority of collective interests has to be expanded to govern not only the individual-collective but also the unit-collective relationship. Similarly, the principle of reciprocity has to be expanded to govern not only interpersonal but also interunit relationships. However, in actuality, these principles are more often than not violated on account of conflicting interests existing among units at various echelons within a collective, or between a unit and the collective as a whole. For instance, interfamily feuds threaten the solidarity of the clan; tribal rivalries are detrimental to the realization of nationhood; familism-clanism, tribalism, and nationalism are all antithetical to ecumenical ideals (cf. Ho, Xie, Liang, & Zeng, 2012). The ideals of total collectivism are not easily and rarely attained.

It is clear that collectivism cannot be fully characterized without considering the kind and hierarchical structure of collectives. Multiple levels of analysis, corresponding to different echelons of a hierarchical structure, are indicated. In addition to structural analysis, individual differences in how a person construes the structural and interpersonal relationships within a given collective have to be considered. Multiple informal groupings of individuals based on psychological needs, affiliation, and identification may be formed. These groupings do not necessarily correspond to the units defined structurally within the collective. As social psychologists know, the reference group with which an individual identifies is not always the same as the group to which an individual belongs by virtue of formal membership.

Confining Analysis to a Target Group

Adding to all this complexity is the fact that an individual may belong simultaneously to different collectives or to different units within the same collective. The distribution of responsibilities, obligations, and conflicting interests among individuals within a social system is likely to be immensely complicated.

An analysis may be simplified if it is confined to a target group within a given collective. A target group rooted in collectivism may be defined as one to which a grouping of individuals in the collective owe their primary allegiance; its interests are identical or nearly identical to the interests of the collective, and its identity is interwoven with the identity of the collective. Thus defined, the target group is an in-group that conforms to the two principles of the collectivistic organization stated above. Again, membership in the target group is psychologically based, and does not necessarily correspond to that defined structurally (as in the case of a clan comprising people with the same surname) or formally (as in a political party with card-carrying members). It is vital, therefore, to begin the analysis with the target group being identified.

Dialectical Synthesis

The psychology of self-contained individualism has sometimes been developed to an extreme or even absurd degree, where the group is no longer regarded as relevant to the analysis of individual behavior. For example, one psychologist asserts in a prestigious journal that, in the case of self-contained individualism, "groups and collectives do not influence persons"; hence the group and collective levels of analysis have no relevance. But how can any person, self-contained or otherwise, be free from the influence of groups or collectives? The assertion denies the very social character of human existence.

A dialectical view insists that both the individual and the group derive its meaning from the coexistence of the other: Without individuals, there is no group to speak of; without the group, the very notion of individual identity loses meaning.

Organization is an intrinsic property of all groups and more generally of societies, individualistic or collectivistic. It varies according to the degree of emphasis placed on the sharing of leadership and responsibility, altruism, public morality, group discipline, harmony, hierarchical structure, and so forth. To be sure, the nature of the social organization rooted in individualism differs from that rooted in collectivism. Nevertheless, analyzing the distribution of responsibilities, obligations, and conflicting interests within target groups is no less a necessary step to an understanding of social organization based on individualistic values.

Are individualism and collectivism diametrically opposing concepts? Does the acceptance of one necessarily entail the rejection of the other? I question the presumed mutual exclusiveness or conflict between personal and in-group interests implied in the individualism-collectivism dichotomy.

Even a brief excursion into the intellectual history of individualism and collectivism is sufficient to reveal their complexity. Two main conclusions emerge.

1. The two constructs should not be construed as opposite ends of a continuum or continua. Rather, they are distinct concepts; one is not reducible to be simply the antithesis of the other. There is no necessary contradiction in holding individualistic and collectivistic views at the same time.
2. Individualism and collectivism have different implications for social organization. In both instances, it is necessary to analyze the distribution of responsibilities, obligations, and conflicting interests among individuals within defined target groups.

Empirical Evidence: Dubious Comparisons between Americans and Chinese

In cross-cultural studies employing the individualism-collectivism construct, Chinese subjects are typically classified as "collectivists," to be compared with other groups (frequently American) classified as "individualists." There is a temptation to explain, all too readily, the group differences found on the basis of cultural differences on the individualism-collectivism dimension. It would be wise to resist this temptation and to reflect on the intellectual traps of invoking individualism-collectivism as an explanatory construct.

In its crudest form, the explanation reduces to: If Chinese are different in their behavior from, say, Americans, it is because they are more collectivistic (and less individualistic) in their orientation than are Americans; and this is because Chinese culture is more collectivistic than American culture. To avoid the fallacy of circularity, even in this form, it is essential to establish that the two cultures indeed differ on the individualism-collectivism dimension, an assumption upon which predictions of the group differences are based.

Such explanations may be faulted on conceptual, methodological, and empirical grounds. Conceptually, it does no justice to the complexity of the two concepts, individualism and collectivism, each of which comprises a number of interrelated component ideas. The two are distinct concepts: One is not reducible to be simply the antithesis of the other. Methodologically, therefore, they should not be construed as opposites of a continuum or continua. Empirically, the evidence casts doubt on the indiscriminate characterization of Chinese culture as exemplary of collectivism. Thus the rug is pulled out of the logical basis upon which the behavioral differences between Chinese and other groups are predicted.

Treating Individualism and Collectivism as Multidimensional Constructs

This author and his associate (Ho & Chiu, 1994) have conducted research on individualism, collectivism, and social organization in Chinese culture. Individualism and collectivism are treated as multidimensional constructs; each embodies a constellation of component ideas. Five major components pertaining to both individualism and collectivism are identified.

1. Individualistic Values (e.g., individuality)/Collectivistic Values (e.g., the supremacy of the group or collective).
2. Autonomy/Conformity.
3. Individual Responsibility/Collective Responsibility.
4. Individual Achievement (e.g., via competition)/Collective Achievement (e.g., via cooperation).
5. Self-Reliance/Interdependence.

Three main conclusions may be reached on the basis of empirical results obtained. First, overall Chinese culture is indeed more collectivistic than individualistic. For instance, cooperation is affirmed but competition is not. However, individualism is by no means uniformly negated across component ideas. In fact, individuality and self-reliance are both strongly affirmed. The strength of affirmation or negation may vary greatly across the five major components.

Second, the evidence consistently supports the contention that Chinese collectivism is specific to role relationships. A person's individualistic or collectivistic orientation depends on the self-other relationship involved and is not predictable from his global attitudes toward traditional values. Furthermore, it does not appear to be associated with personality functioning. The evidence suggests that voluntary and instrumental relationships are gaining ascendancy, while relationships based on blood or marriage ties or on residential location are waning—a reversal of the traditional pattern.

Third, Chinese culture places a strong emphasis on altruism and the maintenance of harmony, values presumed to be conducive to integrative social organization.

Collectivist Harmony or "A Pile of Loose Sand"?

We are now better prepared to confront the paradox stated at the beginning of this essay: How can the Chinese people be collectivists and yet behave like "a pile of loose sand"? By making the distinction between collectivism and integrative social organization explicit in the first instance. Collectivism does not ensure integrative organization and integrative organization is not necessarily grounded in collectivism. Stressing harmony would by no means guarantee that it can, in fact, be maintained.

Research evidence indicates that Chinese collectivism is specific to role relationships or target persons (Ho & Chiu, 1994). Thus, the behavioral orientation toward strangers or outsiders may differ sharply from the spirit of mutual help among insiders. And loyalty to the family or clan at the expense of the country violates the priority of collective interests, thus contributing to the nonintegrative tendencies of Chinese society as a whole (cf. Ho et al., 2012 on familism-clanism and the lack of public-versus-private demarcation).

To many observers, Chinese social organization seems to be characterized by nonintegrative tendencies: lack of sharing of responsibility, public morality, civic-mindedness, and group discipline. Chinese history, in itself a rich source of empirical data, bears testimony to the prevalence of fractional tendencies at various strata of society. Investigations into the extended family reveal that it too is fraught with internal strife: sons fighting over an inheritance, quarrels between the wife and her mother-in-law, and tension between the father and his children. Thus, the Confucian ideal of harmony runs afoul of reality in family dynamics (see Ho, 2019b, Chapter 5.5 "Therapeutic Intervention for Families in Distress").

The Confucian view of social order stresses the maintenance of harmony and the negation of conflicts (see Ho, 2019a, Chapter 4.3 Face in Diverse Cultures: Is Face Saving Just an Asian Preoccupation?). However, it may be argued that expressions of conflicts serve an integrative function; moreover, insisting on maintaining harmony, without giving opportunities for conflicts to be voiced and resolved, sows the seed for nonintegration. The Confucian view is static; it does not recognize the value of conflicts and provides no channels for their resolution. The result is pseudoharmony. When underlying conflicts do erupt into the open, as they have periodically in Chinese history, they tend to assume violent forms.

Two Ways of Life

In Table 1, I attempt to summarize Chinese-Western differences in terms of two ways of life. I am mindful that such an attempt is subject to the pitfalls of oversimplification and overgeneralization. The table is meant to be read as a didactic device for stimulating critical thoughts and reflections, not as the presentation of "truths."

Concluding Thoughts

In this chapter, I have attempted to summarize Chinese-Western differences in terms of two ways of life. I clarify the meanings of individualism and collectivism. In cross-cultural psychology and management studies, typically Chinese are classified or characterized as collectivists and Westerners individualists. I have reasons, both theoretical and empirical, to cast doubt on such a simplistic classification. An exciting possibility for a creative synthesis exists, once we realize that individualism and collectivism need not be construed as mutually exclusive. Individuality is not necessarily lost within the confines of the collective good; individualism without regard for the needs of the collective can easily go rampant.

Table 1. Contrasts Between Western and Chinese Ways of Life

Western	Chinese
Fundamental values	
Individualistic values: intrinsic worth of the human person, self-realization, individuality, individual identity, individual-centeredness	Collectivistic values: the supremacy of the group or collective, collective actualization, uniformity, collective identity, relational orientation
Autonomy / Conformity	
Self-direction; individuation, uniqueness; values solitude; right to personal privacy	Conformity to societal norms, compliance; uniformity (emulation of models); prefers the company of others; collective regulation of individual thoughts and action
Locus of responsibility	
Individual responsibility: The individual actor alone bears responsibility for his actions	Collective responsibility: The whole group may bear responsibility for actions taken by one of its members
Achievement	
Individual achievement via competition and individual efforts	Collective achievement via cooperation and group efforts
Independence / Interdependence	
Self-reliance; fulfillment of individual needs, self-interests, aspirations; rights-preoccupied; security sought in individual efforts	Mutual support; fulfillment of collective goals and interests; obligations-preoccupied; security grounded in group solidarity
Political orientation	
Democracy, human rights	Authoritarianism, individual rights secondary to collective prerogatives
Ethical-legal orientation	
Anchored in the person-God relationship; derived from abstract concepts (e.g., justice); codified as law, absolutistic, independent of personal connections; the rule of law, equality before the law	Anchored in human relationships; good and bad judged on the basis of effects on the social network; rewards and punishments dependent on personal connections; the rule of personal authority invested in the leader or ruler

Table 1. Continued

Western	Chinese
Temporal orientation	
Future orientation: Younger generations will surpass past generations; future generations are "in front of us"; belief in innovation, progress	Past-orientation: Younger generations follow the footsteps of older generations; past generations are "in front of us"; traditionalism, conservatism
Conception of the life cycle	
A single, linear life cycle	Cyclical lives (reincarnation, especially for Buddhists)
Conception of human nature	
Christian conceptions are dominant: humans are made in the image of God, perfectible, endowed with a soul and free will; they are God's favorite creations, to have dominion over other creatures; born with original sin since the fall of Adam and Eve, to be redeemed through God's transfiguring love; sinful, especially sexual, impulses have to be controlled.	Influenced by Confucian, Daoist, and Buddhist traditions. According to Confucianism, human nature develops in the context of interpersonal relationships. In Daoism, human nature is interwoven with the cosmos. In Buddhism, the individual self is but an illusion; "true" human nature is realized only through ridding oneself of this illusion. Sexuality is negated in neither Confucianism or Daoism.
Humankind's relation with nature	
Discontinuity with nature, animals, God; conquest of nature (Promethean); being human is the measure of all things, distinctive in the universe	Continuity (fluid boundaries between human and nonhuman entities); harmony with nature; humans viewed as integral to the cosmos
Guiding principles for action	
Self-expression is paramount	Self-control; securing a place in the social order takes precedence over self-expression
Self-assertion; ideally, conflicts to be resolved within legal-institutional constraints	Submission to authority; maintenance of harmony, avoidance of open conflicts

(*Continued*)

Table 1. Continued

Western	Chinese
Accent on seeking social approval, popularity	Accent on the avoidance of ostracism, losing face, social disapproval
Psychological orientation: respect for individual needs, emotions, and aspirations	Panmoralism (pervasive tendency to apply moral judgments): emphasis on proper conduct
Family and kinship	
Nuclear families	Extended families
Dominance of the husband-wife relationship	Dominance of parent-child relationships
Child-centeredness	Elder-centeredness

15

Growing Up in the People's Republic of China: Culture, Ideology, and Policy

What would a social world in which you don't have siblings, aunts or uncles be like?

Socialization in mainland China demands urgent research attention for good reasons. First, it concerns how children are transformed into adults in the world's largest geopolitical community—also one with the longest unbroken cultural heritage.

Second, radical ideology and policies have been introduced since the founding of the People's Republic of China (PRC) in 1949, resulting in tumultuous social changes. Ideologically, inculcating socialist values is proclaimed the guiding principle for parenting.

Two policies demand particular attention. One is the open-door policy that opens the door to Western influence; like a tidal wave, this influence is bound to have psychosocial consequences of gigantic proportions. The other is the one-child policy, enacted as a legislative decree in 1971 (replaced by the two-child policy in 2015 and the three-child policy in 2021), which amounts to social engineering of such radical nature and unprecedented magnitude that the world has never before seen. What is the impact of these policies on child development?

Continuities and Departures from Tradition

In a review of the literature, Ho (1989; see also Ho, Peng, & Cheng-Lai, 2001) found a remarkable continuity with the traditional pattern of parenting, particularly with respect to the care of infants and young children, and the emphasis given to impulse control, obedience, moral training, and academic achievement (excepting the years during the Great Cultural Revolution). However, discontinuities in socialization were also evident. Public educational institutions and peer relations played a greater role in socialization beginning early in life, resulting from the massive placement of young children in nurseries and kindergartens.

Breaking with the past was pronounced as the official ideology. The national purpose was to translate socialist values into educational practice, not just for children but also for adults; thus, emphasis was placed on socialization beyond childhood as well. Uniformity of views concerning the ideals of socialization was officially maintained throughout the country. However, the goal of translating these ideals into practice was far from realized, especially in rural areas. Significant urban-rural differences remained in parenting, as in other aspects of social life.

Empirical research (Ho et al., 2012; see also Ho, 1996, in press-b) indicates that the traditional values of filial piety and child training in Hong Kong and Taiwan are on the decline and no longer command the same degree of absolute observance they did before. These traditional values are held much less strongly among younger people in families of high socioeconomic status.

Temporal data gathered in Hong Kong in 1970 and 2011 show a moderate decrease on the Folk Values Scales, which measures beliefs and values stemming from the mass culture; but no significant difference on the Ideal Values Scale, which measures core values such as filial piety and culturocentrism-traditionalism stemming from the ethical traditions of high culture. In contrast, temporal data gathered in mainland China in 2003 and 2011 show a moderate increase on the Folk Values Scale, and a fairly large increase on the Ideal Values Scale. This supports the view that continuities with traditional values appear to be remarkably resilient in mainland China, despite radical changes in official ideology.

"Little Emperors"?

There is an alarmist view that, on account of the one-child policy, China is producing a generation of spoiled "little emperors." Not surprisingly, some of these little emperors, overprotected at home, become scared rabbits at school. No less attention should be devoted to what I would describe as the male "cocooned-child syndrome," commonly found in financially privileged families. This syndrome conjures up the image of a male child sitting on the lap of his mother, superdependent, shielded from hardships and lacking in problem-solving abilities—a pattern that is continuous with the traditional upbringing of children, especially male, from rich families .

A review of research studies show that only children appear to enjoy advantages in environmental and health conditions, and tend to have broader interests, better cognitive development, and higher intellectual ability than children with siblings (Ho et al., 2001). However, results in the areas of personality and social functioning have been rather inconsistent. Falbo and Poston (1993) found that, where differences were present, only children were taller and weighed more than others and were most likely to outscore others in verbal tests. Very few only-child effects were found in personality evaluations. This study, based on representative samples of 1,000 schoolchildren from four provinces, is comprehensive and methodologically rigorous. Hence more weight may be given to its findings.

From a methodological point of view, it is important to consider interaction effects between the rural-urban and only-nononly factors. In terms of demographics, only children come disproportionately from urban areas. Because of large rural-urban differences, as a group, only children would have a larger size, higher academic skills, and less desirable personalities (lacking in traditional virtues such as selflessness and enthusiasm for manual labor). This may contribute to the stereotype of only children, held by naive observers who fail to consider rural-urban differences. That is, rural-urban differences may have been mistaken to be only-child effects. Another methodological point is that extensive nursery and other school experiences may modify home influences.

Most important to be considered is that family size has been reduced drastically. This means that only-child effects are restricted to those derived from comparisons between only children and those who have very few siblings. So, instead of talking about only-child effects, we should be addressing the effects of reduced family size, which are more likely to be pronounced.

Investigative Research

Most research studies conducted have been synchronic rather than diachronic. To assess changes through time, we have conducted investigative research whenever opportunities arise for us to search for answers to intriguing questions about parenting in the PRC. Described by Ho, Ho, and Ng (2006), investigative research is a method integrating investigative reporting and ethnographic research. Although it does not preclude other techniques for gathering data, this method tends to rely on disciplined, naturalistic, and in-depth observations over prolonged periods in diverse settings.

Investigative research has the advantage of bringing the investigator to observe closely and directly the phenomenon of interest. It is particularly suitable for uncovering, understanding, and reporting social phenomena that may be hidden from or not easily accessible to observers. In our case, sources of information include observations of parent-child interactions, mostly unobtrusive, at home, in school or other educational settings, and in public places (e.g., in the street, waiting rooms, and eateries); unsolicited or spontaneous expressions by, and conversations with, children, parents, educators, and allied professionals (e.g., child psychiatrists).

What stands out from my investigative research is that ideology pales in comparison with changing socioeconomic realities in determining parental attitudes and behavior. Tradition has survived the onslaught of radical ideology, but will be tested to the limit in the face of changing socioeconomic realities stemming from both internal and external forces at work. The most potent of internal forces stems from structural changes in population consequential to the one-child policy. External forces come from increasing exposure to the outside world, an unavoidable consequence of the open-door policy.

Parents are responding to these forces. Their interest in popular psychology concerning child rearing and development reaches a level unheard of in the past. Children are now valued, even pampered, by their parents and grandparents more so than ever before. Chinese society is showing signs of becoming less age centered and more child centered. My observation is that child centeredness leads to the ascendancy of individualism: placing greater value on personal autonomy and self-interests. In turn, this will add momentum to cultural change.

Increasingly, parents are placing emphasis on the development of competence. In particular, academic success reigns supreme in the scale of parental values. A common belief is that, to ensure success, it is vital to start early by getting the child admitted into a prestigious kindergarten or even nursery school. Some mothers even practice antenatal training in the hope of producing superbabies that will sail through the educational system.

Preoccupation with getting the child to do homework can become a nightmare. The subject of homework invariably appears in the many workshops on parenting I have conducted in mainland China. The resulting mutual torture between parents and children sometimes reaches tragic proportions. Xu Li,

17 years of age, struggled to meet his mother's demand that he be placed within the top 10 of his class. He managed the 18th place; his mother refused to let him play football with his friends and threatened to break his legs. In a moment of rage, the quiet and well-behaved youngster bashed her head with a hammer. Of course, reading too much into a single case of violence should be avoided. Nonetheless, the case of Xu Li has touched a raw nerve, prompting all of China to talk about education, bearing testimony to the fact that the homework problem has reached national consciousness.

Socioeconomic and Psychological Costs of the One-Child Policy

Launched by Deng Xiaoping in 1980, the one-child policy amounts to social engineering of such radical nature and unprecedented magnitude that the world has never before seen. (This policy has been replaced by the two-child policy in 2015 and the three-child policy in 2021.) This population policy has altered fundamentally familial and more generally interpersonal relationships. Chinese society is based on kinship.

Now imagine a social world in which you don't have siblings; both of your parents are only children, and so you don't have aunts or uncles; as a child, six adults (four grandparents and two parents) may well be constantly competing for your attention and affection if physical and financial conditions allow.

The world has never before encountered such a social "experiment" conducted on such a massive scale, at such a rapid pace. I use the imagery of a tidal wave of megatsunamic proportions to characterize the gravity of psychosocial consequences that the population policy has brought.

There Will Not Be Enough Babies

Policymakers often are poorly informed on or show a disregard for relevant social science knowledge. A well-known worldwide pattern is that when incomes increase, family sizes tend to decrease. Many industrial nations have long faced the twin problems of a shrinking workforce and an aging population.

Under the autocratic leadership of the late Lee Guan Yew, Singapore once launched "love boats" onto which (only) male and female college graduates were invited at the government's expense. The purpose was simple: to induce young adults to get married and produce babies. Predictably, the "love boats" policy failed to deliver. Apparently, Lee failed to realize that women cannot be "persuaded" to do something to their bodies they do not want, not even by authority figures.

In China, the demographic trend shows clearly that its workforce is shrinking and the population is aging rapidly. According to official estimates, there will be 1.3 workers for each retiree by 2050, compared with 2.8 in 2018. Thus, policies that cling to birth restrictions defies social science.

As a result of strong, even ruthless, enforcement of the one-child policy, fertility rates dropped below replacement levels in the 1990s and have continued falling. However, changes in population policy may have little or no effect on increasing fertility rates. In a generation that grew up without siblings, a one-child mindset may have already been deeply entrenched. A survey in 2016 by the All-China Women's Federation found that only 20.5% of families wanted a second child; 53.3% of respondents with one child did not want a second. Eventually, China will learn, painfully, what many other countries have learned—that it is much more difficult to induce women to have more babies than the other way around.

The implications for economic development are grave. There will not be enough babies born to meet workforce requirements in the not-too-distant future, leading to a slowdown of economic growth. Jobs will be chasing after workers, fundamentally altering employer-employee relationships and hence individual attitudes and behavior in education, career aspirations, and personal development. My prediction is that the ascendancy of individualism will accelerate at an unprecedented pace.

When Deng launched the one-child policy, he said, "We must do this.... Otherwise, our economy cannot develop well and people's lives won't improve." There is clear irony in this. Clearly, China is in dire need of paying more attention to population psychology.

The "Hidden Babies"

We also must not forget the children born "illegally" to couples who defied the government's family-planning edicts based on the one-child policy. These were China's secret children without an official identity, numbering in the hundreds of thousands, if not millions (no one knows for sure). Their parents faced the threat of hefty fines, forced adoptions, or dismissal from public-sector jobs. Many entrusted their "unplanned" child to relatives or neighbors to avoid getting caught for having given birth to more than one child.

The development of normal parent-child relationships, needless to say, comes under extraordinary strain under these circumstances. For obvious reasons, one can hardly find studies of the secret children, if any, in Chinese journals of psychology. Who would dare to do such a thing?

In the 35 years since China instituted its one-child policy, 120,000 children—mostly girls—have left China through international adoption, including 85,000 to the United States. Kay Ann Johnson, a China scholar and mother to an adopted Chinese daughter, spent years talking with the Chinese parents driven to relinquish their daughters during the brutal birth-planning campaigns of the 1990s and early 2000s. The resulting publication is *China's Hidden Children: Abandonment, Adoption, and the Human Costs of the One-Child Policy* (Johnson, 2017; see also Rascovsky, 1995, on filicide).

It is generally assumed that this diaspora is the result of China's approach to population control, but there is also the underlying belief that the majority of adoptees are daughters because the one-child policy often collides with the traditional preference for a son. Johnson paints a startlingly different picture: The decision to give up a daughter, she shows, is not a facile one, but one almost always fraught with grief and dictated by fear. Were it not for the constant threat of punishment for breaching the country's stringent birth-planning policies, most Chinese parents would have raised their daughters despite the cultural preference for sons.

With *China's Hidden Children*, Johnson reveals the complex web of love, secrecy, and pain woven in the coerced decision to give one's child up for adoption and the profound negative impact China's birth-planning campaigns have on Chinese families. With clear understanding and compassion for the families, Johnson describes their desperate efforts to conceal the birth of second or third daughters from the authorities. As the Chinese government cracked down on those caught concealing an out-of-plan child, strategies for surrendering children changed—from arranging adoptions or sending them to live with a rural family to secret placement at carefully chosen doorsteps and, finally, abandonment in public places.

In the twenty-first century, China's so-called abandoned children have increasingly become "stolen" children, as declining fertility rates have left the dwindling number of children available for adoption more vulnerable to child trafficking. In addition, government seizures of locally—but illegally—adopted children and children hidden within their birth families mean that even legal adopters have unknowingly adopted children taken from parents and sent to orphanages.

The image of the "unwanted daughter" remains commonplace in Western conceptions of China. There is data to support such an image. In present-day China, the sex ratio among newborns in mainland China reaches the highest disparities in the world: 120 boys to 100 girls; in provinces that allow rural couples a second child if the first is a girl or in cases of hardship, a whopping 143 boys for 100 girls among children born second. These figures, based on data from a 2005 census, tell a horrible tale of untold proportions and portend social disruptions on a scale beyond imagination. Young men by the millions, about one in five, will not be able to find a wife, for instance. How would a society cope with such skewed demographics?

The preference of males over females may contribute to a sinister social problem. Child trafficking involving the abducting and buying of male children is common in some rural areas. The "happiness" of the foster parents who buy the child is built upon the misery of the biological parents. And the grownup kidnapped victims are often torn between justice for their biological parents and love for the foster parents who raised them.

Conclusion

The case of the PRC compels us to alter our thinking about the role of culture in parenting. We tend to think of culture as being conservative in nature: enduring, resilient, and largely resistant to alteration. However, the rapid pace with which changes have taken place in the PRC means that the temporal dimension becomes salient: Culture can no longer be treated as a static variable in research, as if it were frozen in time. Another point is that we cannot consider the role of culture in isolation. Both official ideology and policies constitute an onslaught on cultural tradition. Ideology directs parents to bring up children with a socialist worldview, which in large measure clashes with traditional values. Population policies undermine the traditional kinship fabric on which Chinese society is based, redefining the parent-child relationship in the process. The open-door policy leads to an acceleration of cultural change. In sum, culture is intertwined with socioeconomic realities in producing effects on parenting.

16

The Oedipal Myth and Family Pathology in Literature

Filicide is far more typical than patricide: The house of Oedipus is a history of family violence over generations.

Legendary tales provide a rich source for exploring the cultural definition of family relationships. In the West, the Oedipal myth has long been the object of intensive psychological exploration and theorizing. By comparison, the psychological implications of Chinese legends have yet to be explored in depth.

In this chapter, I explore family dynamics through literature, focusing on intergenerational relationships as they are reflected in Chinese as well as Western novels, stories, opera, legends, and myths. The psychological implications with respect to family dynamics and pathology are explored.

After a comparative survey of intergenerational violence in Western and Chinese literature, a discussion focusing on two themes follows: pathogenic demands of culture; and the universal question of how the father-son relationship and, more generally, authority relationships are to be resolved.

Reinterpreting the Oedipal Myth

Western mythologies capture the theme of danger and violence in humankind's quest for knowledge and self-assertion. Greek mythology, in particular, is rich in the tragic hero's spirit of defiance in his quest for knowledge. Prometheus, the creator of mankind, was punished savagely for stealing fire from the gods. Oedipus defied fate dictated by the Delphic oracle; the denouement of his quest for the truth about his own history and destiny was a high point in Greek tragedy. Both Prometheus and Oedipus were tormented tragic heroes who paid dearly for their actions. Yet, their actions were expressions of daring and creativity, bearing testimony to the defiant human spirit.

From these mythologies spring the seminal ideas of individualism, that the individual is a responsible, autonomous, and self-directed being; of existentialism, that the exercise of freedom gives meaning to life; of a worldview that posits the possibility of progress, even mastery over fate, through individual action; and of the love of knowledge, for which people like Socrates are prepared to die. Thomas Jefferson follows this tradition of defiance in declaring eternal hostility to all forms of tyranny over the freedom of thought.

An issue of special importance concerns the interpretation of the Oedipal myth. Freud's interpretation is focused on the sexual rivalry between father and son for the mother. But a broadened interpretation demands no less our attention: The Oedipal myth poses the universal question of how the father-son relationship and, more generally, authority relationships are to be defined. This definition entails the problem of handling intergenerational rivalry and conflicts.

It should be noted that the Oedipal myth begins with attempted filicide: In one version, the father wants to kill his son by having him exposed in the wilderness, after piercing his feet with a nail and binding them together (hence the name Oedipus, "swollen foot"). Moreover, the history of the house of Oedipus is a history of family violence, with filicide being far more typical than patricide over generations (Rascovsky, 1995). Many psychologists, including those of the psychoanalytic persuasion, are unaware of this fact. In the Freudian interpretation, the theme of filicide is neglected. This, in itself, is a topic worthy of investigation. Because of Freud's towering influence, patricide has become the dominant theme in standard interpretations of the Oedipal myth. It is time to redress this bias.

Patricide Versus Filicide and Violence Toward Children

Filicide is far more common than patricide in Chinese stories. For an obvious reason: Patricide is the antithesis of filial piety, regarded as a heinous crime under any circumstances in Confucian-heritage societies. Patricidal impulses must be repressed, rarely given literary or artistic expression.

In cases of patricide, typically it is the foster father, not the biological father, who is killed. In classic Chinese opera, the victim is the foster father in all cases of patricide. The stories all make the foster father responsible, in one way or another, for the death of the biological father. This provides the rationalization, in the name of filial piety, for the son to kill his foster father.

As a popular saying puts it, "There is no place under the sun for both oneself and the mortal enemy of one's father." Filial duty toward the biological father takes precedence over whatever feelings of attachment there may be toward the foster father: The "real" father's death must be avenged. In contrast, in stories where the father kills the son, the son is the biological son.

The Legend of Xue Rengui: A Counterpoint to the Oedipal Myth

Xue Rengui is a historical figure of the Tang dynasty. However, the popular legend about Xue is a superb example of a mythologized historical figure—a collective product of folk imagination.

Synopsis

A soldier of great martial skills during the Tang dynasty, Xue was assigned to military duty on a distant frontier and achieved great victories. His story has been incorporated into the standard repertory of Beijing opera. *At the Bend of the River Fen* is based on the story of Xue's return and reunion with his wife. He had not seen her and had not written her a single letter since he left her pregnant 18 years earlier to join the imperial service.

There are different versions of the story. In one version, on his way home, Xue saw a lad shooting wild geese at the bend of the River Fen. Impressed with the lad's skill, he challenged the lad to a contest of marksmanship, claiming that he could shoot two geese with a single arrow. The lad accepted the challenge, whereupon Xue shot him instead of the geese. Xue exclaimed: "I could have spared the lad, but a soldier like me could never let another person live if he was superior in marksmanship with the weapons in which I excel."

Xue finally reached home and saw his wife Liu Yingchun. Uncertain about her fidelity, he set a fidelity test. He did not reveal his true identity until he was satisfied that his wife had remained faithful to him during his long years of absence. Just as they were about to enjoy their reunion, his doubts and jealousy were aroused when he discovered a pair of men's shoes under a bed. Xue was about to kill her. His wife Liu demanded an explanation. Xue pointed to the shoes. Liu proved to be his rival. She teased him and thus provoked Xue to an intensified transport of jealousy. The following is my translation of the passage depicting the intensity of their encounter.

> **Liu** (Soliloquy) What was it all about? It's about my son's shoes. All right, let me also goad him to anger.... (To Xue) The person who wears these shoes is much stronger than you!
>
> **Xue** Naturally, stronger than me.... You don't like me anymore.
>
> **Liu** Not only stronger than you. Since your departure, I also have to rely on him to eat.
>
> **Xue** Of course. If you were to rely on me for 18 years, you would have starved....
>
> **Liu** I eat together with him every day. At night, I embrace him and sleep together.
>
> **Xue** You really don't have face. How can you say such a thing? Good, if you don't go to die, let me do it!

After the teasing, Liu told Xue that the shoes belonged to his son Xue Dingshan, who was born soon after he left home. The denouement was the tragic realization that the lad Xue had killed was none other than his own son, born shortly after he left home 18 years ago.

Interpretation

There is no intermediate between comic and tragic scenes on the Chinese stage: A comic scene may turn into a tragic one suddenly.

The dramatic encounter between husband and wife after a separation of 18 years is a counterpoint to that of Ulysses and his wife Penelope in Homer's epic poem *Odyssey*. The Penelope motif is very popular with Chinese audiences. It is exploited in many dramas, of which *At the Bend of the River Fen* is the most famous. The heroine Liu Yingchun remains a model of conjugal devotion to this day.

Xue's jealousy leaps out the pages of *At the Bend of the River Fen*. Note his remark, "You really don't have face," suggesting that his rage has more to do with feelings of dishonored manhood than with love. There is no self-reflection or acceptance of responsibility: The fault lies squarely on the wife. In contrast, Liu's psychological sophistication and strength of character are evident. She knows what husbands fear the most: The wife becomes sexually attracted to a younger, stronger man as they grow old. The Oedipal theme looms large in the triad of father, mother, and son.

Had the Medieval chastity belt (which is another myth) been available to be used, Xue could have saved himself from unnecessary worries about his wife's unfaithfulness. Actually, he had something far more potent working for him: The weight of Confucian moral doctrines that prescribe harsh limitations on women's sexual behavior and expressions.

Not to be missed, however, is a direct contrast between the Oedipal myth and the Xue legend: Whereas patricide is committed in the Oedipal myth, it is filicide that is committed in the Xue legend. To a Chinese audience, the Xue legend sends a threatening message that challenging authority can be fatal.

Novels, Legends, and Children's Stories from China

The *Twenty-Four Exemplars of Filial Piety* is a collection of stories of exemplary sons and daughters, meant as models to be emulated. For centuries, these stories formed an integral part of standard educational materials, familiar to almost every Chinese child. Their immense influence on parenting and more generally patterns of thought and action can hardly be overemphasized.

Filial Piety Moves Heaven

The legend of the Sage-King Yu Shun, entitled *Filial Piety Moves Heaven*, ranks first among the 24. It is a superb example of a historical figure mythologized—a collective product of folk imagination. Yu Shun personifies the Confucian model man, extolled by both Confucius and Mencius (see, e.g., *Doctrine of the Mean*, 17; *Mencius*, 4A:28, 5A:1).

Without question, Shun is among the most celebrated Chinese that ever lived; he is also the model man to more people than any other since the dawn of civilization. His name appears in a poem by Mao Zedong, *Song Wen Shen* (*Away with the Daimon of Plague*):

> Six hundred million in this Divine Land,
> Each and all, match Shun and Yao.

This poetic sentiment echoes the Confucian belief in human perfectibility. As stated in *Mencius*, "Every man may be Yao and Shun."

It is ironic that a simple story of one man in the third millennium BC, about whom we know so little, should have had such great impact on Chinese culture. Like those of other sage-kings, the story of Shun is shrouded in legendary beliefs whose historical authenticity is in doubt. We have only fragmentary accounts of Shun's life in various classical texts. From these accounts, I attempt to piece together a coherent story.

Shun was born to a blind, brutish man in the Eastern Barbarian region. As a young man, he was already renowned for his filial devotion. His father, however, rejected him in favor of his younger half-brother Xiang. At that time, the aged ruler Yao was searching for a successor to his throne.

Having heard of Shun's reputation, Yao wanted to give him a trial to assess his suitability. His method of assessment, undoubtedly one of the world's oldest, may claim to have more validity than psychological testing in modern times. He arranged to marry his two daughters to Shun and sent nine sons to stay with him, so as to observe his character. He also assigned governmental duties to Shun and put him through rigorous tests to assess his ability.

But Shun's condition in his family did not improve. His family still plotted to get rid of him. On one occasion, they set fire to a granary after he had gone inside. On another, they sent him down a well and then covered it with stones and mud. On yet another, they tried to get him drunk in order to kill him.

As stated in *Mencius*, "Xiang made it his daily business to slay Shun." Xiang coveted his brother's possessions: "Let my parents have his oxen and sheep. Let them have his storehouses and granaries. His shield and spear shall be mine. His lute shall be mine. His bow shall be mine. His two wives I shall make attend for me to my bed." Shun knew his brother wanted to kill him, but that did not detract him from his sincere brotherly love toward him: "When Xiang was sorrowful, he was also sorrowful; when Xiang was joyful, he was also joyful."

With the help of his two wives, Shun managed to escape death each time. He continued to take care of his half-brother and showed reverence to his father and stepmother. Such steadfast filial devotion led to a measure of moral transformation and improved relations within his family. The *Classic of Filial Piety* states: "His parents became pleasant, and his brother more conciliatory and virtuous." Eventually, Shun succeeded Yao to become one of the most celebrated sage-kings in Chinese history. As recorded in the *Book of History*, "The sovereign said, 'Come, you Shun. For three years I have consulted you on all affairs, examined your words, and found that they can be carried into practice. Now you can ascend the throne.'"

Shun's legend is revealing not only by what it says but also by what it does not. It is not known why Shun was rejected by his family. In the *Book of History*, we are only told that his father was "obstinately unprincipled"; his stepmother was "insincere"; his half-brother was "arrogant." There was no analysis of Shun's family dynamics; nor was there any exploration of Shun's emotional life or his state of mind. Again, we are only informed in the *Book of History* that Shun "daily cried with tears to compassionate heaven and to his parents, taking to himself all the guilt and charging himself with their wickedness."

Mencius explained why Shun was full of sorrow and "felt like a poor man who has nowhere to turn to": All his possession of beauty, riches, and honors was insufficient to remove his sorrow, which could be removed only by getting his parents to be in accord with him. Mencius also gave a hint for understanding his depression: "Shun would say, 'What can there be in me that my parents do not love me?'" Shun thus blamed himself, and not his family, for being rejected; he attributed the cause of rejection to his own imperfection, and not to the wickedness of his father and half-brother.

A picture of clinical depression emerges from Shun's feelings of being rejected and abandoned (having "nowhere to turn to"), inability to "remove his sorrow," and especially self-blaming ("taking to himself all the guilt"). Anger and aggression are directed to the self, not to external aggressors. A psychoanalytic interpretation based on the internalization of aggression suggests itself. But it is alien to Chinese culture.

Shun's legend embodies a number of messages that have profound implications for Chinese patterns of thought and action. First of all, the legend is a statement of optimism and triumph: Filial piety has the power to transform tragedy into a story with a happy ending. Furthermore, Shun's triumph was not based on defiance of parental authority; rather, it was achieved through unwavering filial devotion. Whereas the Xue legend is a tragic tale of horror about filicide, the Shun legend is a tale of triumph over filicide-cum-fratricide. The moral is that exemplary filial devotion can touch heaven, just as in the West it is said, "Faith can move mountains."

However, the Shun legend contains a strong element of wishful thinking: that Heaven be moved. If heaven remained unmoved, and Shun's family persisted in its hostile rejection of him, what would his unwavering filial devotion lead to? Consider others confronted by dangers similar to those to which Shun was exposed: What is the likelihood of their survival?

One can hardly miss the Western parallels or similarities found in biblical accounts of intrafamily violence, such as the stories of Cain and Abel, Esau and Jacob, and Joseph and his brothers; all these are surpassed by the dramatic violence, adultery, and incest in the house of David.

Burying One's Son for the Sake of One's Mother

The legend of Shun shares a common theme with another story from the 24 entitled *Burying One's Son for the Sake of One's Mother*: the danger of being killed by one's own father. A poor man, Guo Ju, was prepared to bury his three-year-old son so that his mother would no longer need to share her portion of food with the child. He said to his wife: "It is possible to have a son again, but not possible to have another mother." She dared not disobey. While digging a ditch, he found gold, with a written message that it was meant to be a gift from heaven to him as a reward for his filiality. The gold saved his infant son. Typically, the story unfolded without any mention of the wife's wishes or feelings.

The peril of being buried was not confined to infants from poor families. In an earlier version of the story, Guo was not poor at all but well-to-do. After his father passed away, he distributed all the family fortune to his two brothers and took on the task of providing for his mother by himself alone. The son about to be buried had just been born. Guo's motive for burying the infant son was the anticipation that raising him would jeopardize fulfilling his filial duty to provide for his mother in her old age.

Given the frequent occurrence of famines, infanticide is salient in the Chinese collective experience. A Marxist interpretation would attribute the rise of the filial ethic, the "superstructure," to conditions of scarcity, its "economic base." But this interpretation does not account for why infants, rather than the aged, should be sacrificed. Rather, filial piety rationalized infanticide made necessary by starvation.

Masochistic and Self-deprecating Behavior

A good many other stories from the 24 provide a rich source of thought in the realm of cultural pathology. The filial acts were sometimes extreme to the point of unreasonableness, even cruelty: A man divorced his wife because she failed to show reverence toward wooden statues that he had carved in the image of his deceased parents.

Masochism seemed to be present in a number of the filial sons who subjected themselves to great personal indignity, physical suffering, the risk of life, or self-sacrifice to satisfy parental demands. An eight-year-old boy named Wu Meng deliberately let mosquitoes feed on himself each summer night in order to prevent his parents from being attacked. Despite ill-treatment by his stepmother, a boy laid himself on a frozen river in order to catch fresh fish, which she desired to eat. On the advice of a physician, a man tasted his sick father's excrement; when the result of this "medical test" indicated a dire prognosis, he prayed that he would die in place of his father.

In another story, the filial devotion suggests excessive, perhaps even pathological, attachment to the mother: A poet and calligrapher was said to have watched his sick mother for a whole year without leaving her bedside or taking off his clothes and who, despite his high social position, performed the most menial tasks, like washing the stool, for her.

Collectively, these are stories of heroic deeds and self-sacrifice: The more torturous, masochistic, or self-destructive the deed is, the more laudable it would be. In the name of filial piety, the filial son would not hesitate to put his health, even life, in peril.

Variations on a Theme

The stories recounted above differ from one another, of course, in some important respects. In the Shun legend, the protagonist is old enough to fend for himself. In *Burying One's Son for the Sake of One's Mother*, the infant is completely helpless.

Guo Ju was motivated by filial considerations, to ensure having enough to eat for his mother. When you are an infant, there is not much you can do. But when you are considered old enough to understand things, you are held responsible for acknowledging your indebtedness to your parents and putting their well-being ahead of your own. In particular, under conditions of scarcity or hardship, you would not want your parents to suffer or be deprived on account of you. Moreover, you would not want your parents to be exposed to the painful situation of having to decide whether to sacrifice your well-being or theirs. Therefore, you would preemptively sacrifice your well-being for their sake. In psychological terms, external cultural demands are now internalized.

In *Dream of the Red Chamber*, written in the 18th century AD and reputedly the greatest Chinese novel that was ever written, the protagonist Jia Baoyu was almost beaten to death by his father. On one occasion, his father was infuriated by reports of Baoyu's misdeeds, one compounded on another to add fuel to his fury. Beside himself with rage, he shouted to the pages, "Gag his mouth. Beat him to death." Baoyu was beaten with a flattened bamboo sweep. Not satisfied that his executioner was hitting hard enough, his father himself administered the beating with savagery. Baoyu was in serious danger of life and limb. He might have died if the womenfolk did not intervene in time. Baoyu showed no spirit of defiance but only passive resistance. He remained fearful of his father, like "a mouse seeing a cat." His case is representative of many Chinese children.

The savage beating also has a basis in filial piety. If Baoyu grew up to be a spoiled, useless person, his father would have failed in his filial duty toward his ancestors, to educate his son properly and thus to protect the good name of his family. In the case of Shun, the father had no good reason to kill his son at all. Thus, different circumstances and motivation underlay the fathers' actions. Nonetheless, all their actions that imperiled the lives of their sons were intentional. Shun was an exemplar of filiality. But Baoyu must be judged, by Confucian standards, an unfilial son for having failed to meet his father's expectations of proper conduct.

Paternal brutality is nothing new. A popular saying states, "The filial son comes from caning." Baoyu's experience must have been shared by countless Chinese children since ancient times. Even today, many seniors may recall the horror of paternal punishment they received during childhood.

A Summation

Regarding intergenerational violence, in virtually all instances the violence is directed from the father to the son in Chinese literature—in contrast to the Oedipal myth.

We may marvel at how deeply ingrained filial values are in Chinese culture. Carried to its logical conclusion, filial piety leads to self-sacrifice for the sake of one's parents, not of one's children. However, it must be made clear that self-destructive behavior per se is unfilial, as is exposing oneself to danger unnecessarily (e.g., participating in a motor car race) in general. Suicide is decidedly unfilial because it breaks the continuity of the parent-child relationship and perhaps even the family line. Self-destructive acts are condoned only when they are performed for filial purposes.

In sum, filial piety takes precedence at the expense of everything else. Sensitivity to human needs, personal aspirations, and growth toward independence are all repressed. Even dubious or wrongful acts may be condoned, even praised, if they are done with filial intentions: A six-year-old child pocketed two of the oranges offered him by his host and, when discovered, explained that they were intended for his mother back home.

Pathogenic Demands of Culture

What are the psychological effects of filial piety on child development? Consider as an example the case of Wu Meng who let mosquitoes feed on himself in order to prevent his parents from being attacked. We have no information on how well-adjusted or maladjusted Wu Meng was. Such a question was simply not a matter of concern in any of the *Twenty-Four Exemplars of Filial Piety*.

However, in terms of social adequacy or meeting the primary requirements of society, Wu Meng must be judged to have been highly successful. Having learned to accept his filial obligations, he prepared himself well for his later roles in life. The reputation he had earned as a filial son brought not only praise and respect for himself but also honor to his entire family. Thus, he secured for himself a worthy position within his social order. In other stories, filial actions were amply rewarded, in material terms or ascendancy in social status.

Nevertheless, Wu Meng's success was achieved at a considerable cost to himself, physical and in all likelihood psychological as well. Does it not raise the question that the requirements of social adequacy and psychological well-being are not always compatible? Certain age-honored ways of socializing children may be quite insensitive to their psychological needs. Consequently, successful adaptation to their cultural milieu can be achieved only at the price of suffering various psychological disturbances.

Thus, we must come to grips with the question: What happens when the demands of a culture are in themselves pathogenic? Given the overriding importance attached to filial piety in traditional Chinese society, what could the child do but conform? What room was there for the social innovator? The rebellious or nonconforming child would have an awfully hard time.

Pathogenic cultural demands are not unique to China. Suppose we substitute religious piety for filial piety, and ecclesiastical authority for paternal authority, we have a picture of Europe during the Middle Ages, which conjures up imageries of mass madness, demonology, exorcism, witch hunt, and the Inquisition. This is to admit that certain cultural aspects may be pathogenic, not just in China but also in the West.

The notion of pathogenic cultural demands that I have introduced imputes cross-cultural validity to the importance of parent-child relationships in the pathogenetic process. Childhood psychopathology may be viewed as a price to be paid for "adapting" to parental demands that embody the pathogenic aspects of culture.

The recognition and treatment of childhood psychopathology depend on how childhood and the parent-child relationship are conceptualized, circumscribed in both the temporal and spatial dimensions by the prevailing ethos and state of knowledge. Culture casts the frame within which the child's behavior is perceived and evaluated. It preconditions the perceiver to be sensitized to certain aspects and sets up mental blocks against other aspects.

Thus, a body of knowledge of childhood psychopathology could not have arisen within Chinese culture, given its moralistic, rather than psychological, orientation toward childhood. In particular, it would be quite inconceivable for a pathogenetic theory that implicates parental responsibility to have been developed. Filial piety acts to create and maintain cultural blind spots against the awareness of childhood psychopathology and its connection with parent-child relationships. The cultural belief expressed in the saying, "There are no wrong (or bad) parents under the heavens," shows how deeply the Chinese conception of parenthood is rooted in filial piety.

After reviewing the empirical evidence, Ho (1996; see also Ho, 1989, 1994, in press-b; Ho et al., 2012) concludes that the psychological consequences of *traditional* filial piety appear to be consistently negative from a contemporary perspective on human development. The evidence implicates filial piety in the development toward authoritarian moralism, cognitive conservatism, and prejudice toward outgroups in Chinese societies. It also indicates, in particular, that the father-son relationship tends to be marked by affective distance, even tension and antagonism. Clearly, more research attention should be paid, therefore, to the negative, pathogenic aspects of culture.

The Perils of Challenging Authority

Defining the father-son relationship entails the problem of handling intergenerational rivalry and conflicts. Both father and son are bound to resolve potential conflicts between them within the confines that their culture allows. For the father, the problem concerns the limits of paternal authority and tolerance of the son's defiance. For the son, a basic developmental task is to internalize societal control over aggressive impulses, accomplished largely through learning how to handle conflicts with the father and other authority figures. A balance between self-assertion and submission to authority is reached upon the successful completion of this task.

As great tragedies of familial relations, both patricide and filicide strike a common chord in the human experience. They remind us of the reality of intergenerational violence within the family. The message embodied in both Greek and Chinese legends is clear: You challenge authority at your own peril.

Why, then, is there a lack of valuing the defiant, innovative thinker in Confucianism? The answer, I submit, is ideological conservatism: Challenging authority, particularly paternal authority, is not only forbidden but also morally undesirable. The tragic hero is extolled only when he is defending established moral principles in conformity with Confucian ethics, in which filial piety and loyalty are central values.

Monkey King in *Journey to the West*

There is no tradition of romanticizing the daring, rebellious hero in acts of exploration or self-assertion in Confucianism. Romanticization finds expression only outside of orthodox Confucianism, in opera, novels, and stories. The best-known example is *Journey to the West*, a novel about the Monkey King who accompanied his master in search of Buddhist scriptures in India. Not disposed to subservience, Monkey King wreaked havoc in the heavenly palace of the Jade Emperor. .

Such a novel is not to be taken seriously by Confucian scholar-teachers. Yet, *Journey to the West* is most popular with both children and adults alike. Monkey King is resourceful and endowed with magical powers; he is an entertaining character; he is not subservient to anyone, except his master. Monkey King has both human and monkey nature.

The tension between submission and self-assertion is a central theme underlying *Journey to the West*. Psychologically, I interpret Monkey King as the projection of an assertive adolescent boy onto a young alpha monkey. Both the boy and the monkey have to be subdued, tamed by their superiors in the process of growing up. Indeed, Monkey King was tamed by powerful figures, including the Goddess of Mercy and the supreme Buddha. Eventually, he reached Buddhahood himself—at which point, however, his spirit of defiance is no more.

The Universal Question: To Submit or to Defy

To achieve a balance between being subdued and remaining defiant, that is a major developmental task that cannot be avoided by adolescents. Challenging authority may be hazardous to your life, regardless of where you live. The dilemma facing the individual is self-assertion versus submissiveness.

To submit or to defy authority, that is the universal question that confronts all of us in the process of growing up. In this regard, the Christian and the Confucian traditions provide dramatically divergent definitions of authority relations, with far-reaching psychological consequences.

The Confucian definition of the father-son relationship allows for no solution to the Oedipal conflict other than total submission. The father's authority remains absolute. In the Judeo-Christian tradition, the biblical commandment, "Honor thy father and thy mother," was God's law conveyed to the Jewish people through Moses. Ultimately, Christian ethics is God-centered, whereas Confucian ethics is anchored in human relationships. The richness of biblical accounts of family violence and pathology, lacking in Confucian orthodoxy, suggests that there is room for thinking and confronting more openly the universal question I have posed.

Concluding Thoughts

This chapter brings up topics that may arouse both curiosity and discomfort in the reader. Curiosity aroused is required to reinterpret the Oedipal myth and explore new frontiers of knowledge. And discomfort because patricide and perhaps ever more filicide arouse horrors deep in our psyche, normally not something that we want to think, let alone talk about; the idea of "pathogenic cultural demands" is disrespectful of cultural traditions that people have long upheld, even glorified. A universal question concerning submission versus defiance has been posed. I won't provide an answer for the reader. But I trust that this chapter has been informative on how readers may come up with an answer by themselves.

Thematic Group 4
Spirituality Versus Spiritual Emptiness

I look into the mirror and see a spiritual void. I then realize what spirituality means to my existence.

The theme of self-encapsulation versus transcendence reverberates throughout the present volume. Transcendence may be manifest in various ways: moving from my Chinese cultural identity to being a world citizen (see Chapter 1), from individual-in-isolation to individual-in-communion, from the closing of the mind to openness, from surrendering self-ownership to self-mastery, from spiritual emptiness to spiritual fulfillment.

This thematic group goes from madness to dignified existence and spiritual development. In Chapter 17, I argue that madness has no necessary connection with violence or evil; I advance the thesis that it is possible to retain a measure of madness in dignified living (madness-in-dignity) and of dignity even in a state of madness (dignity-in-madness).

In Chapter 18, I affirm the coexistence of spirituality and spiritual emptiness, in keeping with our dialectical stance. A strategy for the transcultural assessment of spirituality and spiritual emptiness in terms of component pairs is provided. The result is the Multidimensional Evaluations of Spirituality (see Appendix A for details).

17

Transforming Madness for Dignified Existence

> *We have seen enough of human misery that malignant madness wedded to evil has wrought. But there is hope: Benign madness devoid of evil or violence may be harnessed to enhance human dignity.*

Many people yearn for and actively seek extraordinary experiences, good and bad. William James (1920/2008) once wrote to his family:

> I'm glad to get into something less blameless, but more admiration-worthy. The flash of a pistol, a dagger, or a devilish eye, anything to break the unlovely level of 10,000 good people—a crime, murder, rape, elopement, anything would do. (p.43)

"A devilish eye, elopement, and rape" conjure up romantic-sexual fantasies, in an ascending order of salaciousness. Fantasies of a violent nature are also abundant; "anything would do" is really scary.

To associate madness and violence seems natural enough. Have we not seen enough of mass shootings by mentally disturbed individuals in America, for instance? I will, however, argue that this association is misconstrued. And what does madness have to do with human dignity? My answer is, "Everything." The world has long wanted to expunge madness from dignified existence. But is it possible? And even if the answer is yes, which I doubt, is it desirable?

Advocates of human dignity have long championed the rights of the disadvantaged or disenfranchised, minority or ethnic groups subject to systemic abuse or violence by another, and so forth. In comparison, people with mental disorders have not received the attention they deserve in human dignity and humiliation studies. Throughout history, mentally disordered persons have suffered systemic stigmatization, ostracism, and ill-treatment. What is lesser known is the mistreatment they have received, yes, at the hands of psychiatrists (e.g., overmedication, lobotomy, indiscriminate use of electric shock therapy).

To pay greater attention to the plight of the mentally disordered, I will draw on my firsthand experiences from both being a "doctor" (clinical psychologist) and "patient." I have had my share of extraordinary experiences, which I did not actively seek. They simply occurred spontaneously, inexplicably, and unpredictably during 22 episodes of mood disorder I have had—all of exuberance and none of depression. In terms of psychiatric nomenclature, my condition may be characterized as a unipolar disorder with only hypomanic and/or manic episodes. This condition is highly atypical; common mood disorders are characterized by episodes of depression, or by bipolar mood swings alternating between unusual elevation and depression. (Incredibly, the occurrence of a hypomanic episode coincides with the writing of this manuscript).

I cannot switch the episodes on or off at will. But I continue to value them as life-enriching experiences. After the occurrence of so many episodes of "madness," it is hardly surprising that the question should arise: "Am I mad or enlightened?" Johnson and Friedman (2008) have discussed the challenges psychological diagnosticians face when dealing with religious, spiritual, or transpersonal experiences that may range from healthy to psychopathological. The present rejoinder adduces evidence from my own self-studies (Ho, 2014a, 2014b, 2016) to spell out the conditions under which madness may be rendered benign, even transformed in the service of human dignity.

The connection between madness and evil has already been clarified in Chapter 10. Making a distinction between benign madness and malignant madness is based on ethical, rather than psychiatric, grounds. Malignant madness causes suffering to the sufferer and those around him. If wedded to evil, as in the case of Hitler and his gang of psychopaths, it has no redeeming value; it serves only to magnify suffering and threaten human dignity.

The present chapter defends the thesis that benign madness devoid of evil and violence may be harnessed to enhance dignified existence. In what follows, first I clarify the key construct of human dignity. To justify the claim that human dignity is ecumenical and all inclusive, an excursion into the debate between cultural-ethical universalism and relativism is unavoidable. This debate informs the arguments advanced in which the implicit tensions between universalism and relativism pervade (see "Cultural Relativism and the Definition of Abnormality" in Chapter 9).

Second, I refute the claim that madness and violence are necessarily connected; mentally disordered or disabled persons are more likely the recipients, rather than perpetrators, of humiliation or violence.

Finally, I introduce arguments that summate to support my thesis that it is possible to retain a measure of madness in dignified living (i.e., madness-in-dignity) and of dignity even in a state of madness (i.e., dignity-in-madness).

Construct Explication

The focus here is to clarify the use of three major terms: madness, violence, and human dignity. Obviously, I am using the term *madness* rather loosely. Madness is a nontechnical term that refers, in a broad sense, to mental disorders or abnormal conditions. It lacks specificity and does not refer to a specific disorder. Madness connotes insanity, frenzy, and severity: For instance, psychosis is madness, but typically we would not refer to a common anxiety disorder, which is mild in relative terms, as madness. In sum, without further specification, madness is used broadly to refer to the more severe forms of mental disorders.

The expression of violence takes many forms: subtle-indirect or open-direct; verbal, physical, or both; individual or collective; occasional or repetitive; planned or unplanned; random or institutional. Violence is especially vicious when it is targeted toward a specific cultural or ethnic group, intentionally, systemically, and systematically (e.g., genocide, ethnic cleansing). Against such an extreme affront to human dignity, humanity has declared, "Never again"!

Even when it is expressed in lesser forms, violence humiliates and, therefore, threatens human dignity. In this chapter, we are more concerned with collective, systemic, and institutional (though not necessarily planned) than with individual forms of violence. Accordingly, analysis at the macro sociopolitical level is more applicable than at the micro-psychological level.

To explicate the key construct *human dignity* is essential to the development of my arguments. Here, I simply state that human dignity is characterized by the following five defining attributes.

1. Human dignity is an inalienable right, based on the intrinsic worth of the human person. Therefore, no one should be deprived of dignity. Unlike social status, prestige, face, and the like, it does not have to be earned. It is not respect because, without self-respect, respect by others can hardly be taken for granted. It is not entitlement, the right to be guaranteed benefits under a government program, because human dignity goes beyond tangible benefits. More fundamentally, human dignity does not derive from governmental authority; rather, the exercise of governmental authority itself has to be based on respect for human dignity.
2. Human dignity is a cardinal or core value underlying diverse aspects of life. A loss of dignity would result in a significant decrease in the overall quality of life, and a gain in dignity would give greater substance to a good life. What would life be like without dignity?
3. Human dignity is relational. It is not anchored in the isolated individual person, but in relations between persons: If your dignity is threatened or damaged, so would mine be; equally, if your dignity is secure, I would feel more secure about mine. An important implication follows: Collectively, the total gain or loss of human dignity for humankind is greater than the summation of human dignity over individuals.
4. Human dignity is all inclusive. It is applicable to all without exception, without regard to age, gender, ethnicity, disability or incapacitation, physical or mental condition.
5. Human dignity is universal, based on belief in the unity of humankind. Universality does not negate but allows for ethnic-cultural pluralism. Accordingly, we acknowledge that concrete expressions of human dignity may vary in different ethnic-cultural contexts. However, universality does negate social norms and practices (e.g., ethnic cleansing) that, under specific historical, political, or cultural conditions, result in great harm to human dignity.

Minimal material conditions (e.g., food, shelter, safety) have to be met for dignified living. Threats to dignified living may come from natural calamities, from human action or inaction, or from a combination of natural and artificial causes. For instance, human activities may lead to natural calamities through environmental disregard; and inaction may fail to prevent unnecessary loss of dignity after the occurrence of calamities. Accordingly, conservationist values are essential to the preservation of collective human dignity. They constitute an extension of civic virtues from society to nature, simply because the destruction of the environment on a global scale by human activity will eventually erode the foundation of civil societies.

Universality or ecumenicity is one of the cardinal principles underlying the affirmation of human dignity. Yet, we must make a critical point explicit here: Ecumenicity must not degenerate into the kind of pluralism that allows for "anything goes." Inherent in pluralism is the dialectical tension between two tendencies: diversity and unity. Diversity without unity leads to factionalism; unity without diversity is boring uniformity.

I have stated categorically that human dignity is universal. This invites disputation because many may argue that, as a value, human dignity is subject to various historical and sociocultural interpretations (revisit the age-old debate between universalism and particularism in Chapter 9). A major task lies ahead of us: to identify and catalog commonalities as well as differences in conceptions of human dignity among the world's philosophical, religious, and cultural traditions.

Are Madness and Violence Necessarily Connected?

Does mental disturbance or abnormality necessarily lead people to become prone to violence? Let me first draw on my experience in a huge state mental hospital where I lived and worked as a clinical psychologist for some five years in the 1960s (Ho, 1965; see also "Engineering a Social Revolution in a Mental Hospital" in Chapter 1). Back then, state mental hospitals were places of hopelessness, where inmates were locked up in smelly wards and given no effective treatment.

The one I worked in was a monstrosity with more than 5,000 inmates. My experience led me to question if there was a pervasive or necessary connection between madness and violence. Contrary to common perception, the hospital was a quiet, peaceful place. I saw little physical violence among patients, but mostly passivity, resignation, and despair that resulted from being institutionalized to the hospital milieu. The patients were not perpetrators of violence; rather, they were victims of humiliation and institutional "violence"— an affront to human dignity.

Such institutionalization is common to *total institutions* (e.g., armies, prisons, ecclesiastical institutions) in which workers or inmates perform most of their daily functions within the same geographical location under an authoritarian social structure (Goffman, 1961). Typically, the mentally disordered who are not (or not yet) institutionalized receive no better treatment either.

Elsewhere, American society is full of physical violence (e.g., bullying and gang fights), in contrast to the hospital grounds I have described. The violence seems everywhere, in virtual reality as in real life, among normal people. Mass shootings by the mentally disturbed do occur, with alarming regularity. But to attribute the loss of lives to madness is to turn a blind eye to a more fundamental question: Does the loss of lives result purely from the mad people who have guns, or more from the normal people who oppose gun control? This line of questioning leads to an uncomfortable thought: Human tragedies result more from failures of the normal to prevent their recurrence than from actions of the abnormal.

Madness-in-Dignity and Dignity-in-Madness

My firsthand experiences during episodes of madness lend further credence for negating the putative connection between madness and violence (Ho, 2014a). Rather, they point to a dialectical relation between madness and spirituality: Each may transform, and be transformed by, the other.

In terms of a dialectical relation, the transformation of spirituality entails harnessing the creative forces of madness; and the transformation of madness entails receiving the healing effects from spirituality. The idea of harnessing goes beyond coexisting with madness. Coexistence is like living at the foot of an active volcano, not knowing when it will explode. Harnessing madness is more radical: The creative forces of madness are made subservient to spirituality to drive its further development. The healing forces of spirituality temper the volatility of madness and keep it from causing harm or destruction. Self-reflection and self-monitoring, both indicative of metacognitive functioning, play a crucial role in this dialectical process.

Even in the depth of madness, I would frequently ask myself, "Am I mad or enlightened?" This has helped me greatly to deflate my supreme self-confidence, keep in touch with reality, and avoid causing more harm to myself or others.

In this way, spirituality and madness coexist in a dialectical relation. Spirituality without a measure of madness is devoid of energy; madness without spirituality loses its redeeming value. Spirituality derives creative energy from madness to reach new heights; madness receives the healing, calming effects of spirituality to become benign. Thus, it is possible to achieve a measure of madness in dignified living and of dignity even in a state of madness.

This dynamic conception means that madness may continue to be intertwined with spirituality, not something to be expunged from the mind. A dialectical relation entails tension and conflict. Many psychologists (e.g., Carl Rogers) tend to regard inner conflicts as negative and self-consistency as positive for mental health. Self-consistency is manifest in congruence between the real self and the ideal self. By this count, ironically, psychopaths are the most congruent and thus mentally healthy! The notion of self-consistency may lead to a sterile conception of human functioning in which conflicts have no place. Conflicts are, however, a source for change, adaptation, and creativity in the process of their resolution.

I am humbled by how arduous the process can be; failures persist even after having had plenty of opportunities for learning from 22 episodes of madness. When spiritual forces prevail, unpleasant memories do lose their destructiveness and madness becomes more benign. Thus, I have had limited success: experiencing moments of serenity, most ironically, during episodic madness, and when spiritual forces augmented during madness carry into normal times. These extraordinary experiences have informed me on spirituality in clinical practice (Ho, 2014b).

Eros Versus Thanatos in Madness as in Normality

In Western psychology, the healthy self is conceived as stable over time; it is a coherent, integrated, and unitary whole. In Eastern thought, Daoism and Buddhism in particular, the notion of selflessness is central to the conception of selfhood (Ho, 1995). During episodes of madness, there were moments when I experienced transcendent states of emptiness in which the self appeared to have vanished.

Buddhist ideas of self-emptying or no-mind emptiness refer in a positive light to a state of mind emptied of self and its thoughts and cravings (Ho, 1995, 2014a), and should not be confused with spiritual emptiness. Moreover, differences in conceptions of selfhood between the East and the West entail the need to guard against viewing extraordinary experiences (e.g., selfless self) solely in pathological terms. I would argue further that expanding our conceptions of selfhood opens more doors to life enrichment in the West as well.

To experience the selfless self or the empty mind is to go beyond, not supplant, the normal and healthy. In a similar vein, the achievement of impulse control is a prerequisite to experiencing the extraordinary, which implies overcoming repression and gaining access to the unconscious. If what comes out are unchecked rampant impulses and raw destructiveness, the result would be horror.

Digging deeply into my own self during episodes of abnormal mood elevation, I see a preponderance of positives (e.g., love of humanity) over the negatives (e.g., hateful violence), and I foresee no horror when impulses are expressed in magnified intensities. Early in one of my episodes of madness, I wrote in my diary that Eros without Thanatos is "safe." But a reversal of this preponderance raises the specter of madness wedded to evil. Witness the horrid destructiveness to the world that mad psychopaths, exemplified by Adolf Hitler, have wrought.

To Think the Unthinkable

It is important to distinguish between thoughts, words, and deeds in terms of impulse control. This is especially important when repression vanishes, as in my case, and access to the unconscious is unhindered. Impulses are harmless as long as they remain in the domain of thought.

This is a fundamental viewpoint in psychoanalytic theory—in sharp contrast with Confucian ethics, which insists on keeping thoughts "correct" and "pure." As long as we exercise adequate control over the expression of our impulses in words or in deeds, madness may be rendered benign. And the attainment of an ideal, madness-in-dignity as well as dignity-in-madness, may be in sight. According to Ho (2019a), when nothing is unthinkable there is no boundary to creativity.

The contrast between Confucianism and psychoanalysis is most explicit with regard to thought control. Psychoanalysis is predicated on the total eradication of *all* restrictions on thought: Nothing is unthinkable. Now, to dare to think the unthinkable is the fountainhead of creativity. Thought control suffocates it.

Summary and Conclusions

This chapter acknowledges that the plight of mentally disturbed, deviant, or "mad" persons demands due attention in human dignity and humiliation studies. The construct of human dignity is defined in terms of five attributes: as being (1) an inalienable right, (2) a cardinal value underlying diverse aspects of life, (3) anchored in the relations between persons, (4) all inclusive, and (5) universal. Universality and total inclusiveness, in particular, implies that dignity is applicable to all without exception—without regard to disability or incapacitation, physical or mental condition.

Two main conclusions emerge in this chapter. The first is that the belief in a necessary connection between madness and violence is false. The second is that madness may be not only rendered benign but also harnessed to retain a measure of madness in dignified living and of dignity even in a state of madness.

The creative energy of madness may be harnessed for dignified existence, given that several preconditions are met (Ho, 2016). The first is the capability for self-reflectiveness that enables one to be aware of and monitor the extraordinary state in which one finds oneself. The second is an intact sense of self, without which, paradoxically, selflessness can hardly be attained. The third is adequate impulsive control, without which the destructive forces of madness may get out of control. Finally, most important of all is the preponderance of love over hate, for its reversal would raise the horrid specter of madness wedded to evil. Even when these preconditions are met, sustained effort is needed to transform madness in the service of life enrichment. And without ever having been mad, there may be a limit on how such transformation can be accomplished.

18

Spirituality and Spiritual Emptiness: Toward Transcultural Applicability

Discontent with ordinary existence is the mother of spiritual development.

The idea of spirituality was born when the first *Homo sapien* stumbled on the question, "What will become of me after I am dead?" For humanity, this question has driven the rise of religions, absorbed the intellectual energy of countless thinkers, and shaped the course of human development. It has become the perennial question: Like no other, it compels us to reflect on the time-limited nature of our existence. Spirituality, however, is concerned with much more than death and what happens after death. It informs humanity about the meaning of life and ways of living one's life. Nourished in values in diverse cultures, spirituality represents a distillate of ecumenical wisdom.

In my conception, discontent with ordinary existence is the mother of spiritual development. The reason is that spiritual fulfillment goes above and beyond ordinary existence conditioned by the biological and sociocultural givens in which a person is situated. It entails reaching for the highest ideal, that is, the realization of human potential to its fullest.

It finds expression in different religious-philosophical traditions: in Christianity, to be Christ-like and bear the sufferings of humankind on one's shoulders; in Buddhism, to have "the heart of a bodhisattva," filled with compassion; in Daoism, to be sage like, selfless, spontaneous, living in harmony with nature and society; in Confucianism, to reach self-realization as the ultimate purpose in life through continual self-cultivation; and in Marxism, to struggle for the liberation of humankind from social injustice in the form of class exploitation and oppression. In sum, the paths to spirituality are many, grounded in different beliefs and ideals.

Of course, lofty ideals may be beyond the reach for most of us; so expectations have to be lowered. Although spirituality is marked by the desire to reach for the higher goals of existence, success is not a necessary condition for spirituality. Furthermore, success in one aspect of life may be mixed with failures in other aspects. A spiritual journey can be rewarding in itself, adding color to all aspects of life. The goal of spiritual fulfillment is attractive and the process in search of fulfillment itself is exciting. I would go as far as to say spirituality is built into human nature: We have no choice but to seek it out; the failure to do so violates our being.

In recent decades, psychological studies of spirituality have expanded immensely in both volume and diversity of theoretical perspectives. One special source of influence on this development may be discerned: The rise of cross-cultural psychology that has helped mainstream psychology to be more aware of non-Western traditions rich in conceptions of spirituality, such as Buddhism and Daoism. Still, spirituality is an exceedingly elusive construct to define. Imposing the goal of achieving transcultural applicability makes evaluation doubly more difficult. In this vein, Ho and Ho (2007) have explicated the spirituality construct, differentiated it from religiosity, stipulated the requirements of ecumenicity, proposed strategies for achieving transcultural applicability, and recommended operational procedures of measurement.

The Multidimensional Evaluations of Spirituality (MES)

In this chapter, a conceptual framework for constructing the Multidimensional Evaluations of Spirituality is articulated. The constructs of spiritual fulfillment and spiritual emptiness are explicated, with fulfillment and emptiness conceived in terms of a dialectical relation. Two strategies are adopted for achieving transcultural applicability: (a) extracting commonalities across the world's major philosophical-religious traditions and (b) maximal inclusiveness. Approaches to evaluation rely on (a) diverse sources of data, (b) multidimensional measures, (c) construct pairs, and (d) representing each of these construct pairs on two unipolar continua.

In what follows, I take on the task of constructing the MES. Because of its receptivity to universalistic ideals, MES promises to have transcultural applicability, which has rarely, if ever, been achieved. It would provide researchers and practitioners of spiritual counseling with a comprehensive conceptual framework for working with people from different cultural, religious, or ideological backgrounds.

My conceptualization is universalistic in orientation, not biased toward or anchored in a particular religion or ethical tradition. It does not rest on claiming that there are universal spiritual values that remain invariant across different historical, religious, or cultural contexts; or on claiming that the "true" values are those located at the top of a hierarchy of spiritual values. But it does rest on the claim that commonalties may be found among spiritual values in diverse contexts.

In keeping with pluralism, universality allows for, even welcomes, cultural or religious diversity (Ho, 2014a; see also Chapter 17). This conceptualization resonates with the participatory approach that embraces a pluralistic vision of spirituality.

Explication of the spirituality construct is the first step toward construction. Delineating the essential attributes of spirituality is necessary for defining a set of inclusion-exclusion criteria, which would direct researchers' attention to appropriate target patterns of thought and action. The criteria spell out the conditions for a candidate item to qualify as measuring spirituality, or at least a component of it. This helps to constrain overinclusiveness, which would dilute a construct's utility. Accordingly, I first explicate the construct of spirituality in the following propositions.

1. Spirituality addresses existential or transcendent issues, such as those concerning one's relations with others and one's place in the cosmos. Conviction that life is meaningful and purposeful is quintessential to spirituality.
2. Spirituality is located in the domain of cardinal or supraordinate values underlying all aspects of life, such as respect for life and love of humanity.
3. Spirituality is characterized by self-reflectiveness, and is hence metacognitive in nature.

Collectively, these propositions make clear that spirituality is a subset of psychological phenomena. Spirituality and religiosity are distinct, though overlapping, constructs. It is possible for a person to be religious without being spiritual or spiritual without being religious, be both, or be neither.

Dialectics of Fulfillment and Emptiness

Spiritual fulfillment and spiritual emptiness are not reducible to merely opposites of each other. They may coexist, alternating at different moments, under different conditions, in a person's lifetime. Thus, the attainment of spirituality is a dynamic process in which struggle, change, and self-transformation are central. Spiritual emptiness results not so much from frustrations or failures of existential quest as from inaction, being lukewarm or noncommittal, or, worse, giving up altogether.

When life becomes purposeless, directionless, and meaningless, eventually spiritual emptiness sets in, characterized by the cardinal symptoms of estrangement and alienation. Life would be stagnant, unfulfilled and unfulfilling; symptoms of burnout or feelings of embitterment may appear. In brief, we may conceive spiritual emptiness as a state of impoverishment or deprivation, going below the level of ordinary existence conditioned by biological and sociocultural givens.

Two important points should be added here. First, viewing life as purposeful or meaningful is not necessarily an indication of spirituality. Otherwise, we may find ourselves caught in an uncomfortable position of having to admit ideological fanatics (e.g., Hideki Tojo, Adolf Hitler, Pol Pot), whose singularity of purpose have led to acts of extreme evil against humanity, as being spiritual. Thus, an additional condition has to be present: The purposive actions must not be taken with expressed aims that violate commonly accepted humanitarian principles. Such actions include, but are not limited to, crimes against humanity (e.g., genocide, ethnic cleansing, and terrorism). Here too, I have to admit frankly that my conception is ultimately based on ethical, rather than scientific, judgments.

Second, it is important not to confuse spiritual emptiness with the Buddhist ideas of self-emptying or no-mind emptiness, which refer in a positive light to a state of mind emptied of self and its thoughts and cravings (Ho, 1995, 2014a).

Strategies for Transcultural Applicability

Following Ho and Yin (2016; see also Ho, 1995, 2023; Ho & Ho, 2007), I adopt two strategies based on universalistic ideals freed from theocentric traditions for achieving transcultural applicability (see "Ambivalence Toward Christianity" in Chapter 6): (a) extracting commonalities at a high level of abstraction across the world's major philosophical-religious traditions, and (b) maximal inclusiveness (or minimal exclusiveness).

The strategy of extracting commonalities presupposes that there are core values and precepts shared by different philosophical-religious traditions, although their concrete expressions may take different forms. For instance, suffering presents opportunities for acts of courage, forbearance, or kindness, as well as for strengthening one's faith. This notion is inherent in Buddhist as well as Christian beliefs. Extraction at a high level of abstraction then affirms suffering as an avenue to spirituality—but leaving open what that avenue may entail.

The strategy of maximal inclusiveness states that a core value or belief originating from a major philosophical-religious tradition may be accepted as a candidate item if it is not absent, negated, or disavowed in any other. For instance, pursuing truth, striving to reach higher goals, and valuing human life all qualify for inclusion, because to our knowledge they are upheld in all traditions and are negated in none. In contrast, extending the regard for human life to all living creatures is specific, though not necessarily unique, to Buddhism; atonement for original sin is specific to Christianity. Therefore, these do not qualify for inclusion.

Maximal inclusiveness implies not limiting spirituality to a theistic worldview, which most researchers (e.g., Richards & Bergin, 1997) follow. Such limitation would exclude large portions of humanity, including those who hold nontheistic (e.g., Confucian), atheistic, or agnostic worldviews.

Problems of Measurement

A major problem is that researchers on religiosity or spirituality have relied almost exclusively on paper-and-pencil self-report measures (Hill & Pargament, 2003, p. 70). I have grave doubts about whether such measures are capable of reflecting the richness and complexity of spirituality. Accordingly, we need to have a flexible framework aimed at accommodating innovative techniques that make use of diverse sources of data in the development of the MES. In the same vein, Ho and Ho (2007) have made a case for using diverse sources of data:

> We argue for relying more on (a) qualitative, open-ended, experience-near techniques . . .; personal diaries and phenomenological accounts . . .; (b) nonverbal, expressive measures (e.g., music, drawings, movement analysis); (c) life histories, clinical or observational data, peer reports, reports by significant others;

and (d) videotaped information, narrative analysis, thematic categorization and coding for content analysis. (pp. 71–72)

The MES uses multidimensional measures to reflect the effects of spiritual fulfillment and spiritual emptiness in diverse domains of life. For each dimension, construct pairs are used, with one construct pertaining to a component of spiritual fulfillment and the other to a corresponding component of spiritual emptiness. This allows for covering both positive and negative functioning, and would thus facilitate studying spirituality and its negation as a dynamic process.

Dimension is distinguished from polarity. As stated before, spiritual fulfillment and spiritual emptiness are not viewed as reducible to merely the opposites of each other. For instance, Self-Actualization and Alienation are not construed as merely opposites of each other along the same bipolar continuum; rather, they are represented on two unipolar continua. This representation allows for the possible coexistence of self-actualization and alienation. Similarly, across components within each dimension construct pairs are not viewed as polar opposites on a continuum. Representation on two unipolar continua is better equipped to capture the process of spiritual development in which struggle, ups and downs, are involved.

From Theory to Content Generation

I have articulated a conceptual framework for the construction of the MES. But the framework remains empty until it is filled with contents, by which I mean construct or item pairs grouped into various dimensions. Again, all item pairs must meet the inclusion-exclusion criteria already stipulated. The generation of contents presents, therefore, the next challenge to construction. Besides consulting the relevant literature, I have drawn heavily on knowledge of Eastern and Western intellectual-religious traditions (Ho, 1995; Ng, Ho, Wong, & Smith, 2003) as well as clinical experiences in multicultural settings. My spiritual discoveries (Ho, 2014a, 2014b, 2016; see also Chapter 4) have informed the development of the MES. Episodic encounters with "madness" were highpoints in my journey, during which I experienced heightened literary-esthetic sensitivities; enhanced empathy and creativity; and extraordinary feelings of magnanimity. These experiences have contributed immensely to the generation of candidate items of the MES.

Dimensions of the MES

The MES may be used to evaluate a person's spiritual condition in part or in whole because each dimension forms an autonomous unit that may be used alone. Practitioners using the MES may rely on diverse sources or types of data, including interview data; other-report, report by others (e.g., friends and relatives), observational data, case history, test data, written data by the person concerned (e.g., diary), and documentary evidence (e.g., medical records). Users should make their judgments based on the totality of available evidence, especially when unusual pieces of information or data are encountered (see Appendix A for detailed information on usage). The MES comprises 32 construct pairs, grouped into 7 dimensions.

1. Reflectiveness-Decentering versus Dogmatism-Egocentricity (2 items; cognitive)
2. Heightened Sensibilities versus Psychic Numbing/Turmoil (7 items; affective)
3. Acceptance versus Denial (3 items)
4. Humility versus Arrogance (4 items)
5. Existential Quest versus Hedonistic-Materialistic Pursuits (6 items)
6. Transcendence versus Self-Encapsulation (5 items)
7. Self-Actualization versus Alienation (5 items)

Reflectiveness-Decentering Versus Dogmatism-Egocentricity

This cognitive dimension of MES comprises two components:(a) Reflective Metacognition versus Dogmatism and (b) Psychological Decentering versus Egocentricity.

Reflective Metacognition Versus Dogmatism

Metacognition means thinking about the process of thinking itself (Efklides, 2008). Thinking about important questions concerning life is characterized by metacognitive, reflective thought that involves doubt or struggle. It does not fall back automatically on stereotyped or superstitious beliefs, blind faith, religious dogmas, doctrinaire beliefs for ready answers to important questions concerning life. Spirituality tends to be characterized by higher levels of metacognitive reflectiveness.

As explained in Ho (2012) and Ho and Wang (2009), cognitive construals and perceptions differ in *degrees of complexity*: Construals about an object (e.g., oneself) are first-degree construals; metacognitive construals (metacognition) are second-degree construals; construals of metacognitive construals (meta-metacognition) are third-degree construals; and so forth ad infinitum. In short, any construal may be itself the object of the next higher degree construal. Examples are "I live from day to day; I don't think about tomorrow" (1st degree); "That means a lack of purpose in life" (2nd degree); "When I realize I lack purpose in life, I decided to take action" (3rd degree). Higher degrees are indicative of greater reflectiveness. This provides an operational scheme to delineate more precisely the cognitive aspects of spirituality: Degrees of complexity may be used as an index of Reflective Metacognition.

Psychological Decentering Versus Egocentricity

Being psychologically decentered is a hallmark of the selfless—an effective antidote to cognitive biases and prejudices (Ho, 1995). The self is decentered from the core of the individual's psychological universe. Not situated at center stage, the self no longer perceives the world through it alone. It is now capable of perceiving from other perspectives, freed from the constraints of its own perspective or frame of mind. Correspondingly, there is now greater freedom of action. The decentered self respects the interests of other people, and acts without selfish concerns. In contrast, egocentrism refers to perceiving the world from the perspective of the self alone. It is the absence of psychological decentering and the antithesis of selflessness.

Psychological Decentering may be indexed by the numbers of distinct *perceivers* and *perceiver alterations* in a unit of analysis (as explained in Ho, in press-a). For example, the therapist's verbalization "(the client knows what (God thinks of (him)))" (third degree) involves three perceivers (therapist, client, God) as well as two alterations (from therapist to client and from client to God). The larger the numbers of perceivers and perceiver alterations, the greater the psychological decentering tends to be.

Heightened Sensibilities Versus Psychic Numbing/Turmoil

This aesthetic-affective dimension refers to the capacity for experiencing depth of feelings, both positive and negative. A spiritual person is not happy all or even most of the time, and may even experience anguish at times. Positive feelings and affect predominate in Heightened Sensibilities.

Extreme forms of Heightened Sensibilities are mystical experiences, dramatic conversion experiences, and the like, within or without a religious context

(Miller & C'deBaca, 1994). They are intense, profound, and transcendent, yet difficult to describe. We may view them as extraordinary experiences (e.g., ecstasy, flash of insight, self-cosmos connectedness) that accompany the most dramatic forms of self-transformation, rather than as mystical (at least not in the sense of being unexplainable). Scales of mysticism (Hood, 1985; Hood, Morris, & Watson, 1993) are available; also, the Peak Experiences Scale (Mathes et al., 1982).

The inability to feel/negative affect and feelings predominate in Psychic Numbing/Turmoil. A person may fluctuate between numbing and turmoil. The aesthetic-affective dimension comprises seven components.

Aesthetic Sensibilities Versus Sensuous Overstimulation

Aesthetic sensibilities are heightened in the visual, kinesthetic, or musical, as well as the linguistic, modalities. Michelangelo's Pietà and Bach-Gounod's Ave Maria evoke spirituality, sometimes, even in people who lead their lives in spiritual emptiness. The majesty of nature, the vastness of the cosmos, artistic expressions, beauty in all its variegated forms are aesthetically felt; deep emotions are evoked. Heightened aesthetic sensibilities touch the core of one's being.

In contrast, seeking excitement through sensuous overstimulation is symptomatic of spiritual emptiness. It should be distinguished from aesthetic insensibility, which is simply the absence or lack of capacity to note, experience, and be moved by things of beauty represented in different forms, media, or modalities. (Aversion to particular representations, such as modern art, does not mean absence or lack of aesthetic sensibility; rather, it may simply reflect individual differences in taste.)

Contentment Versus Discontent

Empirical results suggest that spirituality and contentment are positively related (Poage, Ketzenberger, & Olson, 2004). Spiritual persons tend to be content with what they already have, freed from greed; they show gratitude to nature's bounty, God. As expressed in a Chinese saying, "Constant happiness comes from being content." People filled with discontent direct their attention to what they do not have. They register loss, not gain. They see only a bottle half empty.

Delight Versus Embitterment

People delighted in living delight others in their company, and delight in their delight. They have the capacity for experiencing simple, unabashed delight or joy at ordinary moments, or in just being alive.

Embitterment is characterized by (a) accumulation of anger, resulting from prolonged frustration, feelings of being repeatedly and unfairly treated or harmed; (b) external attribution (e.g., blaming others for one's own failures), at least in part; (c) a strong sense of injustice or unfairness; and (d) feelings of undeserved defeat, or of unreached goals. It differs from depression in that guilt, dysphoria, and self-rejection are not essential features (cf. Linden, 2003). Embitterment extinguishes joy like covering a blanket over fire. It is written on one's face.

Depth of Feelings Versus Psychic Numbing

Spiritual persons have the capacity for experiencing depth of feelings, both positive and negative. They are not happy all or even most of the time, and may even experience anguish at times. The antithesis of depth of feelings is not just shallow feelings, but psychic numbing, inability to feel happiness or unhappiness. Indeed, we may regard the inability to feel unhappiness or psychic pain (an instance of emotional numbing) as a symptom of spiritual emptiness. As a Chinese adage states, "There is no greater sadness than the death of feelings from the heart." In place of delight, joy, and exuberance, despondency appears. Habitually sullen, dejected, or despondent people make poor company.

Serenity Versus Turmoil

Serenity is tranquil composure that suggests imperviousness to agitation or turmoil. It is akin to the Buddhist idea of maintaining a temperate (or usual) state of mind in the face of challenging circumstances. A tranquil person feels in harmony with others, at home in the cosmos. Tranquility emerged as one of three factors of spirituality in a study by Ng, Yau, Chan, Chan, and Ho (2005). Turmoil is the antithesis of serenity: It is a state of confusion or agitation. It means more than lack of serenity or disturbed composure.

Spontaneity Versus Inhibition

Spontaneity is freedom from restraint, inhibition, or stagnation. Unencumbered by overregulation, spontaneous persons are playful and humorous. This does not mean that they show indiscriminate disregard for social convention, norms, or moral standards. A champion of spontaneity is the Daoist philosopher Zhuangzi. Inhibited persons lack spontaneity, and tend to be overly self-conscious or ill at ease. They are overregulated, externally by social convention, and internally by impulse control. Inhibition may be manifest in not only affective expression or emotional reactivity, but also the language of the body (e.g., posture).

Affect-posture inhibition emerged as one three factors of the Stagnation Scale (Ng, Chan, Ho, Wong, & Ho, 2006).

Warmth Versus Frigidity

Adamovová and Stríženec (2004) find warmth positively correlated with cognitive orientation toward spirituality. One does not have to be a psychologist to tell a warm person from one who is chronically frigid, angry or, worse, hostile. Most people gravitate toward the warm and friendly, and avoid emotional refrigerators or volcanoes.

Acceptance Versus Denial

This dimension comprises three components: Acceptance versus Rejection of Biological Givens, Acceptance versus Nonacceptance of the Inevitable, and Acceptance versus Nonacceptance of the Unchangeable.

Acceptance is quintessential to spirituality: of self, others; of things and conditions that cannot be changed; of inherent limitations, both personal and human; and of death. It goes beyond forbearance, the capacity to endure pain and suffering, which has no necessary foundation in spirituality. However, in an important sense, acceptance does not preclude taking heroic actions of defiance: to change what appears to be unchangeable.

In Christianity, such actions are extolled as a mark of steadfast faith, to "hope against hope." In Chinese culture, a similar idea is expressed in the saying, "Do the things that you know cannot be done." Acceptance is not fatalism, the belief that one's life condition is fixed, regardless of what action is taken to change it. Acceptance has clinical benefits: For instance, Singer and Dobson (2009) find recovered depressed persons higher on the cognitive style of acceptance show greater reduction in negative mood. Nonacceptance is denial and negation of the reality of life. It is manifest in many ways: self-rejection, rejection of others; stubborn persistence in trying to change the unchangeable; failure to recognize and accept limitations; excessive fear of death.

Classically defined in psychoanalytic theory, denial is a defense mechanism: unconscious and maladaptive. It is not deception, but self-deception. It does not refer to conscious attempts to "deny" the seriousness of the plight in which one finds oneself. Denial should be distinguished from cognitive avoidance, which refers to a conscious attempt to avoid thinking about something. Empirical evidence in support of the psychoanalytic view is unequivocal. Baumeister, Dale, and Sommer (1998) obtained evidence to suggest that denial can be an adaptive defense mechanism. Cooke, Myers, and Derakshan (2003) found denial unrelated with anxiety among asthma patients.

Humility Versus Arrogance

This dimension comprises four components: Personal Limitations versus Personal Strengths or Achievements, Human Imperfection versus Collective Achievements, Higher Principle versus Human Supremacy, and Humility versus Self-Importance.

The conceptualization and measurement of humility require more research attention. In my conceptualization, humility stems from gauging oneself against the collective accomplishments of humankind, the vastness of the cosmos, infinity, some higher being or principle. Humility reflects inner attitudes rather than outer social convention (e.g., maintaining face). For instance, behaviors in face dynamics calculated to show one's modesty in front of others do not qualify. Humility does not imply an absence of pride; however, it does imply an absence of arrogance.

Humility is espoused across the world's philosophical-religious traditions. It results from insight into the insuperable limitations of the human mind and, ultimately, the impossibility of comprehending the infinite by the finite. This insight activates the wisdom to accept human limitations, and it is the mother of humility in a deeply spiritual sense. It is metacognitive in nature: "I know my inherent limitations." In line with Tangney (2000), spiritual growth parallels depth of humility, following the discovery and acceptance of human ignorance and limitations. Humility may also be related to forgiveness, another traditional positive quality (Powers, Nam, Rowatt, & Hill, 2007). Modesty, a lower form of humility, refers to behaviors that negate arrogance: not showing off one's achievements, not seeking the limelight, not expecting others to treat oneself as "special."

Existential Quest Versus Hedonistic-Materialistic Pursuits

This dimension comprises six components: Existential versus Hedonistic-Materialistic Interests, Higher versus Hedonistic-Materialistic Goals, Spiritual versus Materialistic Values, Spiritual versus Addictive Activities, Moderation versus Addictiveness in Material Possessions, and Regulated versus Wanton Pursuits of Pleasure.

Spirituality entails an existential quest for a sense of direction; to answer questions about life and death, being and nonbeing. Of course, different people obtain different answers: The crucial thing is to quest for some higher goal in life, and principles that serve as a guide to leading the good life. Available relevant measures include The Purpose in Life Test (Crumbaugh & Maholick, 1969) and the Spiritual Well-Being Scale (Paloutzian & Ellison, 1991). More recently, Van Pachterbeke, Keller, and Saroglou (2012) have developed a scale measuring existential quest.

To many, hedonistic-materialistic pursuits are more attractive than existential quests. Primacy of hedonistic-materialistic values: Materialism (excessive regard for worldly concerns) and hedonism (pursuit of or devotion to pleasure, especially to the pleasures of the senses) occupy high priority in their scale of values. Excessive hedonistic-materialistic pursuits are symptomatic of spiritual emptiness. In this connection, empirical evidence indicates that materialistic people are negatively stereotyped (Van Boven, Campbell, & Gilovich, 2010).

Transcendence Versus Self-Encapsulation

Transcendence has proven to be a construct that is hard to define and operationalize. Prior refinement in theory is necessary. My conceptualization recasts transcendence as *relational spirituality*, reached through transcending egocentrism. Relationships are integral to one's meaning and purpose in life. The antithesis of transcendence is self-encapsulation, in which the self derives meaning and purpose solely or primarily from its own individual existence, without reference to a larger context. Self-encapsulation is a form of egoism or self-contained individualism. The following five pairs of component ideas further describe contrasts between transcendence and self-encapsulation.

Self-in-Relations Versus Self-Containment

Transcendence entails viewing oneself in a relational context (e.g., self-in-cosmos, personal relationship with God), thus conferring meaning and purpose to one's life. It defines one's relationships with others, society, humanity, nature, cosmos; and (to religious believers) some higher, divine, sacred, or supreme being or beings. The importance of relational contexts, in which the person-in-relations or relational self functions, has been articulated in Ho and Wang (2009; also Ho, 1995). In self-containment, attention is focused on one's own individual existence from which meaning and purpose is derived, without reference to a relational context.

Compassion Versus Hard-heartedness

Acts of kindness typically include giving favors and doing good deeds for others, helping and taking care of people in need. However, kindness does not always entail compassion: We may be kind to people who are not in misery. Compassion goes deeper. It occupies a key position in Buddhism: Deep feeling for the suffering of others, extended to humankind. Devoid of compassion, a person becomes hard-hearted, callous, uncaring, and unfeeling. Compassion includes self-compassion. In a meta-analytic study, MacBeth and Angus (2012) found a substantial negative association between self-compassion and psychopathology.

Selflessness Versus Egoism

A selfless person puts the interests of other people above his own, and acts without selfish concerns. The notion of selflessness is central to Daoism and Buddhism (Ho, 1995). The Daoist philosopher Zhuangzi says, "The perfect man has no self." Selflessness must be distinguished from absence of selfhood. The formation of a healthy self is a precondition for the emergence of selflessness. For the healthy self is the womb within which selflessness is nurtured. The antithesis of selflessness is to act in ways that are motivated solely or primarily by self-interests. Egoism does not necessarily entail selfishness. Egoistic actions are not necessarily illegal or immoral, and do not necessarily infringe on the rights of others.

Altruism Versus Selfishness

Altruism is selfless concern for the welfare of others (cf. Richards & Bergin, 1997, p. 218). It may involve great personal sacrifice, even one's life. Selfishness hardly requires commentary. It is not only the absence of altruism, but also the proclivity toward taking actions that benefit oneself at the expense of others.

Universal Love Versus Misanthropy

Universal love is the lodestone of ecumenicity. It finds expression in the Greek idea of agape, the Confucian ideas of *ren* (benevolence) and *boai* (universal love), the Buddhist idea of *daai* ("big love"), the Christian ideas of caritas and love-feast. At root, it champions the intrinsic value of human life and cherishing care for one's fellow man.

Universal love, more than anything else, is the hallmark of spirituality. It is not just love for specific individuals (e.g., friends and relatives) or groups (e.g., one's countrymen), but the extension of love to all of humanity. Christianity stresses the extension of love to strangers, even enemies. Confucianism also teaches the ethic of extension, though to a lesser extent than Christianity: "To care for the aged of mine as well as those of others; to nurture the young of mine as well as those of others." Buddhism goes to an extreme and extends the regard for life to all living creatures.

Misanthropy is the antithesis of the love for humanity. However, a misanthrope does not necessarily seek to exploit, harm, or destroy his fellowmen. A psychopath does; his actions, therefore, mean an extreme negation of universal love.

Self-Actualization Versus Alienation

This dimension comprises five components: Social Connectedness versus Isolation, Closeness versus Estrangement, Meaningfulness versus Meaninglessness, Normativeness versus Normlessness, and Agency versus Powerlessness.

From a spiritual perspective, the antecedents of self-actualization are acceptance, humility, existential quest, and transcendence. Empirical results confirm the importance of spirituality for self-actualization, meaning in life, and personal growth initiative, regardless of whether it is achieved through religious participation (Ivtzan, Chan, Gardner, & Prashar, 2013). Alienation is a cardinal symptom of spiritual emptiness. It is also a central concept in the humanism of the early writings of Karl Marx (1932/1964). According to Marx, alienation is fundamentally self-alienation because it is human creative activity itself that has created the conditions, economic in particular, for impersonal forces over which humanity is powerless to control.

In his classic study of alienation, Seeman (1959) identified five components of alienation: social isolation, self-estrangement, meaninglessness, normlessness, and powerlessness. Based on Seeman's study, a psychometric measure of alienation with 10 self-report items achieved satisfactory reliability and validity (Cheng, Ho, Xie, Wong, & Cheng-Lai, 2013). Alienation predicts poor general health, maladaptive coping, and social-familial nonengagement among nonengaged youth.

In the present undertaking, I use the term estrangement, rather than self-estrangement; the purpose is to extend the construct to include estrangement from nature or divine being(s). It is important to note that a person may be socially isolated and yet experiences no alienation subjectively. Equally, a person may experience alienation in terms of social isolation at some point in his life, and yet no estrangement from the cosmos or the divine. This is particularly applicable to religious luminaries, such as Hebrew prophets—again, an illustration of how spirituality and its negation may coexist.

Discussion

The conceptual framework articulated above has provided methodological guidance for the present undertaking. Together, the two strategies I have adopted for achieving transcultural applicability, extracting commonalities and maximal inclusiveness, acknowledge that the paths to spirituality are many and are grounded in different values and beliefs across philosophical-religious traditions. However, commonalities may be extracted at a high level of abstraction and with maximal inclusiveness. A theistic or atheistic worldview is neither necessary nor sufficient for spirituality.

In terms of measurement, I have relied on (a) innovative techniques that allow for using diverse sources of data, (b) using multidimensional measures to cover diverse domains of life, (c) using construct pairs to reflect both spiritual fulfillment and spiritual emptiness, and (d) representing each of these construct pairs on two unipolar continua to allow for the possible coexistence of fulfillment and emptiness.

These approaches to measurement are propelled by the general discontent over self-report measures in personality assessment that has been expressed by researchers (e.g., Ho, 2010; Kenny, 1994, p. 194). They constitute, I submit, methodological advantages over paper-and-pencil self-report measures. Hence, making the MES available to researchers will add fresh impetus to generate empirical research into the domains of spirituality and spiritual emptiness.

The Place of Exceptional Cases in Science

The MES derives largely from the author's extraordinary firsthand experiences of "madness" (Ho, 2014a, 2014b, 2016; see also Chapter 3), without which I believe the end product would have been impoverished. The construction of the MES has been highly personal. I am both a creator and a consumer of the MES: Creator, in the sense that I have used my self-study of madness to advance research; and consumer, because I have applied the MES to myself, using diverse sources of data (e.g., diaries, correspondence with friends and colleagues) assembled in my self-study. Through these self-revelations, I hope to demonstrate that extraordinary experiencing is amenable to scientific investigation in the public domain.

My self-study is a truly exceptional case. By definition, an exceptional case is one that does not fit into regularities in a body of knowledge that researchers have commonly accepted at a given period of time. Precisely for this reason, it is invaluable for providing impetus to challenge prevailing scientific beliefs.

But how will the MES be viewed in the scientific community as a personal undertaking? I am not in a position to answer this question, except to say that there has long been a tradition of idiographic research in psychology, including biographical or autobiographical studies of mystics and "mad" religious figures, past or present.

Future Developments

The next research step is to develop the MES empirically, resulting in an omnibus instrument that is (a) multidimensional, (b) reflective of the dynamics between spirituality and its negation, (c) accommodating of diverse sources of data, and (d) transcultural in terms of applicability. This would represent an advance over past research, most of which are grounded in a theistic, particularly Christian, worldview. The methodological and operational challenges are formidable, far exceeding those involved in the development of self-report scales. However, there is no choice but to meet these challenges, if the objective is to capture the richness of spirituality and spiritual emptiness.

Researchers (e.g., MacDonald & Friedman, 2013) have favored the use of well-established, rather than custom-made, measures for an orderly development of science, with research built upon the fruits of earlier investigators. This is a stance with which I agree. Additionally, Ho, Ho, and Ng (2007) express the view that quantification, though not essential to qualification as a science, confers potent advantages to research.

Nonetheless, two points must be made clear. First, psychometric self-report measures do not have an exclusive claim to quantification; diverse sources of data derived from innovative techniques are also amenable to quantification. Second, some qualities may not be appropriately quantified numerically, in terms of means, variances, and so forth; they may be more appropriately described in terms of some other branches of mathematics, such as symbolic logic. An example of this is the formal system of symbolization I have used to characterize Reflective Metacognition and Psychological Decentering.

The MES may be used as a research or counseling instrument. But it should not be viewed merely as an instrument. Rather, it provides a comprehensive conceptual framework for probing into the dynamics of spiritual fulfillment versus emptiness in different domains of life, all of which are cardinal in importance and none of which are trivial, at different developmental periods.

An inviting research agenda to advance our understanding of spirituality and its negation would include investigations into (a) interrelations among the dimensions or scales of the MES; (b) relations between MES dimensions and more generic psychological constructs such as authenticity, self-mastery, openness, creativity; (c) spiritual development at different stages of life; (d) implications for holistic health; and (e) trajectories of posttraumatic adjustment, particularly resilient, even self-transformative, functioning following a life-threatening event or illness. In short, developing the MES to fruition would bring scientific research closer to unraveling the highest domain of human existence, namely, spirituality.

Appendix A

Multidimensional Evaluations of Spirituality (MES)

The Multidimensional Evaluations of Spirituality (MES) is a guide to the self-evaluation of spirituality and spiritual emptiness. It serves like a map for spiritual travelers. It will help you to reflect on your spiritual condition in diverse domains of life, all of which are of cardinal importance and none of which are trivial. The MES makes use of concept pairs; in each pair, one concept pertains to a component of spiritual fulfillment and the other to a corresponding component of spiritual emptiness. This facilitates dynamic analyses of both positive and negative functioning, relying on diverse sources or types of information (e.g., life history, diaries). The MES is a flexible, omnibus tool. It may be used in whole or in part. You may use it regardless of your cultural, religious, or ideological background. The MES comprises 32 concept (or item) pairs, each of which may be used to assess contrasting components of spiritual fulfillment versus spiritual emptiness. These concept pairs are grouped into seven dimensions.

1. Reflectiveness-Decentering versus Dogmatism-Egocentricity (2 items; cognitive).
2. Heightened Sensibilities versus Psychic Numbing/Turmoil (7 items; affective).
3. Acceptance versus Denial (3 items).

4. Humility versus Arrogance (4 items).
5. Existential Quest versus Hedonistic-Materialistic Pursuits (6 items).
6. Transcendence versus Self-Encapsulation (5 items).
7. Self-Actualization versus Alienation (5 items).

Self-exploration is an essential step to be taken on any spiritual journey. I invite or, to put it more strongly, challenge my fellow traveler to a spiritual self-examination: "Take a good look at yourself in the mirror. In what respects and to what extent do you experience spiritual fulfillment, and spiritual emptiness?"

The following is an invitation to a self-exploration of your thinking about spirituality. This will lead you to reexamine your own thinking. You may turn to the tables below as a guide for further exploration.

> People have different ways of thinking about questions such as faith, their relationship with God (or the divine), their place in the world, and so forth. What are your own thoughts?
>
> I would like you to talk about not only what your thoughts are, but also the way you think about the questions I mentioned. For instance, how have you arrived at your present beliefs? What do other people think about them? What are your thoughts on other people's beliefs?
>
> What does spiritual emptiness mean to you? Again, I would like you to put the emphasis on the way you think about this question; in other words, please talk about not just the answer, but how you arrive at the answer.
>
> What is your thinking on the human-divine relationship? To you personally, is love reciprocal or one-sided in the relationship? How does your thinking on the human-divine relationship impact your interpersonal relationships and vice versa?
>
> Is there anything you like to add or clarify? Please feel free to elaborate further. You might have left something out; now is the time to add to what you have already said.

Reflectiveness-Decentering Versus Dogmatism-Egocentricity

This cognitive dimension of the MES comprises two component pairs: Reflective Metacognition versus Dogmatism, and Psychological Decentering versus

Egocentricity. The focus is placed on how, rather than what, you think about spirituality.

Consider this statement, which illustrates both metacognition and psychological decentering: "I attend to not only what others are thinking, but also what others are thinking about what I'm thinking. I also expect others to do the same thing." And this one, "For now we see through a glass, darkly; but then face to face: now I know in part; but then shall I know even as also I am known" (1 Corinthians 13:12). To know myself is demanding enough; to know myself "even as also I am known [by God]" entails knowing something about the mind of God!

Love is central to religious conceptions of the human-divine relationship. It is important to recognize that there are two distinct directions in this relationship: human-to-divine and divine-to-human (see Table 1A). Tension arises from a lack of reciprocities: "I love God, but God doesn't love me"; or "God loves me, but I can't love him because of awful things he has allowed to happen in my life." The benefits of reducing such tension may be generalized to other relationships (e.g., between yourself and your friends).

Table 1A. Directional Components of Human-Divine Love

Directional Love	Illustrations of Invitation
Love between the spiritual traveler and God (direction not specified)	Tell me something about your thinking on the love between you and God.
Perception in the human-to-divine direction	What about your thoughts on your love toward God?
Metaperception in the human-to-divine direction	Do you think God perceives that you love him?
Perception in the divine-to-human direction	What about your thoughts on God's love toward you?
Metaperception in the divine-to-human direction	Do you perceive that God is determined in his mind that he loves you?

Notes: Metaperception means the perception of another perception (e.g., one's own perception, God's perception). Wordings may be altered to suit the traveler's religious background. For instance, for Muslims Allah may be substituted for God.

Reflective Metacognition Versus Dogmatism

Metacognition means thinking about the process of thinking itself. Thinking about important questions concerning life is characterized by metacognitive, reflective thought that involves doubt or struggle. It does not fall back automatically on stereotyped or superstitious beliefs, blind faith, religious dogmas, doctrinaire beliefs for ready answers to important questions concerning life. Spirituality tends to be characterized by higher levels of reflectiveness. Observe the increasing level of metacognitive reflectiveness among these three statements, from one to the next.

1. I live from day to day; I don't think about tomorrow.
2. That means a lack of purpose in life.
3. When I realize I lack purpose in life, I become unhappy and I want to change.

Psychological Decentering Versus Egocentricity

Being psychologically decentered is a hallmark of the selfless—an effective antidote to biases and prejudices. You are decentered from the core of your psychological universe. You are now capable of perceiving from other perspectives, freed from the constraints of your own perspective or frame of mind. Correspondingly, there is greater freedom of action. Your decentered self respects the interests of other people and acts without selfish concerns. In contrast, egocentricity refers to perceiving the world from the perspective of the self alone, characterized by a lack of capacity to perceive the world from multiple perspectives. It is the antithesis of psychological decentering and of selflessness (see Table 1B).

Table 1B. Psychological Decentering versus Egocentricity

Concept pair	Reflectiveness-Decentering	Dogmatism-Egocentricity
General idea	Cognitive dimension of spirituality	Cognitive dimension of spiritual emptiness
Item 1	**Reflective Metacognition** Thinking about important questions concerning life is characterized by reflective, metacognitive thought; involves doubt or struggle.	**Dogmatism** Falls back automatically on stereotyped or superstitious beliefs, blind faith, religious dogmas, doctrinaire beliefs for ready answers to vital questions concerning life.
Examples	"The end of reason is where faith begins. But do not uphold any faith until reason has exhausted itself." "I have sometimes wondered if God exists."	"All the answers are already there, written down. Why bother to think about these questions?" "Generally I simply follow the teachings of my faith."
Item 2	**Psychological Decentering** Perceives the world from different perspectives.	**Egocentricity** Perceives the world solely or primarily from one's own perspective.
Examples	"I know what my friends think about me, in the same way that my friends know what I think about them." [Strong capacity for alternating between perspectives] "America and China share a common challenge: Each side has something from which the other needs to learn (or to avoid)."	"I have no idea of what my friends are thinking at all. There is simply no way to find out what's in the minds of other people." "What do you mean by looking at the world from other peoples' perspectives? We live in this country. People from other countries don't behave as we do."

Heightened Sensibilities Versus Psychic Numbing/Turmoil

This aesthetic-affective dimension of spirituality refers to the capacity for experiencing deep feelings, both positive and negative. A spiritual person is not happy all or even most of the time, and may even experience anguish at times.

Positive feelings and affect predominate in Heightened Sensibilities. Extreme forms of Heightened Sensibilities are mystical experiences, dramatic conversion experiences, and the like, within or without a religious context. They are intense, profound, and transcendent, yet difficult to describe. We may view them as extraordinary experiences (e.g., ecstasy, a flash of insight, self-cosmos connectedness) that accompany the most dramatic forms of self-transformation, rather than as something unexplainable.

The inability to feel predominates in Psychic Numbing; negative affect and feelings predominate in Psychic Turmoil. You may fluctuate between numbing and turmoil. The dimension of Heightened Sensibilities versus Psychic Numbing/Turmoil includes the following seven components (see Table 2).

Aesthetic Sensibilities Versus Sensory Overstimulation

Aesthetic sensibilities are heightened in the visual, kinesthetic, or musical, as well as the linguistic, modalities.

Michelangelo's Pietà and Bach-Gounod's Ave Maria evoke spirituality, sometimes, even in people who lead their lives in spiritual emptiness. The majesty of nature, the vastness of the cosmos, artistic expressions, beauty in all its variegated forms are aesthetically felt; deep emotions are evoked. Heightened aesthetic sensibilities touch the core of your being.

In contrast, seeking excitement through sensory overstimulation is symptomatic of spiritual emptiness. It should be distinguished from aesthetic insensibility, which is simply the absence or lack of capacity to note, experience, and be moved by things of beauty represented in different forms, media, or modalities. (Aversion to particular representations, such as modern art, does not mean absence or lack of aesthetic sensibility; rather, it may simply reflect individual differences in taste.)

Contentment Versus Discontent

Freed from greed, spiritual persons tend to be content with what they already have; they show gratitude to nature's bounty, God. As expressed in a Chinese saying, "Constant happiness comes from being content." People filled with discontent direct their attention to what they don't have. They register losses, not gains. They see only a bottle half empty.

Delight Versus Embitterment

People delighted in living delight others in their company, and delight in their delight. They have the capacity for experiencing simple, unabashed delight or joy at ordinary moments, or in just being alive. Embitterment is characterized by accumulation of anger, resulting from prolonged frustration, feelings of being repeatedly and unfairly treated or harmed; external attribution (e.g., blaming others for one's own failures), at least in part; a strong sense of injustice or unfairness; and feelings of undeserved defeat, or of unreached goals. It differs from depression in that guilt, dysphoria, and self-rejection are not essential features. Embitterment extinguishes joy like covering a blanket over the fire. It may be written on your face.

Depth of Feelings Versus Psychic Numbing

Spiritual persons have the capacity for experiencing depth of feelings, both positive and negative. They are not happy all or even most of the time, and may even experience anguish at times.

The antithesis of depth of feelings is not just shallow feelings, but psychic numbing, inability to feel happiness or unhappiness. Indeed, we may regard the inability to feel unhappiness or psychic pain (an instance of emotional numbing) as a symptom of spiritual emptiness.

As a Chinese adage states, "There is no greater sadness than the death of feelings from the heart." In place of delight, joy, and exuberance, despondency appears. Habitually sullen, dejected, or despondent people make poor company.

Serenity Versus Turmoil

Serenity is a tranquil composure that suggests imperviousness to agitation or turmoil. It is akin to the Buddhist idea of maintaining a temperate (or usual) state of mind in the face of challenging circumstances. A tranquil person feels in harmony with others, at home in the cosmos. Turmoil is the antithesis of serenity: It is a state of confusion or agitation. It means more than a lack of serenity or disturbed composure.

Spontaneity Versus Inhibition

Spontaneity is freedom from restraint, inhibition, or stagnation. Unencumbered by overregulation, spontaneous persons are playful and humorous. This does

Table 2. Heightened Sensibilities Versus Psychic Numbing/Turmoil

Concept pair	Heightened Sensibilities	Psychic Numbing/Turmoil
General idea	Positive feelings and affect predominate: heightened aesthetic sensibilities and depth of feelings; tranquility; spontaneity.	Negative feelings and affect predominate: discontent, embitterment; psychic numbing; turmoil; or inhibition.
Item 1	***Aesthetic Sensibilities*** Aesthetic sensibilities are heightened in visual, kinesthetic, musical, linguistic or other modalities.	***Sensory Overstimulation*** Seeks excitement through sensory overstimulation.
Item 2	***Contentment*** Content with what one already has; count one's blessings; gratitude to nature's bounty, God.	***Discontent*** Driven by greed: Directs one's attention to what one does not have; registers loss, not gain; sees a bottle as half empty, rather than half full.
Item 3	***Delight*** Capacity for experiencing simple, unabashed delight; joy at ordinary moments, or in just being alive; enthusiastic.	***Embitterment*** Accumulated anger, feelings of being repeatedly and unfairly treated or harmed; blaming others; a strong sense of injustice of unfairness; feelings of undeserved defeat, or of unreached goals.
Item 4	***Depth of Feelings*** Capacity for experiencing depth of feelings, both positive and negative.	***Psychic Numbing*** Psychic numbing, inability to feel happiness or unhappiness. Sullen, dejected, despondent; apathetic.
Item 5	***Serenity*** Experiences harmony, serenity, tranquility, or inner peace.	***Turmoil*** Experiences agitation, confusion, or disorganization; inner turmoil.
Item 6	***Spontaneity*** Freedom from constraint, unencumbered by overregulation, social convention; playfulness, humor.	***Inhibition*** Overly self-conscious, ill at ease; affective or postural inhibition; feelings of obstruction, blockage, or stagnation.

Table 2. Continued

Concept pair	Heightened Sensibilities	Psychic Numbing/Turmoil
Item 7	*Warmth* Feelings and inner emotions toward people characterized by warmth.	*Frigidity* Feelings and inner emotions toward people characterized by frigidity, anger or hostility.
Examples	Mystical or transcendent experiences (e.g., ecstasy, a flash of insight, self-cosmos connectedness). "I experience emotions so intense that tears flow from my eyes." [Item 4]	Indulgences in excitement (e.g., driving fast cars), bombardment by light, color, or sound. "I feel empty inside, so I need some excitement." [Item 1]

not mean that they show indiscriminate disregard for social convention, norms, or moral standards. Inhibited persons lack spontaneity, and tend to be overly self-conscious or ill at ease. They are overregulated, externally by social convention, and internally by impulse control. Inhibition may be manifest in not only affective expression or emotional reactivity but also the language of the body (e.g., posture).

Warmth Versus Frigidity

You do not have to be a psychologist to tell a warm person from one who is chronically frigid, angry or, worse, hostile. Most people gravitate toward the warm and friendly, and avoid emotional refrigerators or volcanoes.

Acceptance Versus Denial

Acceptance is quintessential to spirituality: of self, others; of things and conditions that cannot be changed; of inherent limitations, both personal and human; and of death. It goes beyond forbearance, the capacity to endure pain and suffering, which has no necessary foundation in spirituality. It is not fatalism, the belief that your life condition is fixed, regardless of what action is taken to change it.

Denial is nonacceptance or negation of the realities of life. It is manifest in many ways: self-rejection, rejection of others; stubborn persistence in trying to

Table 3. Acceptance Versus Denial

Concept pair	Acceptance	Denial
Item 1	***Acceptance of Biological Givens*** Accepts one's biological givens (e.g., sex, race), physical characteristics (e.g., appearance). Understands that biological givens do not determine one's destiny.	***Rejection of Biological Givens*** Rejects one's biological givens (e.g., sex, race), physical characteristics (e.g., appearance). Feels embarrassed or ashamed.
Item 2	***Acceptance of the Inevitable*** Accepts the inevitable facts of life, such as aging, death.	***Nonacceptance of the Inevitable*** Preoccupied with or worries excessively over the inevitable facts of life, such as aging, death.
Item 3	***Acceptance of the Unchangeable*** Accepts other conditions or realities that cannot be changed through individual or collective effort. (Differs from fatalism, believing that it is futile to change conditions or realities that may indeed be changed with effort.)	***Nonacceptance of the Unchangeable*** Denial of other conditions or realities (other than those in Item 1) that cannot be changed; stubbornly persists in trying to change the unchangeable.
Example	"I have been told that I have six months to live. I accept the fact with calmness and dignity." [Item 2]	"All the doctors say that I have a serious disease, but I just don't believe what they say." [Item 3]

change the unchangeable; failure to recognize and accept limitations; excessive fear of death (see Table 3).

Classically defined in psychoanalytic theory, denial is a defense mechanism: unconscious and maladaptive. It is not deception, but self-deception. It does not refer to conscious attempts to "deny" the seriousness of the plight in which you find yourself. Denial should be distinguished from cognitive avoidance, which refers to a conscious attempt to avoid thinking about something.

Is denial or cognitive avoidance good or bad? That depends on many factors, including frequency, intensity, duration (temporary versus prolonged, entrenched), and the situation(s) or occasion(s) in which you engage in denial or cognitive avoidance. You are in denial when you say (and genuinely think) you are not afraid, but are seen by all to be shivering, sweating, and so forth. So are you when you have a life-threatening illness and refuse to accept medical opinion (consistently expressed by reputable physicians). These are bad.

Suppose you have a terminal illness, understand and accept medical opinion, but say to yourself, "I remain optimistic; I shall endure." You are not in denial; rather, you may be expressing a sentiment of hope, courage, fortitude in the face of great misfortune. You come close to acceptance. Good.

In literature, Faust sold his soul in exchange for youth. In life, the quest for turning back the biological clock now falls on medicine. Advances in medicine (especially genetics and biotechnology) fuel demands for pushing the frontier of life preservation, even life improvement, to new heights. But humankind will not be satisfied until the gods of death are vanquished. Patients will demand more, even the impossible, from medical practitioners. Insatiable demands, however, signify a lack of acceptance—and of wisdom.

Humility Versus Arrogance

Humility stems from gauging yourself against the collective accomplishments of humankind, the vastness of the cosmos, infinity, some higher being or principle (see Table 4). Humility reflects inner attitudes rather than outer social convention (e.g., maintaining face). For instance, behaviors in face dynamics calculated to show your modesty in front of others do not qualify. Humility does not imply an absence of pride; however, it does imply an absence of arrogance.

Humility is espoused across the world's philosophical-religious traditions. It results from insight into the insuperable limitations of the human mind and, ultimately, the impossibility of comprehending the infinite by the finite. This insight activates the wisdom to accept human limitations, and it is the mother of humility in a deeply spiritual sense. It is metacognitive in nature: "I know my inherent limitations." Spiritual growth parallels depth of humility, following the discovery and acceptance of human ignorance and limitations.

Modesty, a lower form of humility, refers to behaviors that negate arrogance: not showing off your achievements, not seeking the limelight, not expecting others to treat you as "special."

Table 4. Humility Versus Arrogance

Concept pair	Humility	Arrogance
Item 1	**Personal Limitations** Aware of and accepts personal imperfection and limitations.	**Personal Strengths or Achievements** Arrogance; shows off one's strengths or achievements. (Should not be confused with pride.)
Item 2	**Human Imperfection** Acknowledges human imperfection and limitations.	**Collective Achievements** Arrogance in the collective achievements of humankind or of a particular group (e.g., racial superiority)
Item 3	**Higher Principle** Acknowledges the existence of some higher being or cosmic principle.	**Human Supremacy** Meeting the needs of humankind is the guiding principle for action, without due consideration for other life forms or conservation
Item 4	**Humility** Sense of humility: Feels humble against the collective accomplishments of humankind, the vastness of the cosmos, infinity, some higher being or principle.	**Self-Importance** Inflated sense of self-importance: Seeks the limelight, or expects others to treat oneself as "special."
Examples	"The more I know, the more I know how much I don't know. I feel humbled." [Item 1] "The finite recoils in the face of the infinite." [Item 4]	"Hong Kong people are superior to the backward peoples of Asia. That's why we import domestic helpers." [Item 2] "Given our advances in technology, there isn't any environmental problem that Americans can't solve." [Item 2]

Table 5. Existential Quest Versus Hedonistic-Materialistic Pursuits

Concept Pair	Existential Quest	Hedonistic-Materialistic Pursuits
Central idea	Primacy of spiritual values: Existential quest occupies a high priority in the person's scale of values. (Whether or not spiritual fulfillment is actually attained is not the central issue here.)	Primacy of hedonistic-materialistic values: Materialism and hedonism occupy a high priority in the person's scale of values.
Item 1	***Existential Interests*** Interested in existential questions: Why am I here, where will I go? What happens to me when I die? How may I overcome my fate?	***Hedonistic-Materialistic Interests*** Interested primarily in questions pertaining to hedonistic-materialistic pursuits, to the exclusion of existential questions.
Item 2	***Higher Goals*** Quest for some higher goal in life or principles that serve as a guide to leading a good life.	***Hedonistic-Materialistic Goals*** Guiding principles concern primarily reaching hedonistic-materialistic goals, or exclude the idea of leading a good or better life.
Item 3	***Spiritual Values*** Spiritual values are more important than amassment of personal wealth. (Unlike Item 1, which pertains to interest and curiosity, this one pertains to the priority of values that guide action.)	***Materialistic Values*** Excessively materialistic: preoccupation with amassment of personal wealth.

(Continued)

Table 5. Continued

Concept Pair	Existential Quest	Hedonistic-Materialistic Pursuits
Item 4	***Spiritual Activities*** Devotes free or leisure time and energy to activities for spiritual inspiration (e.g., acquiring knowledge about spirituality through reading, discussion, or formal study; engaged in expressive-artistic activities that evoke spiritual experiences; traveling to spiritual places of spiritual significance; engaged in actions for the betterment of humankind that has a spiritual dimension to the person).	***Addictive Activities*** Devotes free or leisure time and energy to unproductive or, worse, addictive activities (e.g., surfing the Internet; not directly aimed at amassing wealth or consumer products).
Item 5	***Moderation in Material Possessions*** Possession of consumer products or other material objects is subject to control and regulation by the person's values and principles.	***Addictiveness in Material Possessions*** Preoccupation with possession of consumer products or other material objects; addictive consumer behavior.
Item 6	***Regulated Pursuits of Pleasure*** Pursuits of pleasure are subject to control and regulation by the person's values and principles.	***Wanton Pursuits of Pleasure*** Preoccupation with pursuing pleasure; pursuits take on a wanton or obsessive-compulsive quality.
Examples	"I invest emotional or intellectual energy and attach great significance to beliefs concerning human existence." [Item 1] "I devote time and energy to activities such as reading books or attending workshops on spirituality, listening to music or doing artwork, traveling to places for spiritual fulfillment." [Item 4]	"The only things I care about are those I can touch and feel, like sex, drinking, eating good food." [Item 1] "I spend my free time surfing the Internet, playing pachinko or computer games." [Item 4] "I shop until I drop dead, purchasing all kinds of things I don't really need." [Item 5]

Existential Quest Versus Hedonistic-Materialistic Pursuits

Spirituality entails an existential quest for a sense of direction; to answer questions about life and death, being and nonbeing (see Table 5). Of course, different people obtain different answers: The crucial thing is to quest for some higher goal in life and principles that serve as a guide to leading the good life. To many, hedonistic-materialistic pursuits are more attractive than existential quest. The primacy of hedonistic-materialistic values: Materialism (excessive regard for worldly concerns) and hedonism (pursuit of or devotion to pleasure, especially to the pleasures of the senses) occupy a high priority in their scale of values. Excessive hedonistic-materialistic pursuits are symptomatic of spiritual emptiness.

Transcendence Versus Self-Encapsulation

Transcendence is relational spirituality, reached through transcending egocentrism. Relationships are integral to one's meaning and purpose in life. The antithesis of transcendence is self-encapsulation, in which the self derives meaning and purpose solely or primarily from its own individual existence, without reference to a larger context. Self-encapsulation is a form of egoism or self-contained individualism. The following five pairs of component ideas further describe contrasts between transcendence and self-encapsulation (see Table 6).

Self-in-Relations Versus Self-Containment

Transcendence entails viewing oneself in a relational context (e.g., self-in-cosmos, personal relationship with God), thus conferring meaning and purpose to one's life. It defines one's relationships with others, society, humanity, nature, cosmos; and (to religious believers) some higher, divine, sacred, or supreme being or beings. In self-containment, attention is focused on one's own individual existence from which meaning and purpose are derived, without reference to a relational context.

Compassion Versus Hard-Heartedness

Compassion occupies a key position in Buddhism: Deep feeling for the suffering of others, extended to humankind. Kindness does not always entail compassion: We may be kind to people who are not in misery. Typical acts of kindness include doing favors and good deeds for others, helping and taking care of them. Devoid of compassion, a person becomes hard-hearted, callous, uncaring, and unfeeling.

Selflessness Versus Egoism

A selfless person puts the interests of other people above his own and acts without selfish concerns. The antithesis of selflessness is to act in ways that are motivated solely or primarily by self-interests. Egoism does not necessarily entail selfishness. Egoistic actions are not necessarily illegal or immoral, and do not necessarily infringe on the rights of others.

Altruism Versus Selfishness

Altruism is the selfless concern for the welfare of others. It may involve great personal sacrifice, even one's life. Selfishness hardly requires commentary. It is not only the absence of altruism but also the proclivity toward taking actions that benefit oneself at the expense of others.

Universal Love Versus Misanthropy

Universal love is the lodestone of ecumenicity. At root, it champions the intrinsic value of human life and cherishing care for one's fellowmen. Misanthropy is the antithesis of love for humanity. However, a misanthrope does not necessarily seek to exploit, harm, or destroy his fellow man. A psychopath does; his actions, therefore, mean an extreme negation of universal love.

Self-Actualization Versus Alienation

Self-actualization means the realization of one's potentials, to be the best that one can be. The antecedents of self-actualization are acceptance, humility, existential quest, and transcendence. Having engaged in soul searching, self-actualized persons experience a profound sense of fulfillment and mastery. Alienation is the negation of self-actualization. Its components are social isolation, estrangement, emptiness, meaninglessness, normlessness, and powerlessness (see Table 7).

Table 6. Transcendence Versus Self-Encapsulation

Concept pair	Transcendence	Self-Encapsulation
Central idea	Relational spirituality: Views the self in a larger context; spirituality is reached through transcending egocentrism; universal love.	Views the self as self-contained, without reference to a larger context; encapsulates oneself; misanthropy.
Item 1	*Self-in-Relations* Views the self in a relational context (e.g., self-in-cosmos, personal relationship with God); relationships with others, society, humanity, nature, cosmos, or some higher being or beings are integral to one's meaning and purpose in life.	*Self-Independence* Views the self as independent, self-contained, without reference to a relational context. Attention is focused on one's own individual existence from which meaning and purpose are derived.
Item 2	*Compassion* Being kind to others; deep feelings for the suffering of others, extended to humankind.	*Hard-Heartedness* Hard-hearted, callous, uncaring and unfeeling toward the suffering of others.
Item 3	*Selflessness* Considers the interests of other people, acts without selfish concerns.	*Egoism* Acts in ways that are motivated by self-interest.
Item 4	*Altruism* Selfless concern for the welfare of others; involves personal sacrifice.	*Selfishness* Acting in ways that are motivated by only self-interests, often at the expense of others.
Item 5	*Universal Love* Champions the intrinsic value of human life and cherishing care for one's fellow man; respects life in all its forms.	*Misanthropy* Hatred of humankind; prefers to lead the life of a loner.
Example	"The life of the individual is incomplete. We all need to relate with others, for the welfare of all." [Item 1]	"I do my thing and you do your thing. No one has the right to interfere with my freedom. It's entirely my own business if I choose to risk my life in some dangerous sports." [Item 1]

Table 7. Self-Actualization Versus Alienation

Concept pair	Self-Actualization	Alienation
Central idea	In touch with oneself; feels a closeness to others, nature, divine being(s); regards life as meaningful, purposeful, regulated by norms; has a sense of agency.	Estranged from oneself, others, nature, divine being(s); experiences emptiness, meaninglessness, normlessness, and powerlessness.
Item 1	**Social Connectedness** Feels socially connected with others.	**Social Isolation** Feels socially isolated from others.
Item 2	**Closeness** Feels close to or being in touch with oneself, nature, God; at home in the cosmos.	**Estrangement** Feels estranged from oneself, nature, God; out of place in the cosmos; inward emptiness.
Item 3	**Meaningfulness** Views life as meaningful, purposeful; has a sense of direction; committed to some goal in life.	**Meaninglessness** Views life as meaningless, purposeless; disoriented, lost; not committed to any goal in life.
Item 4	**Normativeness** Views life as regulated or guided by norms and values.	**Normlessness** Experiences normlessness, moral void: Norms and values regulating life are absent or not operational.
Item 5	**Agency** Experiences oneself as an agent acting in control of one's life-activity; has a sense of mastery.	**Powerlessness** Feels powerless, unable to control impersonal forces dominating one's life.
Examples	"For a number of years, I have had feelings of being close to the divine." [Item 2] "Yes, society has to be regulated by norms. Yet, I am a *free* agent." [Item 4, Item 5]	"I feel like a stranger to myself. I don't know what kind of a person I am." [Item 2] "I am lost. I don't know what I want to do with my life." [Item 3] "Like a jellyfish I am, controlled by the currents of the sea." [Item 5]

Appendix B

Strategies of Coping

Below I guide you through an exploration of strategies for coping with life's misfortunes (trauma, major illness, loss, and so forth). I've created a structure involving four pairs of contrasting strategies:

1. Forbearance versus Intolerance
2. Forgiveness versus Vengefulness
3. Hope versus Despair
4. Meaning Reconstruction versus Entrenchment

For each pair, I offer questions for you to consider as part of your self-exploration. Answering the questions will help you determine what coping strategies you use and whether they are helpful or harmful to you.

I have had my share of misfortunes. I have experienced despair and depression. But I've managed to emerge from the depths of despondency with renewed hope and passion for life. Central to my strategy is to direct attention away from my own misery to helping others. That's why I feel the urge to share with fellow travelers my experiences in coping with life's misfortunes.

Next, I engage you in dialogues such that therapeutic movement from the negative to the positive direction may be realized. Invitation to change following self-exploration is always there, gently but surely. The appeals of approaching life's problems based on positive strategies are highlighted. Negative strategies are under attack, relentlessly if necessary. With the aid of tables, I illustrate how techniques of therapeutic intervention may be applied. Note that principles underlie techniques. Emphasis is placed on taking action and on directing attention away from the self, toward others.

I have assumed the role of a counselor in these dialogues. However, in line with Dialogic Action Therapy, nothing would be better than to engage yourself in internal dialogues and thus act as your own therapeutic agent. Let us now see how you may do so across the four pairs of coping I offer.

Forbearance Versus Intolerance

Forbearance is the capacity to endure pain, suffering, or ill fortune without complaint. Often, forbearance is dictated by necessity, as when people fall victim to natural calamities, harsh socioeconomic or political realities beyond one's control, or are threatened, fearful of punishment or retaliation, under duress or, in the extreme, bondage of slavery. Forbearance may or may not entail fortitude, the moral courage to stand up for one's conviction in the face of threat or danger to oneself. Intolerance, in the present context, refers to unwillingness or inability to endure frustration, pain, suffering, or ill fortune, coupled with a tendency to complain.

Invitation to Self-Exploration

People experience pain and suffering at some time or another. How have you reacted to your own experiences?

What if the pain and suffering were inflicted upon you by the deliberate acts of others (e.g., provocation, insults, oppression)? People around you are likely to see that you suffer. How do you deal with this situation?

Suppose you are threatened and you find yourself in danger when you stand up for your convictions (i.e., strong beliefs in some principle). What then? Would you give up your convictions, or endure the pain and suffering? Please consider carefully and explain.

Please feel free to elaborate further. You might have left something out; now is the time to add to what you have said.

Table 1. Forbearance Versus Intolerance

Strategy pair	Forbearance	Intolerance
Central idea	Capacity to endure pain and suffering	Intolerance of pain and suffering
Item 1	Endures pain and suffering due to ill fortune (e.g., sickness, natural calamities, harsh socioeconomic or political realities beyond one's control).	Responds to pain and suffering due to ill fortune (e.g., sickness, natural calamities, harsh socioeconomic or political realities beyond one's control) with impatience, irritability, anger, resentment, or bitterness; tends to complain or whine; blames others, the world, God.
Dealing with impatience, irritability, anger, resentment, bitterness	You have gone through a painful experience. You feel you have suffered enough. . . .. You have also been impatient, irritable, resentful. You complain a lot. You have emotional outbursts. . . .. These responses are not helpful. They make life more miserable for you and others around you. I wonder what's behind them. [Explore and deal with possible feelings of guilt, inadequacy, and the like.] No one is asking you to just rid yourself of negative emotions. You have a right to feel angry, after what you have gone through. But, I am asking you to contain your anger, and prevent it from doing more harm. . . .. Better still, turn your anger into strength, to do something positive. Complaining and blaming have not made things better. So why not do something else more useful. For example.	
Item 2	Endures pain and suffering inflicted upon oneself by the deliberate acts of others such as provocation, insults, oppression. (Reflects an inner attitude, not merely inhibition of outward expression.)	Responds to pain and suffering inflicted upon oneself by the deliberate acts of others (e.g., provocation, insults, oppression) with resentment or bitterness (the outward expression of which may be inhibited due to fear of punishment or retaliation).

(*Continued*)

Table 1. Continued

Strategy pair	Forbearance	Intolerance
Coping with provocation, insults, oppression	You have suffered because *you feel* other people have done something horrible to you. [The first order of intervention is to ascertain if there is a realistic basis for the feeling. We now assume there is.] You feel angry inside. Yet, you dare not show your anger. . . . Of course, showing your anger may be dangerous. You may be punished even more. Understandably, you are afraid. . . . Bottling up your anger is not a good option, because the anger can eat you up and make you feel worse. So, let's talk about other options. . . . [Exercises in self-assertion would be useful here.] [Now comes the hardest part. There is no escape, realistically speaking. This may be difficult for Americans to understand. The fact remains that there are plenty of bullies in the world who inflict pain on others without the slightest compunction and who wouldn't go away.] This is really hard. You suffer, repeatedly, with no end in sight. You can't fight against something that powerful. . . . Does it mean there is nothing you can do? No. At the very least, stop feeling sorry for yourself, because that would compound the suffering. It's not your fault. . . . I would go further: Give yourself credit. You have endured a great deal of pain, more than your fair share. Now, that's strength in its own right.	
Item 3	Directs one's attention to reduce the pain and suffering of others (which may be caused by one's own).	Becomes intolerant of others because of one's own pain and suffering.
Redirecting attention to others	You seem to have become intolerant of others, because of the pain and suffering you have had. In turn, your intolerance may cause pain and suffering to others. This is a vicious cycle. . . . Restore yourself, and reverse the vicious cycle. The best way of doing this is to direct your attention to reduce the pain and suffering of others, to make life better for them. . . . You see, in the end, you make your life by making life better for others. That's the Dao.	

Table 1. Continued

Strategy pair	Forbearance	Intolerance
Item 4	Endures pain and suffering with fortitude or moral courage to stand up for one's convictions in the face of threat or danger to oneself.	Retreats from one's convictions in the face of threat or danger to oneself.
Affirming fortitude	It's hard to hold onto your convictions in the face of such pressures and threats to yourself. Harder still to stand up for them. You may have to pay a heavy price for it. . . .. If you do, however, you will live in the knowledge that you have lived with moral courage, and hold your head up high. . . .. The decision is yours. [Some of you might say that this goes beyond therapy to ethics. No, it is still therapy because clarifying the consequences of different decisions and encouraging ethical deliberations are part of therapy.]	

Approaches and Attacks

Invitation to self-examination and change is always there, gently but surely. No matter what the traveler says or does, invitation sticks onto him like an octopus aimed at its prey. There is really "no way out" of it. This may evoke anger in the traveler, which presents another opportunity for emotional education. Note that principles underlie techniques. Emphasis is placed on taking action and on directing attention away from the self to others. In Table 1, the therapeutic process calculated to enhance forbearance and to reduce intolerance is illustrated.

Forgiveness Versus Vengefulness

Forgiveness has two directions: To forgive someone, and to ask for forgiveness from someone. Forgiving oneself stands in a dialogic relation with both forgiving someone and asking for forgiveness. Forgiving oneself and forgiving others are mutually reinforcing.

Asking for forgiveness from others without forgiving oneself is incomplete forgiveness. Forgiving oneself without forgiving others is a mark of egocentrism; it negates the right to ask for forgiveness.

The antithesis of forgiveness takes two forms. Vengefulness: to harbor resentment or hatred, resort to personal vindictiveness, get even or seek revenge against the offender. Irresponsibility: to admit no responsibility for harm done to another, feel no remorse, and take no action that may undo at least in part the harm done.

Counseling practitioners have not attended sufficiently to self-other dialogic relations in forgiveness: They tend to dwell on forgiving others, and do not give due attention to forgiving oneself, asking for forgiveness, even less to reparation or restitution.

Invitation to Self-Exploration

People react differently to being offended, harmed, or unfairly treated by others. Think of some experiences you have had. Normally how do you react?

Some people pardon or forgive their offenders. Some seek vengeance. What about yourself? What does it mean for you to pardon/forgive/revenge? How would you feel afterward?

Suppose the offence is repeated, again and again. How would you react? What if the offender deliberately inflicts pain and suffering on you? How would you react?

We have been talking about your being offended. What if you are the offender? Think of some experiences you have had. To what extent do you assume responsibility? Repent? What actions have you taken, if any, to make up?

What about forgiving (or refusing to forgive) yourself? What does it mean? How would you feel afterward? What do you think is the relation between forgiving (refusing to forgive) yourself and forgiving (refusing to forgive) others?

Please feel free to elaborate further. You might have left something out; now is the time to add to what you have said.

Approaches and Attacks

It is important to assess the nature of the alleged committed act in question. To ask for forgiveness presumes that a wrongful act, of commission or omission, has indeed been committed, as judged according to prevailing ethical norms. If no wrongful act has been committed, then the real issue relates not to forgiveness, but to feelings of guilt that have no realistic basis. The task is then to reduce guilt, rather than to ask for forgiveness.

Therefore, before talking about forgiving or asking for forgiveness, it is essential to establish if indeed an offence has been committed and clarify the

Table 2. Forgiveness Versus Vengefulness

Strategy pair	Forgiveness	Vengefulness
Item 1	Repentance: Assumes responsibility for one's wrongdoings; feels remorse, contrition, or self-reproach.	Irresponsibility: Refuses to assume responsibility for one's wrongdoings; feels no remorse, contrition, or self-reproach.
Guilt reduction versus Repentance	Before talking about asking for forgiveness, we should examine first what you had in fact done. . . . No one thought what you did was wrong. You yourself have a tough time explaining why what you did was wrong. Yet, you feel guilty. . . . [The task here is guilt reduction, not repentance.] **Sins of Commission** You need to consider that your actions have an effect on how you feel about yourself. . . . It takes courage to repent. . . . I don't think we can go further if you take no action for reparations. . . . **Sins of Omission** You failed to act when action was called for, resulting in causing injury to others. Assuming responsibility is the first step toward a resolution.	
Item 2	Ask for forgiveness from someone from someone whom one has offended.	Refuses to ask for forgiveness from someone whom one has offended.
Asking for forgiveness	You have been troubled by what you did to your friend for a long time. The question is, however, what you have done about it. . . . Have you thought of asking her for forgiveness? . . . You are afraid that she may reject your asking. You may not be able to know for sure. . . . But, if you have the courage to ask, you would have at least done your part. . . . You have done something that is difficult to do for most people. You said sorry and you asked for forgiveness from your friend. Now you feel much better. What else have you learned? . . . How can you make sure that you will not repeat the same error? . . . In what ways have you changed as a person?	
Item 3	Makes reparation or restitution as an attempt to undo, at least in part, the damage done to someone.	Makes no reparation or restitution as an attempt to undo, at least in part, the damage done to someone.

(*Continued*)

Table 2. Continued

Strategy pair	Forgiveness	Vengefulness
Making reparation	Asking for forgiveness may not be enough. You haven't made any reparation to make up for the damage done. ... Making reparation would give substance to your asking for forgiveness. What are you prepared to do?	
Item 4a	Grants a pardon to the offender(s), involving merely permitting the offender(s) to go unpunished.	Refuses to pardon: Tries to get even or seek revenge against the offender(s).
Pardoning the offender(s)	You refuse to pardon the offenders. You want them punished. Does it help to undo what has already been done? Or make things better for yourself? ... It's time to pardon.	
Item 4b	Grants a pardon to oneself, involving merely permitting oneself to go unpunished.	Refuses to pardon: Continues to torment or punish oneself.
Pardoning oneself	You refuse to pardon yourself. You continue to punish yourself. What will that do to yourself and others around you? Does it help to undo what has already been done? Or make things better for the person(s) you have wronged? ... It's time to stop punishing yourself.	
Item 5a	Conditional forgiveness: Excuse the offender(s) from an offence.	Refuses to forgive: Continues to harbor resentment or hatred toward the offender(s); vindictive.
Forgiving the offender(s)	You have been dwelling on the hurt caused by your friend. This bitterness is eating you up. When is the time to let go? ... No, I don't mean forgetting; I mean forgiving. ... At least, give him a second chance. ...	
Item 5b	Conditional forgiveness: Excuse oneself from an offence.	Refuses to forgive: Continues to feel guilty, blame oneself.
Forgiving oneself	You have no hesitation in forgiving others. Yet, the thought of forgiving yourself never occurs to you. Why not? ... It is time for you to learn to be kind toward yourself.	

Table 2. Continued

Strategy pair	Forgiveness	Vengefulness
Item 6a	Full or unconditional forgiveness of the offender(s), in thought and action.	Refuses to forgive: Continues to harbor resentment or hatred toward the offender(s); vindictive.
Forgiving the offender(s) unconditionally	You say you have forgiven your offenders. Yet, deep down you still blame them for what they have done; your attitude is condescending; you wouldn't let go of resentment....	
Item 6b	Full or unconditional forgiveness of oneself, in thought and action.	Refuses to forgive: Continues to feel guilty, blame oneself.
Forgiving oneself unconditionally	You say you have forgiven yourself. Yet, deep down you still blame yourself for what you have done.... It's time to let go of the past, totally.	
Item 7	The act of forgiving occasions moving and inspiring oneself to be a better person.	Refuses to forgive: Continues to harbor resentment or hatred toward the offender(s), vindictive; or to feel guilty, blame oneself.
Inspiring the traveler to be a better person through forgiving	You have taken a courageous step of letting go of your bitterness. You have forgiven your friend, *and* yourself. Where do we go from here? ... Have you let your friend know you have forgiven him? ... What changes have occurred in yourself and in your relationship with him? ... You may even set an example of forgiveness, and inspire others to forgive.	
Item 8	The act of forgiving occasions moving and inspiring the offender(s) to be a better person(s).	Refuses to forgive: Continues to harbor resentment or hatred toward the offender(s); vindictive.
Inspiring the offender(s) to be a better person(s)	You may even inspire your offender(s) to be a better person(s). You may say something like this to him: "There is no need for you to ask for forgiveness. But that doesn't mean no demands are put on you. Are you assuming responsibility for what you have done? Are you sorry? Have you repented? Have you asked for forgiveness? Made reparations? ... What have you learned? What are you going to do to avoid making the same error? In what ways will you change for the better as a person? ... How?"	

apportioning of responsibilities. This point cannot be emphasized enough. There are plenty of people who make a profession of unconditional self-blaming. God, please help our self-blaming fellow travelers when they seek help from religious or pastoral counselors who, overzealous to practice forgiveness, commence counseling on the false presumption of culpability.

It is also important to attend to sins of commission as well as omission (negligence or failure to act when action is dictation by moral obligation or human decency).

If the spiritual traveler is unwilling to forgive, redirect intervention toward letting go of fixations (e.g., of past traumas, revenge) and moving forward in life: "I understand that you are not willing to forgive, at least not yet. But life goes on, and you will not allow bitterness and vindictiveness to lessen the value of your life."

The therapeutic-redeeming aim is often no less than the alleviation, even elimination, of self-torment that has been buried deep within your dialogic self for years. Table 2 illustrates the therapeutic strategies involved.

Hope Versus Despair

Hope is the mother of the will to live and of actions for change. Hope is oriented toward the future: What is bad will pass and what is good will be preserved or restored. It differs from optimism, a general orientation that the future will be better than what it is now. Hope maintains that orientation even in the face of calamity or great adversity. It derives from various sources, including religious faith, political ideology, personal conviction and fortitude, and social support; it may also derive from seeing hope in and through others, one's children, students, friends, humanity. Though future oriented, hope impacts the present. Despair is the archenemy of hope. It is extreme pessimism, believing that all is lost and that there is no way out of the present predicament or misfortune.

Invitation to Self-Exploration

Some people react to misfortune, such as major illness and natural or man-made calamity, with despair; others maintain hope. What about yourself? What does hope mean to you? Despair?

Think of the most serious difficulty you have to face in your life. Is there a way out? Or no way out at all? Will things get better, or worse? What would the darkest moment be like? Do you tend to dwell on the past or look forward to the future?

Table 3. Hope Versus Despair

Strategy pair	Hope	Despair
Item 1	Believes there is a way out of the present predicament.	Believes there is no way out of the present predicament.
Pointing to a way out	Of course, you despair. You believe there is no way out. . . .. Think again. Is there really no way out? . . . There is a way out. Now is the time to explore what that is.	
Item 2	Feels that inner resources are available to confront the present predicament.	Feels that inner resources are unavailable to confront the present predicament.
Activating inner resources	You feel you just don't have what it takes to deal with your present situation. Right? . . . What makes you so sure that you don't? . . . Look to your past where you did have what it took to overcome difficulties. . . .. Feel the inner strength within you. Rekindle it. Let it grow. You need all the strength you have. So just let it grow and grow.	
Item 3	Feels that external support (e.g., family, friends) is available.	Feels that external support (e.g., family, friends) is unavailable.
Accepting external support	***Perception of Unavailable Support May Be Inaccurate*** Family and friends are not here to help you. That's what you think. . . .. They don't want to help you? Or, closer to the truth is that you don't want to accept their help. What makes it so difficult for you? Your family and friends want to help you. That should give you more strength. . . .. Accept their help. Everyone needs support from other people sometimes. ***Perception of Unavailable Support May Be Accurate*** You feel that family and friends are not here to help you. . . .. There are reasons for that. . . .. Right now, the important thing is that there are/may be other people who are ready to help. For example. . . .. Are you ready to accept their help?	
Item 4	"God [bodhisattva or some other divine being] will not abandon me."	Feels abandoned, forsaken by God or some other divine being.

(Continued)

Table 3. Continued

Strategy pair	Hope	Despair
Combating feelings of being abandoned	You feel abandoned. That's a horrible feeling.... But, more important, are you abandoning yourself? Heaven abandons those who have abandoned themselves. Have you thought about that? ... It's great that you no longer feel abandoned. You have faith. Now, will you abandon yourself?	
Item 5	Believes that fortune or some higher or supernatural force is favorable toward oneself: For example, "Heaven has no paths of desperation for people."	Believes that fortune or some higher or supernatural force is unfavorable toward oneself: For example, "I am jinxed."
Combating feelings of being doomed	So, you feel doomed? That would make things worse.... Has your fortune always been unfavorable to you? You count the negatives, and ignore the positives. That would make anybody feel doomed.... So do another counting. Think about the positives.... Now, you no longer believe you are doomed. That's a good feeling. You can move on.	
Item 6	Future orientation (looks beyond the present).	Fixation on the present (does not look beyond the present).
Look beyond the present	You haven't looked beyond the present. Kind of fixated.... There is always another day, tomorrow. Nobody knows for sure what tomorrow will bring. What makes you so sure of yourself? ... What happens tomorrow may depend on what you do today. So, what are you going to do now? ... It's great that you are now looking beyond the present. What does the future hold for you?	
Item 7	Sense of self-efficacy: "I shall overcome."	I can't do anything.
Enhancing sense of self-efficacy	You feel helpless. That's understandable, given what has happened to you.... But do you have to continue to feel helpless? The more you feel helpless, the more you may become helpless.... Think of an example where you were able to handle a difficult situation.... Now, you have more confidence. That gives you more strength.	

Table 3. Continued

Strategy pair	Hope	Despair
Item 8	Optimism: Believes that the future will be better; sense of a bright future; encouraged.	Pessimism: Believes that the future will be worse; sense of a foreshortened future (e.g., does not expect to have a career, marriage, children, or a normal life span); discouraged.
Combating pessimism	You are pessimistic. You are convinced that things will get worse. . . . You sound so sure that you are right. Is this a pattern? . . . Your newfound optimism is very encouraging.	
Item 9	Will to live, to survive.	Will to live, to survive, is lacking or absent; suicidal ideation.
Activating the will to live	You wallow in self-pity. . . .. You want to die. Here, we have emotional honesty, at least. . . .. You owe to yourself to ask the question, "Is suicide the *only* way out?" . . . If you have the guts to kill yourself, you don't mind waiting a bit longer to answer that question. . . .. Give yourself more time. That's not too much to ask for. . . .. I sense you now have a will to live, to survive. Great. That's a key to solutions.	
Item 10	Refuses to give up, continues to struggle.	Giving or has given up; a sense of futility sets in.
Don't give up	You seem to have given up. You think it's futile to keep on struggling. . . .. This may be cruel. But I have to ask what would happen if you really give up. Is it an option? . . . Just don't give up. That's the beginning of finding a solution.	
Item 11	Sees hope in and through other people (e.g., one's children, students, friends, humanity).	Despairs of other people (e.g., one's children, students, friends) and in humanity.

(*Continued*)

Table 3. Continued

Strategy pair	Hope	Despair
Seeing hope in and through others	***Perception of others may be inaccurate*** You despair of other people. You feel they have let you down. . . . Have they really let you down? Do you bear some responsibility? . . . Think of others, even if you no longer care about yourself. . . . ***Perception of others may be accurate*** To despair of other people is an awful feeling. But you still have a choice: to *accept* reality, or to keep on torturing yourself on account of other people's failings. To go a step further, you can still find hope in people, despite their failings. [The idea here is to accept the proclivity to disappoint as part of human nature.] . . . There may still be others who will not fail you. Don't tell me that everyone has failed you, and will continue to fail you in the future. [The task here is to combat overgeneralization.] You can find hope in and through them.	
Item 12	Takes action to help oneself; proactive, engaged.	Takes no action to help oneself; passive, disengaged.
Taking action to help oneself	You haven't taken action to help yourself. There is no cure for laziness, but there is cure for despair. Now you know what you must do. . . . Describe how you have taken action to help yourself. . . . Keep it up.	
Item 13	Takes action to help others; proactive, engaged.	Takes no action to help others; passive, disengaged.
Taking action to help others	One of the best ways of helping yourself is to do something for others. I suggest that you start to help others, not just yourself. If you do, don't be surprised that you will be rewarded. . . . Describe how you have taken action to help others. . . . That can be more powerful than helping yourself.	

What inner resources or external support (e.g., family, friends) is available to help you? Have you felt helpless?

Have you felt jinxed? Abandoned by God (or some other divine being)? Despair of other people? Have you thought that it is futile to continue to struggle? Have you had thoughts of suicide?

What actions, if any, have you taken to help yourself? Or to help others?

Approaches and Attacks

To combat despair, negative feelings and thoughts (as in feeling forsaken by God or some other divine being) are first accepted, rather than being labeled as "irrational" or "superstitious," to be extirpated. Even suicidal thoughts are acknowledged, validated as "honest." However, the basis for the negative feelings and thoughts are attacked through incisive questioning and invitations to reconsideration. In particular, brought to the traveler's attention is the rigidity and absolutism of convictions that underlie his despair. No effort is spared to rekindle, sustain, and magnify hope. This entails activating your moral courage and inner resources to overcome despair and to embrace life again. Table 3 illustrates the therapeutic strategies involved.

Meaning Reconstruction Versus Entrenchment

People reconstruct meaning in response to adverse life events, making sense of what appears to be unfair or, worse, senseless. Unlike forbearance, which entails merely or primarily endurance, meaning reconstruction is a dynamic process that seeks to restore loss of meaning and purpose, even to create new meanings. This process involves cycles of construction, deconstruction, and reconstruction, and the dialectics of thought and action. Entrenchment, in the present context, refers to unwillingness or inability to find new meanings or purpose. Mental conservatism, fixation, or rigidity inhibits meaning reconstruction, and renders entrenchment more likely. The result is that old constructions are left untouched.

Invitation to Self-Exploration

Let's talk about how you respond to adverse life events, and what meanings you make of them. Think of an adverse event or unfortunate experience in your life. What are your thoughts about it now? Talk about your thoughts at different points in time. What factors have contributed to changes/lack of changes? What have you learned?

People attach different meanings to their unfortunate experiences. Looking back, in what ways have you examined the way you previously looked at your own experience? What changes have occurred in the way you look at this experience? When? How? Please explain. In what ways have you made sense of this experience?

Table 4. Meaning Reconstruction Versus Entrenchment

Strategy pair	Meaning Reconstruction	Entrenchment
Central idea	Attempts to reconstruct meaning and purpose in response to adverse life events.	Mental rigidity or fixation on previous or existing meaning constructions; deconstruction without learning or reconstruction, leaving oneself worse off; construction of meanings, though new, represent accentuations of unhealthy or destructive tendencies in previous constructions.
Item 1	Engages in *deconstruction*, examining and altering previous or existing constructions of meaning. Learn from accumulation and summation of experience.	Maintains existing constructions; leaves previous or existing constructions of meaning untouched.
Invitation to deconstruction	You have gone through an ordeal. You have been looking at it in the same old way for a long time.. ... This hasn't been helpful. It continues to trouble you.. ... A misfortune means different things to different people. There are different ways of looking at it. How about a reexamination of how you have been looking at yours? I'm saying that a fixed, entrenched way of looking at the past can be a part of the problem.. ... What can you learn from your misfortune and the way you have been looking at it?	
Item 2	Attempts to make sense of the adverse life event(s); to restore loss of meaning and purpose.	Sees the adverse life event(s) only as unfair, or worse, senseless.
Making sense of adverse life event(s); restore meaning and purpose	You only see what has happened to you as unfair, or worse, senseless. You can't make sense out of it.. ... I bet you are bitter. You say you have lost your purpose in life. Wouldn't that make you even bitterer in the long run? Leading a life without purpose is no way to live.. ... There is no necessary connection between misfortune and loss of purpose. I encourage you to restore meaning and purpose to your life. So, let's start with.. ...	

Table 4. Continued

Strategy pair	Meaning Reconstruction	Entrenchment
Item 3	Seeks to *construct* new, healthy meanings and purpose.	Deconstructs without construction, without learning or benefiting from previous experiences; constructs new meanings that accentuate unhealthy or destructive tendencies in previous constructions.
Constructing new meanings and purpose	Yes, I see that you look at things differently now. You seem to have become gloomier. You have filtered out color from your life. That can't go on. . . .. Now, I invite you to take another look at how you may look at your misfortune. A healthier look this time. . . .	
Item 4	Relates with others differently following the emergence of new meanings.	Maintains previous ways of relating, or getting worse.
Finding new ways of relating	It's great that you have started to explore new meanings about your unfortunate experiences, to restore purpose to your life. How does that translate into new ways of relating with other people? For instance. . . .	
Item 5	Engages in actions prompted by new meanings; acts according to plans.	Maintains previous patterns of action, or getting worse.
Finding new ways of acting	You've been talking about new meanings and purposes. What about new ways of acting?	
Item 6	Meaning *reconstruction*. Evaluates and reflects on new patterns of relating (Item 4) and acting (Item 5), leading to more new meanings, learning, and plans for action.	Existing constructions are entrenched; unhealthy or destructive tendencies strengthened further.
Reflection and reconstruction	Let's reflect on your new patterns of acting and relating. . . . In what ways have they gone astray and made things worse for your life? . . . In what ways have they been helpful, constructive?	

What new meanings to your life, if any, have emerged from this experience? When? How? What are their implications for acting and relating with people? Plans for action?

So how do you relate with others now? In what ways, if any, are you relating differently from before? And how do you act (or behave) now? In what ways, if any, are you behaving differently from before? Are there things you do now that you have never or rarely done before?

What have you learned from these new ways of relating and acting? What new meanings have emerged? In what ways have you changed or not changed as a person?

Please feel free to elaborate further. You might have left something out; now is the time to add to what have said.

Approaches and Attacks

Several principles provide guidance to meaning reconstruction. The first is the need to be sensitive to the pain that reconstruction may bring and to overcome it. The second is to be reminded, again in line with Dialogic Action Therapy, that all the reconstruction will do little if no effective actions follow. The third is to be aware that reconstructed meanings devoid of spiritual values may be negative, thus worsening life. Finally, closure has to be achieved: There should be no unended or unending deconstructions. Table 4 illustrates the therapeutic strategies involved in meaning reconstruction.

Appendix C

Highlights of 22 Episodes of Madness, Diaries, and a Free Association

Chronicle of Outstanding Features or Extraordinary Events

The following table presents a convenient summary of all 22 episodes in a chronological order.

Episode	Salient features
Hypomania 1 lasting 2 weeks	First encounter with hypomanic symptoms. Music figured prominently; I gave it the title "The Conductor Who Couldn't Count."
Hypomania 2 lasting 1 month or longer	Prolonged insomnia. Pronounced changes in social behavior caused considerable anxiety in my family and among my friends and colleagues.
Hypomania 3 lasting 4 days	Brief and mild. No adverse effect on occupational or social functioning.
Mania 1 lasting 1 week or longer	Intensity exceeded previous episodes. Out-of-bound behaviors. Experienced selfless self; dramatic self-healing; androgyny; willful visual hallucinations.

Episode	Salient features
Hypomania 4 lasting 1 month or shorter	Positive tenor; affirmation as a teacher-educator.
Mania 2 lasting 1 month	Major problem was inability to fall asleep; brain fatigue. Recorded a free association. Out-of-bound behaviors; heavy occupational and social costs.
Hypomania 5 lasting 1 week or longer	Cognitive deficits and other scary symptoms. Immersed in dancing in public. Intercultural encounters. Recovery relatively fast and easy.
Hypomania 6 lasting 1 month	Elated mood. Hypomanic symptoms were mild and kept under control. Holistic health and artistic self-expression were intertwined. No adverse social consequences.
Hypomania 7 lasting 1 month	Elated mood. Imbalance: dramatic fluctuations in energy level. Managed to keep episode under control; no adverse social consequences. Engaged in demanding physical activities, such as qigong and Taiji push-hands.
Hypomania 8 lasting 3 weeks	Shaking chills; mental fatigue and confusion, severe enough to require emergency admission to hospital. Outward manifestations of hypomania kept under control. Dared not drive.
Hypomania 9 lasting 4 months	Multiple peaks. Physically and socially very active.
Hypomania 10 lasting 1 month	Infused with *qi* (energy). Alterations in time and sense perception.
Hypomania 11 lasting 1 month	Mild. Prodromal symptom noticed. Dared not drive.
Hypomania 12 lasting 2 months	Able to conduct a series of training sessions. Engaged in audacious acts; telling others I was a "Living Buddha" for a good cause on one occasion.
Hypomania 13 lasting 1 month	Mild. Mental fatigue, coupled with superefficiency in memory retrieval. Dared not drive on some days. Boundary between normal and abnormal states blurred. Remarkable experience being able to suddenly recall the strategies of *Weiqi* (*Go*) grandmasters and thus to compete with advanced players, even in a state of severe mental fatigue.

Episode	Salient features
Hypomania 14 lasting 6 weeks	Very mild. Mental fatigue. Able to sleep. Strong libidinal drive. Affective expressions disinhibited. Social functioning not compromised, but even enhanced.
Hypomania 15 lasting 6 weeks	Very mild. Mental fatigue appearing as the first prodromal symptom, followed by physical and emotional reactivity to music.
Hypomania 16 lasting 4 months	Mild. Practiced expressive dance to music for hours, almost daily. Physically fit enough to dance for whole days to make professional recordings to produce DVD sets.
Hypomania 17 lasting 2 months	Mild. Mental fatigue made it impossible to do any work requiring sustained concentration or arithmetic calculations. Visualized myself lying in a coffin about to be interred, absolute darkness, silence, and nothingness; experienced no fear, a cosmic experience.
Hypomania 18 lasting 2 months	Mild. Marked by high spirits and sociability. Organized a party in my home during which I performed expressive dance to music and entertained my guests with much laughter.
Hypomania 19 lasting 1 month	Mild. Similar to preceding episodes in recent years.
Hypomania 20 lasting 1 month	Fatigue, both mental and physical, is the salient symptom, requiring frequent rests. Sleeps more than usual. Mood elevation is very mild.

Hypomania 1. Lasting two week, this episode was my first encounter with hypomanic symptoms. My music appreciation was dramatically enhanced, even for pieces I had listened to countless times before. I pretended to be a conductor and discovered that I have previously unknown capabilities. As I practiced conducting more, I become more proficient, on the beat. Instead of following the music, I felt as if I were creating it. The more I immersed myself in the process, the less self-conscious I became and the more I enjoyed doing it. As we will see, music figures prominently in later episodes as well.

Hypomania 2. Lasting over a month, this episode brought home to me how prolonged insomnia, fatigue, and energy depletion can tax my body to the limit. Unlike the preceding episode, changes in my social behavior caused considerable anxiety in my family and among my friends and colleagues. The most outrageous thing I did took place in front of a large class of undergraduates: While talking about the June Fourth massacre in Beijing, suddenly uncontrolled (not uncontrollable) emotions took hold of me; tears flowed from my eyes, visible to all. This was the first time I had displayed such emotions in public. Some students were disturbed because my public display was incompatible with their image of a professor.

Hypomania 3. This mild episode is marked by its brief duration of only a few days. I recorded that I "slept for 12 hours [and] completely recovered" in my diary. So I thought that sleep held the key to recovery, as I did in subsequent episodes. There were no adverse effects on my occupational or social functioning in the least. Ironically, I conducted a two-day workshop on depression and suicide prevention just before the onset. On the following day, I attended court as a forensic expert witness. However, at home I was struggling with fatigue, compulsivity, and disturbance of short-term memory.

Mania 1. Though lasting no more than two weeks, this episode is probably the most dramatic. Exceeding the hypomanic episodes, this one was serious in terms of social costs. My behavior exceeded what most other people regarded as the bounds of normality.

Hypomania 4. Lasting only four days, this episode had no adverse effect on my occupational or social functioning. The overall tenor was remarkably positive. I felt more affirmed of my role as teacher-educator than I had ever felt before. I also wrote in my diary that "Suppression of artistic impulses can be hazardous to your health." This realization would evolve into a cardinal drive in subsequent episodes.

Mania 2. Lasting about a month, this episode incurred heavy occupational and social costs. I experienced extreme fluctuations between exuberance and anguish. Heightened literary and aesthetic sensibilities were prominent. I had the capacity to experience simple, unabashed delight in ordinary things (e.g., the root of a tree, the droning sound of cicadas). I experienced serenity and inner peace, but also inner turmoil. One night I woke up suddenly, feeling I was the loneliest person in the world, understood by none and fighting lonely battles all my life. So underneath the mania was a deep sense of anguish, loneliness, and yearning for human contact. Recovery followed after taking two Risperdal tablets, 1 mg each.

Hypomania 5. Lasting over a week, this episode took place on board the *Queen Victoria* cruising around the Mediterranean. Impervious to signs of exhaustion, I danced almost nightly. I surprised myself with how good I was, when I entered into a state of selfless-oblivion. For the first time, I was able to be spontaneous, to move without any inhibition, to enjoy myself, *in public*. Sometimes, when I danced alone, people on the dance floor would stop dancing and watch me. My sociability, love of adventure, and aesthetic capacity were undiminished. I took the initiative to interact with passengers as well as staff on board. One night, I ventured into the grand theatre. Seeing no one there, I took advantage of the occasion, walked onto the empty stage and danced, as if the theatre was full of people—thus to satisfy my aspiration, long frustrated, to be an artistic performer, at least for a while.

Hypomania 6. Lasting about a month, the cardinal symptom of this episode was a prolonged low level of energy, punctuated with frequent bouts of depletion; significantly, racing thoughts or excessive talkativeness was secondary. A major achievement was getting rid of my hunchback posture through exercise. This physical breakthrough ignited a chain reaction in the psychological and spiritual realms (see the section "Caught Between the Challenges and Rewards of Hypomania" in Chapter 2).

Hypomania 7. This episode was separated from Hypomania 6 by only a few months. Also lasting about a month, it was virtually a continuation of the preceding episode.

Hypomania 8. This episode took place after my relocation from Hong Kong to California. Lasting about three weeks, it was kept unknown to all but a few.

Sometimes, while listening to music, I noticed that my tolerance for volume diminished dramatically and that somehow the music did not sound right. Reminded of how brain trauma (e.g., concussion) may result in oversensitivity to noise, I thought that these were signs of a tired brain.

The episode saw me descending into a scary state of severe mental fatigue and confusion. It was so bad that I would get lost while taking a walk around my neighborhood. I was unable to drive for more than a week. The mental confusion was severe enough to require emergency admission to a hospital. The attending doctor decided that hospitalization was not necessary and prescribed risperidone for treatment. Taking three tablets of 3 mg each put me on the track of recovery. Predictably, as my mood elation disappeared, my mundane life resumed.

Hypomania 9. Lasting four months, this episode took place in Beijing, PRC. It had multiple peaks. Physically, I was very active, spending a great deal of time dancing and practicing martial arts.

On several occasions, I had hiccups that lasted on and off for some five hours in the middle of the night. Bewildered, I consulted a Taiji master about what happened. She congratulated me, saying "It's a good thing." True enough, although the process was unpleasant, the end result was beneficial to my health. After the hiccups subsided, I felt a sense of extraordinary well-being; whatever gastrointestinal imbalances or disturbances I had previously were gone.

I found myself practicing a movement technique that I had been trying to perfect, namely, moving both arms independently of each other. There is endless variation in this independence of left-right arm movements. For instance, one may draw a small circle rapidly with the right hand while drawing a large square slowly with the left. Soon, drawing figures developed into virtual calligraphy (writing Chinese characters in the air).

Hypomania 10. Lasting about a month, this episode took place in Macao. It was marked by some unusual perceptual and psychophysical experiences (e.g., feeling a powerful flow of energy or *qi* within my body).

Hypomania 11. This episode took place in California, Macao, and Zhuhai (a city in mainland China). Lasting about a month, it was basically similar to preceding episodes.

Hypomania 12. Lasting about two months, this episode took place partly in Macao where I conducted training workshops for counselors. My audacious adventures in this "schizophrenic city" are described in Chapter 2.

Hypomania 13. Lasting about a month, this episode took place in California. Incredibly, it occurred while I was in the process of writing an academic article. By this time, the benefit of cumulated learning from past experiences amounted to premonition. Prodromal signs appearing about two to three weeks before onset could be read: unexplainable mental fatigue and confusion, fluctuations in energy level, heightened esthetic-literary sensitivities and emotional responsiveness to music.

Hypomania 14. Lasting 6 weeks, this episode took place in California. It was also the mildest I had thus far. Unlike preceding episodes, I was able to sleep well, for at least a few hours on a daily basis. Still, I suffered from severe mental fatigue, which prevented me from performing even simple tasks such as making vacation bookings. Libidinal drive was strong. Affective expressions were disinhibited, even in public. However, these did not compromise my social functioning. If anything, my expressiveness and humor lead to much laughter on social occasions.

Hypomania 15. This mild episode is like a continuation of the last, separated by less than 2 months. Lasting 6 weeks, it took place in California. Incredibly, I was in the process of writing an academic article during its prodromal phase. Unexplainable mental fatigue made it difficult for me to complete the process until recovery.

Hypomania 16. During this mild episode, I practiced expressive dance to music for hours, almost daily. Physically fit enough to dance for whole days to make professional recordings to produce DVD sets.

Hypomania 17. This episode represents a high point of my spiritual journey. On the night of June 21, 2017, I lied down in bed, assuming a "corpse" posture (a yoga technique for utmost relaxation). I then visualized myself lying in a coffin about to be interred. I could hear and feel nails being pounded as the cover of the coffin was closed, quickly. Then there was absolute darkness, silence, and nothingness. Yet I had no fear at all. . ... Soon I sensed a faint shimmering of light, quite impossible to describe. Yes, it was a cosmic experience.

Hypomania 18. This episode is marked by high spirits and sociability. I organized a party in my home during which I performed expressive dance to music and entertained my guests with much laughter.

Hypomania 19. This mild episode is similar to preceding episodes in recent years.

Hypomania 20. Unlike episodes in recent years, this episode is marked by extreme fatigue, physical and mental, rather than mood elevation. The fatigue interfered with the writing of this book. In contrast to Hypomania 8, my tolerance for volume *increased* when listening to music. In all, it makes me feel that the body does work in "mysterious" ways.

Diaries

I have kept diaries written during or around many of the episodes, some of which are included in the main text. Here is an abridged version of my diary written around the end of Mania 1.

> I have had the good fortune of gaining the most extraordinary, mystical experiences, each time during a period of about several weeks. My inner-private and outer-social selves merged. The child inside came out. I became unusually playful, spontaneous, disinhibited—in a sense, more genuine.
>
> In retrospect, I did cross the boundary of social and cultural acceptability. But I retained the master switch: metacognitive awareness and control of my actions. Critical reflectiveness and scientific doubt were fully operative. I was aware that other people viewed my behavior as weird. However, I caused no harm, to myself or to others—only a great deal of worry to bewildered people close to my life. My impulse control was intact. At no point would I do anything that I considered morally wrong or reckless.
>
> My physical condition was characterized by imbalance: My body was near exhaustion, yet my mind remained active, running on fast time. I was mentally

hyperactive. I was thirsty most of the time. I felt hot where others would feel cold. Aware that my energy reserve might be depleted, I moved around slowly. Sometimes, I would half-close my eyes, a conservation technique that I had learned from a yoga master.

My brain's consumption of energy must have been extraordinarily high. Coupled with prolonged sleeplessness, this led to disturbances of cognitive functioning. At worst, I found it difficult to perform even simple arithmetic. I got confused easily. I could perform only one task at a time. I could be extremely forgetful, like forgetting what I had done or where I had put something just a few seconds ago. At times, I could focus on just one thought at a time. While I was staying focused, I would make myriad associations. The next moment, no trace of what I had just been thinking about could be found. The thought was gone. I became obsessive about lost memories—lost in the cosmos forever. I tried to record some of my thoughts on paper or in a computer file before they got lost. At some point, I said to myself, "Let go of lost memories. They will come back. Let my mind rest." That helped to put an end to the obsession.

When my energy level improved, I was unusually focused and efficient. At home, I performed different household tasks very efficiently. Often my hands and legs maneuvered and performed complex tasks without conscious direction, as if the "wisdom of the body" had extended to the executive ego: They accomplished what my mind had intended, without deliberation or being aware of its own intention.

Freed from obsessive-compulsive tendencies, I read rapidly, without worrying that I might have missed something; unencumbered by perfectionism, I wrote fluently. I enjoyed doing even "tedious" tasks, such as throwing the garbage out. Every second of life was enjoyable. Better still, I felt a sense of tranquility, at peace with myself, at home in the cosmos. I have had my share of self-torment, overattachment, compulsivity, embitterment, which I had tried to overcome for decades. All vanished. I achieved shamelessness. I became more tolerant and compassionate. I cherished the simple joys of just being alive. Walking around in the streets, I would say to myself, "Life is wonderful. The world is so beautiful."

I felt humbled by the commanding heights of human achievement, the vastness of the cosmos. The more I knew, the more I became aware of my profound ignorance. Knowledge and humility were like twins. I experienced the near-despair of trying to fathom the infinite with a finite mind.

Clearly, my manic period was marked by extraordinary creativity, heightened aesthetic sensitivity, depth of feelings, and deep humility. These positive, delightful features are significant: They define the nature of my mania. Definitely, racing thoughts, faster than usual, appeared. Sometimes I was obsessed with losing these thoughts, which I couldn't utter fast enough, let alone put down in writing. Speed was also manifest in an extraordinary sensitivity to cues in social interaction. Watching films or TV shows provided delightful occasions for predicting the next scene, what the actors would say and do. My predictions showed uncanny accuracy, as if I had overtaken the role of the director. That was empathy: I and the director became one. Probably I conducted some of my best psychotherapy sessions or workshops, during which my empathy joined forces with the courage to be myself.

Things of beauty appeared in plentiful ways. More precisely, I keenly perceived many things as never before—ordinary things, like people's faces; the sound of running water; tree leaves, through which the rays of the setting sun penetrated. My friends once showed me a Japanese painting, which instantaneously absorbed my attention. In my early days as a graduate student in clinical psychology, I developed an interest in the clinical use of drawings. Now, that interest was elevated to aesthetic appreciation. I talked with my friends about the aesthetic features of the painting, and in so doing also about the artist endowed with the faculty to create it. I surprised myself, because I never thought I had much capacity for appreciating visual art.

Music evoked strong emotions. Reactions to J. S. Bach were total and could not be described as anything short of spirituality. Tears would flow profusely from my eyes whenever I listened to the *Largo* from his *Violin Concerto in G Minor*. This emotional response was specific to this piece of music and to none other. I was in touch with the deepest pathos—without despair. Real catharsis! Listening to music induced spontaneous movements, involving my head (inside and outside), my limbs, my whole body and being. My artistic impulses, long subdued, demanded expression. I rebuked myself:

You coward, where is your courage-to-be?
The artist that you are,
To fulfill your potential
In working, living, and relating?

There were times when the body moved involuntarily. The movements differed from aimless automatism described in neuropsychiatry. They were clearly meaningful, albeit raw, expressions. I liberated myself. I danced. I entered into a state of dynamic meditation. In that state were incorporated elements of hypnotherapy, transcendental meditation, music, dance, and martial arts, which I had learned imperfectly in past years. I experimented with different forms and techniques. For instance, independently one arm might move slowly and softly, draw an imaginary circle of varying size, and so forth, while the other was doing something different. I learned to express myself in ways I had not known before. My body was transformed.

During meditation, at times the self seemed to have vanished. I experienced the no-mind state of emptiness. I felt energy flowing within my body. So I thought of taking advantage of it. Several days before, I injured my left knee; the pain was so bad that I was walking with a limp. I absorbed sunlight outside to magnify the energy flow and directed it to my injured knee. There was a growing sensation of warmth around the injured area. I visualized a volcano around this area, which magnified the sensation further. Finally, there was only light: The body, together with the self, had dissolved. When I came out of this transcendental state, I found the pain gone. I had healed myself—a tangible benefit that was verifiable to several people who knew about my injury.

On other occasions, vivid images appeared, spontaneously or directed at will. The virtual was experienced as the real. I came as close to willful hallucination as I had ever. One unforgettable sequence was seeing myself being nailed on a cross, which was lying on the ground. I wanted it to be raised, so I could see things from a vertical perspective. I felt no physical pain, but intense feelings of pathos for the sufferings of humankind. I felt what Jesus must have felt. All these came as close to a transformative, religious experience I have had in my life—up to now, that is. Another sequence was a transgender experience: turning myself into a woman, feeling and acting like one. It was educational, more powerful than any role-reversal game in psychotherapy. I also experienced androgyny, the yin and the yang, united in one body.

I glimpsed into the mystical-transcendental. But one concern I had was that the combined forces of heightened sensibility and intensified emotionality can be hazardous. I might be too easily fired up by ephemeral ideals and thus act impulsively. Or I might be overly attached to, and hence enslaved by, objects of pleasure or beauty. However, I thought that the Buddhist attitude of nonattachment may keep overattachment at bay: engaged and involved with worldly objects, without being possessive; letting go of fixations. It differs from detachment, which refers to emotional noninvolvement with and disengagement from the world.

A psychoanalyst would say that in my case repression vanished. The unconscious became accessible. Nothing was unthinkable. My mind functioned with holistic oneness, interconnected. This had the effect of enhancing my aesthetic, empathic, and cognitive capabilities.

Retrieval of information and association of ideas were superefficient, so much so that I was overwhelmed by my own outpouring of creativity. I became obsessively attached to ideas and objects, including the self. I had no physically aggressive or destructive tendencies, although direct expressions of verbal aggressiveness sometimes exceeded my normal level.

I have now greater insight into what mystical experiences are like. Here is a question to absorb the interest of those in search of enlightenment. How does one maintain optimal balance for extended periods between creative expressiveness and control? That is, exercise adequate control over impulses without the need for repression; get in and out of manic-like states at will. The person who attains such balance would be sagelike, united in body, mind, and spirit; he lives his daily life in accordance with his inner wishes, and acts without transgression. Destructive forces having been harnessed to serve creative purposes, genuine harmony within the self is achieved.

Sleep held the key to recovery: I knew I would come out of it if only I could get enough sleep for a few days consecutively. Alas, I also feared that, having succeeded, self-torment and other negatives would return, along with normality.

Free Association

In Mania 2, I did a free association, written rather than uttered. Using my computer, I simply typed as fast as I could whatever came to mind. The text is reproduced below exactly as it was written, with the exception of added annotations enclosed within double square brackets.

> Ecumenical but in all cultures ? yes but what the hell is DAT [[see Note 1]], i 've never heard of this therapy don't woryy i have not heard of it either Insomnia cbt ret [[Cognitive Behavioral Therapy, Rational Emotive Therapy]] "I don't engage in such low level activity any more"**not** allowed to change a word anticompulsivetraininguse this as illustration finally i know how to treat read on, all ye who suffer from sleepless nights cunning [not cunt please] go with the folw do not resist and you will fall asleep try it cbt = cognitive so calledbtherapy ret = reticuylar easy therapy? Now laugh those of you who are informed if you are indeed informed

rm donald ? rumsfel [[Donald Rumsfeld]] you don't know what you don't know the most brillian man who ever lived now you are really offended right? Go with the flow don not resist and every vally shall be exalted [[see Note 2]] meaning that in case you don't know what i am talking about this treasure trove = rational emotive therapy the bane of the . . . enough is enough you have suffered long enough please suffer no more if you would only listen to you inner voice and all that crab [note spe] crab by the way you think it's a nme noun? Worong it a verb don't believe me look it up in a dictuionary crab the monarch crab have you eve eaten one? [[see Note 3]] those misguy published editors who think they know it all have already *deleted* this from thyie email you see you can't control your won fingers send ti al the very least to your supervisor otherwise . . . don't say that I didn't warn you now you may delte i know you are very busy i can be compassionate let see who has the last aaugh notice why how already my stuyle changes no english professor can write like i do they will regret it you see highly competive people they don like to see others game of oneupmanship they jealos of their competitors no? i have offended you enough just kidding [i laughing this very moment] send it to your friends just to amuse t them ok they get the laugh of thie life at no expense to you how that for salesmanship who cares?

Do you know where/how/when it tastes very tricky you can taste i am not going to tell you hint ask you austrauilian friends, donw below where the whole continent will drift away fall of from the eath but do you know that many ereons years ago it was part of pangeothe great land mass before you and i were born where were you before you were born of boy if you can answer this q y can live forever in fact you cdan live forever, if you would only believeit **never before has such a bood been written nor eill one be wriiten for a long time to come you see genius appears ohnly once in one's life time of court never once to most** i am really tired can't go on i am going to sleep my apology . . . but you see you have been tricked, i am not going to slppe because i don't whqt you to suffer sleepless not anymore read on because you get this opportunioty only one in your life time the see that falls on bareen soil will not grow be kind to yourself after you have been so creel to all your life read on i beg you sat guanranteed just like the salemen in the United States those blasted psychopaths who sell thir mothers for a dime i you will not be able to put this book down because if you do you screw up you own ficking life it is not my fault [please not that i did mean to write that word, remember xion [[Nixon]] with all his expletives, you president yif you don't remeber, just in case he lived io organge county in CA one of the richest pleacdes i i know because i once talught there some years ago when i was sane] not i am not sure i am SURE you have been tricked again and again i guarantee you innumberable time who is writing all this nonsense? Nonsense you 'll see i am not going to tell ya who wrote this if you can' fingure it out abfter you finish reading this book you are hopless people commit suicide when they feel hopeless serious busines funny professor have been teaching all their life then were students once how come they have never learned to less boring just a little but you think i am curing professuions i was once a PROFESSOR a dime a dozen no i am cursing you the students who allo it to happen respoonsibility Gestalt people kep say it rem perls [[Fritz Perls]] that bastard who treat gloria a real classic!!!!!!!!!!!! rogers carl in case you don'gt rem who he was ... all those great therapists who have problaly done more harm than good all of them not one exception ellis [[Albert Ellis]] was a real idiot rm ho he argued with his client oh i hate that word client client-centred [bristish sp] damn the brits arrogant SABs [SOBs] who not that long ago felt so superiot to americans publishers are just wonderful people they are so helpful you know i shall be indted to them for the rest of my life to get his bo pub i am willing to seel my soul rm faust? Make apack with the devil, man white back raimbow hsipan all ye labour [mozart messah] read on now guess the finish the sentence ... i be damned today is July 4th god bless america but does a really need to be blessed ... by god/allah/what have you sept 11th you were bombed and the rest of the world felt for you alas alone can gb a real presino t his father, ok. Don't get me wrong his fathe was a good man he [[George Bush]] will come down a the worst p in US history asndnow the rest of the world is very very angry with you why becase you had the aufacity to elect an idiot you have only yours to bl American have short mem you are offended right if you are not/yes, read on. . . finish

Rainbow deep major breakthroughs master pupil case study the strangest creature you will ever meet in your life guaranteed yin yang case file

MAN have you note the grandiosity of the title of this book? A book for all seasons in all cultures Life This is not a book about therapy, but life first sentence chinesetelewritinglinquistic experiment Nprograming "I don't know anything about it." PTA [[ProfessionalTraining in Action]] case effecicy of movement mindfulness The mindful mind . . . Electronic submission You may write to me no agent needed megalomanic this is what i m racing thoughts pass through my head a explosion of creativty i predict that these publishers will come running who needs an agen if they ca recognize this as a great book no the greatest goob on therapy ever wirtten they are a hopless bunch east and west north and south thw wisdom acculated since the dawn of human ditory science tech art and scienbce quantum mechanics all in one i was a physicist once bebore i became enlightenedhave you ever been enlighted i bet you have ? i am not going to insult you yes i am goint o insult you to waky up from you rslumberylou have3 ben sleepijg long enopugh

Fire Burning in My Head

The bably of the clas daughters son no in my life don't know how to maria Mkbreakthoughtsd self-transformation use this word throught thebook i really have struglle hard resiscompulsity all my life a good deed a day sarahsingaporeangeuklingivan + girl friend I think she is smarter reminder after a while i get used to it you don't need to understand what this all means, because . . . get it?if you don't get it now, you will never get it [[see Note 4]] remember joyceirish? James, ah, now I recall his name free association authenic movement DMT [[see Note 5]] freud ordinary folks will nbot understand a thing but therapist? They are a hopless bunch counseling never read a book from cover to cover i don't need to the epitomy of boredom germans incapable of experiencing , it was once said, by EG Boring [who's this guy, who tortured me when I was just a humbble grad study even though i didn't know it at the time] enough of boredom dishonesty it is now 4:13 am i am dead tired but i can't let this these thoughts be lost forever without their benef mankind [not i didn't say womenkind]Sexist sexual harassment note spelling this will go on forever never once have you seen anything like iot in print fucking shit [first time in my life, deep apoloty if i have offended you but i don't mind if i had indeed offended you how this book had come to be written put his in the beginning of the book if of what use is a pen to a writer if with his pen he/she cannot beguile gullible wr readers to altar rem **shakespeare** prf of english think they un joce james really i love the irish simply because they ambivlent to englih admit it don't deny it deep donw you still have animosity toward the Brits now excuse me i have to . . . don' ask where i am going i am back i hope i bet you still here becuae you can let this gbokk [[book]] down right wrong i bet my life on itNOW you must be really **confused** good for you i know it

Note 1. Around that time, I was planning to write a book entitled *Dialogic Action Therapy: The Dao of Creative Living in All Cultures*. I also thought of an alternative subtitle *Therapy for All Seasons*.

Note 2. I meant not to force myself to sleep, but to go with the flow; and then, everything will be all right (like Every Valley Shall Be Exalted, from Handel's Messiah).

Note 3. I once wrote a poem about Australia.

Australia

The world's largest monolith,
Mount Uluru bulges
From the continent's navel.

The desert's nipple springs in Alice Springs.
King crabs invite mainlanders to crab
The monarch of Tasmania.
The Great Barrier Reef bars
No tourist invasion.
Koala bears bear their noses.
Kangaroos brain with brainless hops.
Crocodiles tear without tears.
But where have all the humans gone?
Alas, they have little place
In tourism promotion brochures all intend to freak.

An Australian I once asked,
In a language not my own,
"Are you a continent or an island?"
An indignant "neither" I got.
"A nation born of the underclass,
Criminals and rejects, from another—
Has there ever been one in history?" I asked
In naivete. Whereupon interjected a hidebound Brit,
"Yes, Australia." To his train of thought I followed:
"So shiploads of moral imbeciles *decreased*
Standards in both origin and destination."
You've been drifting away from Pangaea,
From us, like a wayward son, far away,
Though in good fortune not as far as Antarctica. . . . . .
After some 180 million years, come back now
To us, unfossilized, appurtenant
To New Zealand, as part of Asia.

Note 4. I was referring to some students with whom I have formed close relationships: a student known to her classmates as the baby of the class (bably of the clas), Maria, a student nicknamed Monkey (Mk), Sarah, Geukling, and Ivan. I have two daughters, but no son.

Note 5. Rainbow, a DanceMovement therapist, refers to movement stemming from the unconscious and hence totally uninhibited as authentic movement. I have developed Dynamic Relaxation and Meditation (DRM), which incorporates elements of meditation, hypnosis, muscle training, music, dance, and martial arts, as an avenue to holistic health.

Commentary

The free association makes clear that I was "**not** allowed to change a single word," as "anticompulsive training"—in accordance with the fundamental rule of free association in classical psychoanalysis. I was "really tired" but could not fall asleep; my strategy was to "go with the folw [flow]" and not to resist. I seemed to enjoy playing tricks on the imaginary reader with opposites, such as "i am not sure i am SURE you have been tricked again and again." Significantly, I told myself to "be kind to yourself after you have been so creel [cruel] to [yourself] all your life"; and I felt "i became enlightened."

Progressing from the beginning to the end, the free association became increasingly free; the outpouring became increasingly uncensored. Discursive thoughts, including flight of ideas, are rampant, and features characteristic of mania may be discerned. There is fragmentation and incoherence, but no confabulation or loss of contact with reality. In the last sentence I wrote at that time, I showed a capacity to anticipate the reader's reaction: "NOW you must be really **confused** good for you i know it." I also displayed a playful attitude while reflecting on my writing style in this passage: "Let see who has the last aaugh notice why how already my styule changes no english professor can write like i do they will regret it you see highly competive people they don like to see others game of oneupmanship they jealos of their competitors no? i have offended you enough just kidding [i laughing this very moment]."

I showed low regard for the counseling profession (not to be confused with disdain for counseling itself): Therapists "are a hopless bunch." I confessed that I never read a book in counseling "from cover to cover," implicating counseling texts as boring, intellectually bankrupt. In all, I had critical-aggressive-hostile as well as lewd impulses: "cunt," "fucking shit [first time in my life, deep apoloty if i have offended you but i don't mind if i had indeed offended you]." Never before have I expressed my lewd or hostile impulses so blatantly in words. I was aware of megalomania and acknowledged the explosion of creativity as I free associated: "Megalomanic this is what i m racing thoughts pass through my head a explosion of creativty." Toward the end, positive themes of struggle with compulsivity, self-transformation, and benefiting mankind appear: "Breakthoughtsd self-transformation . . . i really have struglle hard resiscompulsity all my life 'i am dead tired but i can't let this these thoughts be lost forever without their benef mankind.'"

Appendix D

Expressive Dance to Music: A Royal Road to Holistic Health (Explanatory Notes)

I have always been a lover of classical music. And as Professor of Clinical Psychology, I face the challenge of introducing unconventional (some would say audacious) approaches to holistic health characterized by body-mind-spirit interconnectedness. But what does music have to do with my professional practice?

My life took a sudden turn when I reached the age of 58. Unexpectedly and inexplicably, one day I listened to music in a way that I had never before listened. Emotions ensued far more intensely than usual, penetrating my soul. I began to move, to be a pretend conductor, or dance to the music spontaneously—involving my head (inside and outside), my limbs, my whole body and being. Dancing to music became my royal road to entering into a dynamic state of meditation and to holistic health. This was a momentous discovery. Ever since then, expressive dance to music has played an increasingly vital role in my personal as well as professional life.

Expressive dance allows for maximal freedom and spontaneity, not for any lesser standard in attending to musical rhythm and the composer's intentions. There is no set form, sequence, or choreography; consequently, even performance by the same dancer may differ from one occasion to another.

In subsequent developments, I have incorporated elements of hypnosis, music, movement, dance, Chinese qigong (breath work or vital energy work) and martial arts into a new approach to health enhancement, named Dynamic Relaxation and Meditation (DRM). In the present undertaking, the presence of martial arts may be seen in some of the pieces of music, and the closing movements at the end of each piece illustrate qigong at work.

I may have found the elixir of longevity, professional and chronological. If you want to work and to live long, be a conductor. Witness the longevity that conductors have typically enjoyed. They love their work, which demands great physical endurance. They enter into a state of total concentration akin to dynamic meditation when they conduct. I suspect too that the intimate connection between heartbeat and musical rhythm plays a part. Alas, very few of us can ever aspire to be a conductor. A comforting thought, however, is that expressive dance to music may be the next best thing. I have reached the age of 77 by the time the present DVDs are recorded.

In terms of music appreciation, I am a late bloomer. Expressive dancing to music has helped me greatly to listen to music with interpretive depth. Still, I am fully aware of my limitations as a dancer. I lack the athleticism that younger dancers possess. I try to make up for this deficiency with greater emotional expressiveness. I have been mostly groping in the dark, alone, without external guidance. But I have learned a great deal through experimentation and experiences accumulated over years of practice. With humility, therefore, I offer the present set of DVDs to viewers to appreciate expressive dancing to music and, perhaps more importantly, the potential that it may bring to their holistic health.

How are the pieces of music selected? I have to react emotionally to the music, of course. Pieces that drive my body to move spontaneously upon hearing them for the first time are especially suitable candidates for selection. Collectively the pieces selected should reflect historical, cultural, and musical diversity.

Many of the selected pieces of music have more than one recording and some have different lyrical versions. For instance, many a prima donna has vied for supremacy in the role of Bellini's Norma and put their mark on the aria Casta Diva. I settled for the rendition by Maria Callas, who has to my ears the sexiest voice. I felt compelled to choose Sometimes I Feel Like a Motherless Child sung by Marian Anderson because of both its historical significance and the singer's contralto voice of the century.

Expressive dancing relies on the body to express emotions. The language of music translates into the language of the body. Each piece demands the dancer to resonate with those of its composer. That's interpretation. Good writing is supposed to adhere to the principle, "Show, don't tell." In expressive dancing, the performer simply can't tell.

The range of emotions in the selection is wide indeed, ranging from simplicity to complexity, from anxiety to serenity, and from elation to total despair. Anxiety and apprehension are expressed in Looming Anomaly; serenity in the Largo of J. S. Bach's *Concerto in G minor*. Dejection and despair are expressed in Sometimes I Feel Like a Motherless Child. But hope survives in the midst of these negative emotions. Marian Anderson cries out with conviction, "True believer"! Not so in Schindler's List, where there is nothing but utter dejection and total despair, and where hope has been smothered. But hope is restored in the next piece, Gabriel's Oboe by Ennio Morricone, conveyed through its primitive spirituality. In terms of sequencing, it is also fitting that Ave Maria follows Sometimes I Feel Like a Motherless Child. The Holy Virgin is the universal Mater Dolorosa who feels the pain of all children in the world. To those who embrace her, none is motherless.

DVD1

This comprises nine pieces, six by supreme luminaries of past centuries that require no introduction and three by contemporary classical composers. Here, I comment only on my emotional reactions to specific pieces and perceptions of performance demands they impose.

The program begins with an aria Casta Diva, which throws me into action. In Bellini's opera bearing the same name, Norma is torn between love and duty, destined to die for love—predictably, as in other tragic operas. However, she is not a helpless woman pining for her lost lover, as in other tragic operas such as La Traviata or Madam Butterfly. Norma is a resolute and complex character replete with inner contradictions. The aria is thus demanding for the dancer, no less than for the singer, who must exude the inner struggles and intense emotions of a complex character.

Mozart's genius makes my dancing come naturally. His Romanze from the *Piano Concerto in D minor* speaks for itself. It moved me the first time I heard it and will continue to do so every time I hear it in the years to come.

The dynamism and especially the militancy of Wagner's Ride of the Valkyries are most suited to bring forth elements of martial arts in my performance. I was driven especially by the soprano and contralto voices that embody the supernatural Valkyries' fearless and untamed pagan qualities.

J. S. Bach's music exemplifies spirituality. The Largo in his *Concerto in G minor* has a very special effect on me. For many years, tears would flow from my eyes when I danced to it and entered into a state of selfless-oblivion, in touch with the deepest pathos—but without despair. Real catharsis! This time, tears flowed from my eyes again, in front of crew members doing the video recording, out of my control.

The Largo in Bach's *Double Concerto in D minor* presents a formidable challenge to the solo dancer: how to represent the two violins with a single body. I conceive of it in terms of the interaction between the Yin and Yang. The emotions that are evoked are those of two lovers, a man and a woman who have fallen in love. The first violin is the female with a higher pitch, and the second is the male with a lower pitch. I represent the female with my left and the male with my right arm. That is because generally the left side of my body is relatively agile, whereas the right side is stronger. I have to train hard to identify and follow the interaction of the two violins. To achieve the ideal of "show, don't tell" is extremely difficult. Communication with the audience has to rely entirely on nonverbal means, the language of the body. Demands are put on the viewer too. The explanation in this pamphlet may help the viewer to pay particular attention to this left-right representation.

With Seiji Ozawa conducting the Boston Symphony Orchestra, Beethoven's Egmont Overture presents a different kind of challenge, namely, physical endurance. Its intensity drives my body to perform beyond its limitations, to become oblivious of the signals of physical fatigue, even exhaustion.

DVD2

This comprises 12 pieces categorized into three groups: Inspirational, Intercultural, and New Age Ambient. Some of these pieces are outside of my customary repertoire. A few weeks of intense preparation just before the recording helped me to feel comfortable with expanding into new genres of music, beyond the classical.

Naturally, religious sentiments are prominent in the Inspirational group. With lyrics written by Brendan Graham, You Raise Me Up is sung as a contemporary hymn in church services. I am pleased to have chosen the innovative rendition by artists in Hong Kong, with the sounds of wind and sea waves incorporated in their recording.

Ravi Shankar's Prashanti (Peacefulness) may sound alien to Western ears. The vocalists are Ravi Shankar and S. P. Balasubramanyam. The Vedic prayer (translated into English) that serves as the vocal is reproduced here:

Oh Lord, be benevolent to us.
Drive the darkness away.
Shed upon us the light of wisdom.
Take the jealousy, envy, greed, anger away from us,
And fill our hearts with love and peace.

Yo-Yo Ma is my hero who champions intercultural fertilization in the musical realm. Defune (Setting Sail) is taken from Yo-Yo Ma Plays Japan, an early exemplar of intercultural fertilization. The Silk Road Ensemble he has created is indeed a meeting of strangers who will enrich the musical world across cultures. The piece "Ambush from Ten Sides," a traditional Chinese composition arranged by Li Cang Sang and China Magpie, is a real success in intercultural fertilization. Its militant tenor invites an interpretation with martial arts as a central component.

The Indian piece Shristi (Creation) scares me with its rhythmic complexity. As its composer Sandeep Das explains: "I wondered what would happen if I gave my percussion friends in the Ensemble a huge rhythm canvas to fill with their musical colors while imagining the creation of the universe by Shiva and his drum."

Two pieces, both composed by Nuttavut Chanprasit, are rooted in Thai culture. Proud to Be Thai, with lyrics written by Sukunya Wangsomnuk, expresses joyous ethnic pride. Thai Forest, composed specifically for the present project, exemplifies simple delight upon entering into a forest. Nuttavut also plays an exotic instrument called ranadeak in this recording. Simplicity does not imply easiness. I find it most challenging to catch the spirit of these two compositions originating from "The Land of the Smiling Buddha."

I confess that initially I had little or no idea on how to catch the meanings of Looming Anomaly and Arrival, both composed and performed by my nephew Ken Lee and his collaborator Chris Echols. Ken explains that Arrival is a sequel to Looming Anomaly, and that both are instrumentals created through improvisation. In Looming Anomaly, scientists on earth cannot determine whether an anomaly they have discovered is malevolent or benevolent. But the people on Earth realize that their survival depends on reaching it, no matter what. Arrival is full of hope for the future of humankind, after our spaceships have journeyed vast distances to reach the Looming Anomaly.

My interpretation is that uncertainty, fear of the unknown, and suspense created by mystery dominate the humans' state of mind, until they have summoned enough courage to confront their uncertain destiny. Finally, the sound of the electric guitar played by Ken appears in Arrival, signaling hope. Yes, hope can be a dangerous idea that drives people to do crazy things. I wrote to Ken: "I have finally found my connection to the duo pieces you have created. How? Seriously, by mimicking, even outdoing, the cosmic-comic naughtiness-nuttiness of their composer-cum-performer. Like nephew, like uncle."

To place an order, visit my website at www.EasternTotalHealth.wordpress.com

Appendix E

The Undiscovered Illness: The Opposite of Depression (Excerpts from *Scientific American*, March 2019, reproduced here with permission)

In October 1997, at the age of 58, David Ho had an unusual experience while listening to a recording of Bach. "I began to dance and pretended to conduct," he says. "And as I practiced, instead of following the music, I felt as if I were creating it. I entered into a state of selfless-oblivion, like a trance. My mind exploded. Flashes of insight rained down, and I saw beauty everywhere, in faces, living things and the cosmos. I became disinhibited, spontaneous, liberated."

Ho was in the grips of his first episode of mania. His description sounds like an enviable burst of creative energy, but the symptoms of mania can also include inflated self-esteem, grandiosity, racing thoughts, extreme talkativeness, decreased need for sleep, increased activity or agitation, reckless behavior, delusions, and other psychotic events. Severe episodes can impair day-to-day functions, sometimes enough to require hospitalization.

Perhaps the most surprising thing about such cases is that in the eyes of the psychiatric profession, mania does not exist as a distinct and unalloyed condition. Mania is usually known as the upside of bipolar disorder. For most people, it occurs alongside periods of depression, the downside. But Ho, who has had 20 manic episodes since 1997, has never suffered from depression. Thousands of people in the U.S. share that experience. Unlike those who experience only depression, however, patients with mania alone are lumped with those who have bipolar disorder. This puts psychiatry in the strange position of claiming that depression by itself is different from depression accompanied by mania but that mania by itself is not.

Most psychiatrists agree unipolar mania exists, but there is debate about whether it differs sufficiently from bipolar disorder in important enough ways to warrant a distinct diagnosis. Central to that debate is the tension in psychiatry between fewer, broader categories and more numerous, tightly defined ones. But the missing diagnosis may have consequences for patients: some studies suggest that people with unipolar mania may respond differently to certain treatments. If, as some researchers believe, unipolar mania and bipolar disorder differ in their underlying biology, classifying mania separately could speed development of new treatments that are more personalized and effective. But because unipolar mania is far less common than bipolar disorder, research into the condition has been both scant and equivocal.

As both a patient and a clinical psychologist, Ho is well placed to advance this debate. In 2016 he published a self-study in the journal *Psychosis* cataloguing his symptoms, which include enhanced recall, increased empathy and spiritual experiences. He has suffered some ill effects, including severe fatigue, confusion, and behavior that caused concern among friends and colleagues: he once burst into tears while delivering a lecture. But his professional training has helped him control his impulses and avoid delusional thinking. On balance, he believes that his madness, as he calls it, has enriched rather than damaged his life. "I'm aware my case may be atypical," Ho says. "Precisely for this reason, it challenges prevailing psychiatric beliefs that fail to acknowledge the positive value of mental disorders."

A Modern Illness

Credit for the modern concept of bipolar disorder usually goes to nineteenth-century French psychiatrist Jean-Pierre Falret, who called it folie circulaire, or "circular insanity," for its periods of pathologically elevated and depressed moods, usually separated by symptom-free periods of varying length. This idea became gospel in the early twentieth century, when a father of modern psychiatry, Emil Kraepelin, proposed a historically significant hypothesis.

At the time, psychiatry drew a distinction between so-called reactive psychoses, which were seen as a response to outside events, and endogenous psychoses, which were innate. Kraepelin divided all endogenous psychoses into two broad classes: dementia praecox—now known as schizophrenia—and manic-depressive insanity, now known as bipolar disorder. Endogenous depression was therefore classed as a form of manic- depressive insanity. All mania also fell under the same rubric because mania was thought never to be a reaction to outside events. There were dissenters, notably the renowned German neurologist Carl Wernicke, who held that mania was related to hyperactivity of neural firing and depression to decreased neural activity. But Kraepelin's idea dominated and persists in today's diagnostic system.

The question of what to include under the umbrella of bipolar disorder reignited in 1966. In separate investigations, psychiatrists Carlo Perris of Umeå University in Sweden and Jules Angst of the University of Zurich in Switzerland each studied some 300 patients with either true bipolar disorder or depression alone and more than 2,000 of their close relatives.

Both researchers found that relatives of the bipolar patients had more mood disorders than those of patients with depression alone. They also discovered that although bipolar illness was common in the relatives of bipolar patients, it was no more common in relatives of depressed patients than in the general population. These findings, Perris and Angst argued, suggested that bipolar disorder and depression were genetically different conditions.

As a consequence, when the third edition of the *Diagnostic and Statistical Manual of Mental Disorders*, or DSM, appeared in 1980, it included major depressive disorder as a condition distinct from bipolar disorder. Perris and Angst's studies focused only on depression and did not address mania. "There weren't enough cases of pure mania to do anything reasonable," Angst says.

Whether unipolar mania should have its own diagnosis is complicated by bipolar disorder's clinical diversity. The manic and depressive phases vary in severity and the extent that one or the other dominates. The pattern of episodes varies unpredictably and from patient to patient. Mixed states, involving aspects of opposite mood extremes simultaneously, sometimes occur, too. Indeed, many psychiatrists argue that mood disorders are best thought of as lying on a spectrum, ranging from major depression through various bipolar presentations to pure mania.

In Search of a Subtype

The variability of symptoms, along with findings from large psychiatric genetics studies that implicate numerous biological factors, suggests that bipolar disorder includes a range of subtly different conditions. "One reason we still have limited understanding of bipolar disorder after 50 years of intense research is that it's treated as one entity, and it's clearly not," says psychiatrist Paul Grof of the University of Toronto.

The resistance to subtyping may be the result in part of changes in research funding over the past few decades, as the pharmaceutical industry has taken over progressively more psychiatric research from universities, Grof says. Drug companies generally just want to know if a new drug is better than a placebo, and the larger the patient group, the greater the likelihood of finding a significant difference. Subdividing bipolar disorder into smaller populations would complicate these efforts. The industry also prefers to study diagnoses recognized by the Food and Drug Administration—and unipolar mania is not on its list.

Institutional inertia can also come into play. Every rewrite of the *Diagnostic and Statistical Manual of Mental Disorders* is a laborious process. Each edition is based on the previous one, and any change must be backed by fresh evidence, with papers submitted to committees justifying the decision. The last edition, *DSM-5*, was published in 2013, and in the view of the committee tasked with reviewing mood disorders, unipolar mania was covered by the bipolar diagnosis known as BP-I, which is mania with or without associated depression. "There was very limited discussion as to whether mania should be separate because the onset and course of illness weren't seen as that different from BP-I," says psychiatrist Trisha Suppes of Stanford University, who was a member of the *DSM-5* work group for mood disorders.

The lack of a separate diagnosis may be making evidence harder to gather. The standardized clinical interview used under the DSM to make diagnoses for research studies has no category for unipolar mania, meaning investigating the condition would have to rely on ad hoc techniques that might not align with those used in other studies. Unipolar mania is thus at the hub of a catch-22: the absence of a diagnosis is an impediment to research, and the paucity of research makes creation of a diagnosis less likely.

In studies that do occur, the lack of a formal designation for unipolar mania makes it difficult to compare results. "A major problem is definitions," says Allan Young, a psychiatrist at King's College London. One source of disagreement is the severity of symptoms necessary for a case to qualify as mania. Another is the frequency of episodes. Some studies include anybody who has had at least one episode of mania with no history of depression, whereas others require three or four. Still others stipulate a minimum number of years of illness. These differences have led to widely disparate prevalence estimates for unipolar mania, ranging from 1.1 to 65.3 percent of bipolar patients.

Most of the studies completed so far also have methodological problems. The bulk are retrospective, in which researchers simply ask participants to recount past experiences—a process known to underestimate depression, perhaps inflating estimates of pure mania. Prospective studies that follow patients for years and include periodic assessments are better. "What you really want is someone who's lived their whole life, had multiple episodes of mania, and never had depression," Young says, "The first lady I saw like this died in her late 60s and had her first episode at 21, which is getting on for 50 years, so that's very convincing."

One of the longest prospective studies, led by David Solomon, now at the Warren Alpert Medical School of Brown University, began in 1978 and was published in 2003. It began as a study of 229 bipolar patients, 27 of whom had mania with no history of depression. The investigators followed those 27 patients for up to 20 years; seven of them remained free of depression throughout the period. The results suggest that of the original 229 patients, 3 percent had unipolar mania. Solomon does not advocate the creation of a separate diagnosis for unipolar mania unless future research establishes differences in genesis, prognosis or treatment response. But if the rate reported in the study held for the general population, the number of people with unipolar mania in the United States would be around 100,000—and hundreds of thousands more worldwide.

Psychic Fuel for the Creative Brain: The Mad Genius May Be More Than a Cliché

Of all the tropes of artists and mental afflictions, the most enduring is the one of a genius in the throes of mania. Iconic figures ranging from William Blake to Ernest Hemingway to Kurt Cobain were known or believed to be bipolar. The association has intuitive appeal: the euphoria, abundant energy and racing thoughts of mania are credible fuel for creativity.

Scientific evidence for the association has mostly been inconclusive. Much of the data comes from historical sources, and most accounts are anecdotal. Modern investigative techniques have revealed surprisingly little about what happens in the brain during mania, partly because brain imaging requires minimal head movement, so scanning someone in a floridly manic state is a challenge. As a dynamic process involving the interplay of multiple brain networks, creativity is also difficult to research.

But comparing findings from research into bipolar disorder with certain studies of creativity reveals hints of a link: cognitive "disinhibition" seems to be a feature of both the creative state described as being in the "flow" and altered brain circuits in bipolar disorder.

Brain-imaging studies have found reduced activity in a part of the prefrontal cortex that helps to regulate emotion, which may be linked to impaired impulse control and extremes of mood in bipolar patients. (The prefrontal cortex is the brain's "orchestra conductor" responsible for directing various mental processes.) Some of these studies have also found diminished activity in an area involved in suppressing the kind of spontaneous thought that appears to well up from the unconscious, seemingly out of nowhere.

These results are reminiscent of a 2008 study of improvising jazz musicians and a 2012 study of free styling rappers, conducted by the team of speech neuroscientist Allen Braun, then at the National Institutes of Health, which found reduced activity in the part of the prefrontal cortex that inhibits spontaneous cognition. They also found an increase in activity in a section of the prefrontal cortex that is part of the so-called default mode network, which revs up when a person is not focusing on a task but is rather imagining things or ruminating on the past. The researchers believe what they observed reflects relaxation of focused attention and control, making way for a creative thought process in which inspiration bubbles up from the unconscious. Other studies have found reduced thickness of certain cortical regions in both creative and bipolar brains, which may be linked to altered brain activity and disinhibited cognition.

Another element in the thinking patterns of creative and manic people is the ability to make mental connections that elude others. Neuroscientist Nancy Andreasen of the University of Iowa has found that creative people show greater activity in the so-called association cortices, which are regions tasked with linking related elements of cognition. These brain areas are not devoted to processing specific sensory or motor functions but instead with tasks such as tying together a written word with its sound and meaning. Andreasen believes creative ideas probably occur when these types of associations occur freely in the brain during unconscious mental states, when thoughts become momentarily disorganized—not unlike psychotic states of mania.

This observation resonates with clinical psychologist David Ho, who has experienced racing thoughts and extraordinarily enhanced recall during manic episodes, letting him write without inhibition or self-doubt. "With repression vanished, my mind functioned with holistic oneness," he says. "Creative ideas rained down faster than I could cope." Researchers do not know if the association cortices are more active in mania, but all these findings suggest that at key moments of the creative process, our thought processes flow more freely, with novel combinations of sights, sounds, memories, meanings, and feelings producing insight and originality in creative work akin perhaps to what happens during mania.

Of course, mental illness is neither necessary nor sufficient for creative talent, and severe manic episodes most likely are too debilitating for any kind of sustained activity. But researchers have found that family members of people with bipolar disorder also tend to be more creative than average, supporting the idea that mild manifestations of the disorder may furnish cognitive benefits.

It is important not to romanticize conditions that mainly cause suffering, but evidence that mania can enhance creativity in some people may help reduce the stigma of a diagnosis. "It is possible to retain a measure of madness in dignified living," Ho says, "and of dignity even in a state of madness."

References

Adamovová, L., & Stríženec, M. (2004). Personality-structural correlates of cognitive orientation to spirituality. *Studia Psychologica, 46*, 317–325.

Albee, G. W. (1977). The Protestant ethic, sex, and psychotherapy. *American Psychologist, 32*, 150–161.

Andreasen, N. C. (1987). Creativity and mental illness: Prevalence rates in writers and their first degree relatives. *American Journal of Psychiatry, 144*, 1288–1292.

Andreasen, N. C. (2008). The relationship between creativity and mood disorders. *Dialogues in Clinical Neuroscience, 10*, 251–255.

Andreasen, N. C. (2011). A journey into chaos: Creativity and the unconscious. *Mens Sana Monographs, 9*, 42–53.

Angst, J. (2015). Will mania survive DSM-5 and ICD-11? *International Journal of Bipolar Disorders, 3*, 24.

Angst, J., & Grobler, C. (2015). Unipolar mania: A necessary diagnostic concept. *European Archives of Psychiatry and Clinical Neuroscience, 265*, 273–280.

Beesdo-Baum, K., Höfler, M., Gloster, A. T., Klotsche, J., Lieb, R., Beauducel, A., . . .Wittchen, H.-U. (2009). The structure of common mental disorders: A replication study in a community sample of adolescents and young adults. *International Journal of Methods in Psychiatric Research, 18*, 204–220.

Bowler, K. (2018). *Everything happens for a reason, and other lies I've loved*. New York: Random House.

Case, A., & Deaton, A. (2020). *Deaths of despair and the future of capitalism*. Elizabeth, NJ: Princeton University Press.

Cheng, T. K., Ho, D. Y. F., Xie, W., Wong, H. Y. K., & Cheng-Lai, A. (2013). Alienation, despair and hope as predictors of health, coping, and nonengagement among nonengaged youth: Manifestations of spiritual emptiness. *Asia Pacific Journal of Counselling and Psychotherapy, 4*, 18–30.

Chinese Society of Psychiatry. (2001). *Chinese classification of mental disorders* (3rd ed.). Jinan, Shandong Province, China: Author.

Cooke, L., Myers, L. B., & Derakshan, N. (2003). Lung function, adherence and denial in asthma patients who exhibit a repressive coping style. *Psychology, Health & Medicine, 8*, 35–44.

Crumbaugh, J. C., & Maholick, L. T. (1969). *The purpose in life test*. Chicago: Psychometric Affiliates.

DeLuca, J. (Ed.). (2007). *Fatigue as a window to the brain*. Cambridge, MA: MIT Press.

Dutton, K. (2016, September). Would you vote for a psychopath? *Scientific American*. Retrieved from https://www.scientificamerican.com/article/would-you-vote-for-a-psychopath/

Efklides, A. (2008). Metacognition: Defining its facets and levels of functioning in relation to self-regulation and co-regulation. *European Psychologist, 13*, 277–287.

Ehrenreich, B. (2018). *Natural causes: An epidemic of wellness, the certainty of dying, and killing ourselves to live longer*. New York: Twelve.

Falbo, T., & Poston, D. L. (1993). The academic, personality, and physical outcomes of only children in China. *Child Development, 64*, 18–35.

Freeman, C. (2005). *The closing of the Western mind: The rise of faith and the fall of reason*. New York: Vintage Books.

Goffman, E. (1961). *Asylums: Essays on the social situation of mental patients and other inmates*. New York: Doubleday Anchor.

Greyson, B. (2000). Some neuropsychological correlates of the physio-kundalini syndrome. *The Journal of Transpersonal Psychology, 32*, 123–134.

Hill, P. C., & Pargament, K. I. (2003). Advances in the conceptualization and measurement of religion and spirituality: Implications for physical and mental health research. *American Psychologist, 58*, 64–74.

Ho, D. Y. F. (1965). Staff too can be institutionalized. *Mental Hospitals, 16*(4), 137–138.

Ho, D. Y. F. (1974). Prevention and treatment of mental illness in the People's Republic of China. *American Journal of Orthopsychiatry, 44*(4), 620–636.

Ho, D. Y. Y. (1978). The conception of man in Mao Tse-tung thought. *Psychiatry, 41*, 391–402.

Ho, D. Y. F. (1989). Continuity and variation in Chinese patterns of socialization. *Journal of Marriage and the Family, 51*(1), 149–163.

Ho, D. Y. F. (1994). Cognitive socialization in Confucian heritage cultures. In P. M. Greenfield and R. R. Cocking (Eds.), *Cross-cultural roots of minority child development* (pp. 285–313). Hillsdale, NJ: Lawrence Erlbaum.

Ho, D. Y. F. (1995). Selfhood and identity in Confucianism, Taoism, Buddhism, and Hinduism: Contrasts with the West. *Journal for the Theory of Social Behaviour, 25*, 115–139.

Ho, D. Y. F. (1996). Filial piety and its psychological consequences. In M. H. Bond (Ed.), *Handbook of Chinese psychology* (pp. 155–165). Hong Kong: Oxford University Press.

Ho, D. Y. F. (2010). Pooled peer ratings, self-ratings, and estimated ratings of therapeutic communication and popularity: A relational analysis. *The Humanistic Psychologist, 38*, 317–335.

Ho, D. Y. F. (2012). Therapeutic applications of dialogues in dialogical action therapy. In H. J. M. Hermans & T. Gieser (Eds.), *Handbook of dialogical self theory* (pp. 405–422). Cambridge, UK: Cambridge University Press.

Ho, D. Y. F. (2014a). *Enlightened or mad? A psychologist glimpses into mystical magnanimity.* Lake Oswego, OR: Dignity Press.

Ho, D. Y. F. (2014b). A self-study of mood disorder: Fifteen episodes of exuberance, none of depression. *Spirituality in Clinical Practice, 1,* 297–299. http://dx.doi.org/10.1037/scp 0000040

Ho, D. Y. F. (2016). Madness may enrich your life: A self-study of unipolar mood elevation. *Psychosis: Psychological, Social and Integrative Approaches, 8*(2), 180–185. http://dx.doi.org/10.1080/17522439.2015.1135183

Ho, D. Y. F. (2019a). *Rewriting cultural psychology: Transcend your ethnic roots and redefine your identity.* Irvine, CA: Universal Publishers. Retrieved from http://www.universal-publishers.com/book.php?method=ISBN&book=1627347348

Ho, D. Y. F. (2019b). *Rewriting psychology: An abysmal science?* Irvine, CA: Universal Publishers.

Ho, D. Y. F. (2023). *Laozi's classic of virtue and the Dao for the 21st century: A psychology study.* New York: Peter Lang.

Ho, D. Y. F. (in press). Dialectical thinking: Bridging East and West. In A. Belolutskaya, M. F. Mascolo, & N. Shannon (Eds.), *Routledge handbook of dialogical thinking.* Oxfordshire, UK: Routledge.

Ho, D. Y. F. (2023). Filial Piety Scale and Traditional Chinese Values. In C. U. Krägeloh, M. Alyami, & O. N. Medvedev (Eds.), *International Handbook of Behavioral Health Assessment.* Cham: Springer. https://doi.org/10.1007/978-3-030-89738-3_53-1

Ho, D. Y. F., & Chiu, C.-Y. (1994). Component ideas of individualism, collectivism, and social organization: An application in the study of Chinese culture. In Kim, U., Triandis, H. C., Kagitcibasi, C., & Yoon, G. (Eds.), *Individualism and collectivism: Theory, method, and applications* (pp. 137–156). Thousand Oaks, CA: Sage.

Ho, D. Y. F., & Ho, R. T. H. (2007). Measuring spirituality and spiritual emptiness: Toward ecumenicity and transcultural applicability. *Review of General Psychology, 11,* 62–74.

Ho, D. Y. F., Ho, R. T. H., Ng, S. M. (2006). Investigative research as a knowledge-generation method: Discovering and uncovering. *Journal for the Theory of Social Behaviour, 36,* 17–38.

Ho, D. Y. F., Ho, R. T. H., & Ng, S. M. (2007). Restoring quality to qualitative research. *Culture and Psychology, 13,* 377–383.

Ho, D. Y. F., Peng, S. Q., & Cheng-Lai, A. (2001). Parenting in mainland China: Culture, ideology, and policy. *International Society for the Study of Behavioural Development Newsletter,* No. 1, Serial no. 38, 7–9.

Ho, D. Y. F., & Wang, H. L. (2009). Interpersonal perceptions and metaperceptions in Dialogic Action Therapy: A relational methodological approach to theory construction. *The Humanistic Psychologist, 37,* 799–100.

Ho, D. Y. F., Xie, W., Liang, X., & Zeng, L. (2012). Filial piety and traditional Chinese values: A study of high and mass cultures. *PsyCh Journal, 1,* 40–55.

Ho, D. Y. F., & Yin, Q. (2016). A heuristic framework for multidimensional evaluations of spirituality: Toward transcultural applicability. *The Humanistic Psychologist, 8*(2), 180–185.

Hood, R. W., Jr. (1985). Mysticism. In P. Hammond (Ed.), *The sacred in a secular era* (pp. 285–297). Berkeley: University of California Press.
Hood, R. W., Jr., Morris, R. J., & Watson, P. J. (1993). Further factor analysis of Hood's Mysticism Scale. *Psychological Reports, 3*, 1176–1178.
Ivtzan, I., Chan, C. P. L., Gardner, H. E., & Prashar, K. (2013). Linking religion and spirituality with psychological well-being: Examining self-actualization, meaning in life, and personal growth initiative. *Journal of Religion and Health, 52*, 915–929.
James, W. (2002). *The varieties of religious experience: A study of human nature* (Centenary ed.). London: Routledge. (Original work published 1902)
James, W. (2008). *The letters of William James* [Electronic book]. New York: Cosimo. (Original work published 1920)
Jamison, K. R. (1993). *Touched with fire: Manic-depressive illness and the artistic temperament.* New York: Free Press.
Johnson, C. V., & Friedman, H. L. (2008). Enlightened or delusional? Differentiating religious, spiritual, and transpersonal experiences from psychopathology. *Journal of Humanistic Psychology, 48*, 505–527.
Johnson, K. A. (2017). *China's hidden children: Abandonment, adoption, and the human costs of the one-child policy.* Chicago: University of Chicago Press.
Kaidanovich-Beilin, O., Cha, D. S., & McIntyre, R. S. (2012). Crosstalk between metabolic and neuropsychiatric disorders. *Biology Reports, 4*, 14.
Kenny, D. A. (1994). *Interpersonal perception: A social relations analysis.* New York: Guildford Press.
Korchin, S. J. (1976). *Modern clinical psychology: Principles of intervention in the clinic and community.* New York: Harper & Row.
Kyaga, S., Lichtenstein, P., Boman, M., Hultman, C., Långström, N., & Landén, M. (2011). Creativity and mental disorder: Family study of 300 000 people with severe mental disorder. *The British Journal of Psychiatry, 199*, 373–379.
Lee, B. (2019). *The dangerous case of Donald Trump: 37 psychiatrists and mental health experts assess a new president.* New York: Thomas Dunne Books.
Lee, S., & Kleinman, A. (2002). Psychiatry in its political and professional contexts: A response to Robin Munro. *Journal of the American Academy of Psychiatry and the Law, 30*, 120–125.
Lepore, J. (2018). *These truths: A history of the United States.* New York: Norton.
Linden, M. (2003). Posttraumatic embitterment disorder. *Psychotherapy and Psychosomatics, 72*, 195–202.
MacBeth, A., & Gumley, A. (2012). Exploring compassion: A meta-analysis of the association between self-compassion and psychopathology. *Clinical Psychology Review, 32*, 545–552.
MacDonald, D. A., & Friedman, H. F. (2013). Quantitative assessment of transpersonal and spiritual constructs. In H. L. Friedman & G. Hartelius (Eds.), *The Wiley Blackwell handbook of transpersonal psychology* (pp. 281–299). Chichester, West Sussex, UK: Wiley.
Martínez-Arán, A., Vieta, E., Reinares, M., Colom, F., Torrent, C., Sánchez-Moreno, J., . . .Salamero, M. (2004). Cognitive function across manic or hypomanic, depressed, and euthymic states in bipolar disorder. *American Journal of Psychiatry, 161*, 262–270.
Marx, K. (1932/1964). *The economic and philosophical manuscripts of 1844.* New York: International Publishers. (Released by Soviet researchers in 1932)

Mathes, E. W., Zevon, M. A., Roter, P. M., & Joerger, S. M. (1982). Peak experience tendencies: Scale development and theory testing. *Journal of Humanistic Psychology, 22*, 92–108.

Mehta, S. (2014). Unipolar mania: Recent updates and review of the literature. *Psychiatry Journal.* Article ID261943, 6 pages. http://dx.doi.org/10.1155/2014/261943

Merikangas, K. R., Cui, L., Heaton, L., Nakamura, E., Roca, C., Ding, J., . . .Angst, J. (2014). Independence of familial transmission of mania and depression: Results of the NIMH family study of affective spectrum disorders. *Molecular Psychiatry, 19*, 214–219.

Michael, N., Erfurth, A., Ohrmann, P., Gössling, M., Arolt, V., Heindel, W., . . .Pfleiderer, B. (2003). Acute mania is accompanied by elevated glutamate/glutamine levels within the left dorsolateral prefrontal cortex. *Psychopharmacology, 178*, 344–346.

Miller, W. R., & C'deBaca, J. (1994). Quantum change: Toward a psychology of transformation. In T. Heatherton & J. Weinberger (Eds.), *Can personality change?* (pp. 253–280). Washington, DC: American Psychological Association.

Ng, A. K., Ho, D. Y. F., Wong, S. S., & Smith, I. (2003). In search of the good life: A cultural Odyssey in the East and West. *Genetic, Social, and General Psychology Monographs, 129*, 317–363.

Ng, S. M., Chan, C. L. W., Ho, D. Y. F., Wong, Y. Y., & Ho, R. T. H. (2006). Stagnation as a distinct clinical syndrome: Comparing 'Yu' (stagnation) in traditional Chinese medicine with depression. *British Journal of Social Work, 36*, 467–484.

Ng, S. M., Yau, J. K. Y., Chan, C. L. W., Chan, C. H. Y., & Ho, D. Y. F. (2005). The measurement of Body-Mind-Spirit well-being: Toward multidimensionality and transcultural applicability. *Journal of Social Work in Health Care, 41*, 33–52.

Nurnberger, J. Jr., Roose, S. P., Dunner, D. L., & Fieve, R. R. (1979). Unipolar mania: A distinct clinical entity? *The American Journal of Psychiatry, 136*, 1420–1423.

Paloutzian, R.F., & Ellison, C.W. (1991). *Manual for the spiritual well-being scale.* Nyack, NY: Life Advances.

Perlin, M. L., & Lynch, A. J. (2018) "To wander off in shame": Deconstructing the shaming and shameful arrest policies of urban police departments in their treatment of persons with mental disabilities. In D. Rothbart (Ed.), *Systemic humiliation in America* (pp. 175–194). Cham, Switzerland: Palgrave.

Perugi, G., Passino, M. C. S., Toni, C., Maremmani, I., & Angst, J. (2007). Is unipolar mania a distinct subtype? *Comprehensive Psychiatry, 48*, 213–217.

Poage, E. D., Ketzenberger, K. E., & Olson, J. (2004). Spirituality, contentment, and stress in recovering alcoholics. *Addictive Behaviors, 29*, 1857–1862.

Powers, C., Nam, R. K., Rowatt, W. C., & Hill, P. C. (2007). Associations between humility, spiritual transcendence, and forgiveness. *Research in the Social Scientific Study of Religion, 18*, 75–94.

Rascovsky, A. (1995). *Filicide: The murder, humiliation, mutilation, denigration, and abandonment of children by parents* (S. H. Rogers, Trans.). Northvale, NJ: Jason Aronson.

Richards, P. S., & Bergin, A. E. (1997). *A spiritual strategy for counseling and psychotherapy.* Washington, DC: American Psychological Association.

Rotenberg, M. (1974). The Protestant ethnic versus Western people-changing sciences. In J. L. M. Dawson and W. J. Lonner (Eds.), *Readings in cross-cultural psychology* (pp. 277–291). Hong Kong: Hong Kong University Press.

Roth, A. (2018). *Insane: America's criminal treatment of mental illness*. New York: Basic Books,
Sampson, E. E. (1988). The debate on individualism: Indigenous psychologies and their role in personal and societal functioning. *American Psychologist, 43*, 15–22.
Schweitzer, A. (1913/2011). *The psychiatric study of Jesus: Exposition and criticism* (C. R. Joy, Trans.). Whitefish, MT: Literary Licensing. (Original work published 1913)
Seeman, M. (1959). On the meaning of alienation. *American Sociological Review, 24*, 783–791.
Simmons, S. (2018). Systemic humiliation and practical politics. In D. Rothbart (Ed.), *Systemic humiliation in America* (pp. 75–102). Cham, Switzerland: Palgrave.
Singer, A. R., & Dobson, K. S. (2009). The effect of the cognitive style of acceptance on negative mood in a recovered depressed sample. *Depression and Anxiety, 26*, 471–479.
Steward, K. (2020). *The power worshippers: Inside the dangerous rise of religious nationalism*. London: Bloomsbury Publishing.
Tangney, J. P. (2000). Humility: Theoretical perspectives, empirical findings and directions for future research. *Journal of Social and Clinical Psychology, 19*, 70–82.
Thomte, R. (1948/2009). *Kierkegäärd's philosophy of religion*. Eugene, OR: Wipf & Stock. (Original work published 1948)
Van Boven, L., Campbell, M. C., & Gilovich, T. (2010). Stigmatizing materialism: On stereotypes and impressions of materialistic and experiential pursuits. *Personality and Social Psychology Bulletin, 36*, 551–563.
Van Pachterbeke, M., Keller., J., & Saroglou, V. (2012). Flexibility in existential beliefs and worldviews: Introducing and measuring existential quest. *Journal of Individual Differences, 33*, 2–16.
Yazici, O., Kora, K., Uçok, A., Saylan, M.,Ozdemir, O., Kiziltan, E.,. . .Ozpulat, T. (2002). Unipolar mania: A distinct disorder? Journal of Affective Disorders, 71, 97–103.
Yüksel, C., & Öngür, D. (2010). Magnetic resonance spectroscopy studies of glutamate-related abnormalities in mood disorders. *Biological Psychiatry, 68*, 785–794.

Index

Abnormality 86, 91, 92, 95, 121, 140, 194, 197, 199, 201, 203, 219, 220, 221, 226, 227, 229, 231, 317, 319
Acceptance 35, 41, 67, 131, 132, 148, 150, 153, 187, 221, 222, 224, 225, 241, 248, 284, 303, 301, 335, 336, 339, 343, 351–353, 358
Achievement 23, 41, 51, 63, 67, 68, 96, 145, 159, 160, 176, 198, 215, 231, 248, 279, 285, 288, 292, 321, 336, 353, 354, 383, 386
Aesthetic/artistic-literary impulses/ sensitivities 36, 45, 52, 206, 387
Aggression
  aggressive behavior 228
  passive-aggressiveness 123
Alienation 81, 84, 141, 184, 260, 328, 330, 331, 339, 344, 358, 360
  estrangement 194, 328, 339, 358, 360
  meaninglessness 194, 339, 358, 360
  normlessness 339, 358, 360
  powerlessness 339, 358, 360
  social isolation 76, 147, 258, 259, 339, 358, 360
Americans 27, 39, 41, 62, 101, 114, 225, 228, 242, 243, 245, 259, 264–267, 274, 275, 281, 284, 285, 354, 364, 391
  illusion of unlimited personal freedom 281
Arrogance 67, 80, 331, 336, 344, 353, 354
Attention-Deficit/Hyperactive Disorder (ADHD) 226
Atypicality 15, 95, 188, 204
Authoritarianism 261, 288
Authority 12, 13, 18, 19, 25, 82, 83, 121, 124, 168, 186, 224, 234, 236, 237, 271, 273, 276, 288, 289, 296, 299, 300, 303, 305, 309–312, 318
  authority figures 12, 13, 18, 276, 296, 310
  authority relations/relationships 229, 300, 312
Autonomy 6, 193, 279, 285, 288, 294

Body-Mind-Spirit (BMS)
  interconnectedness 60, 73, 102, 136, 182, 395
  see also holistic health
Brain fatigue 70, 129, 138, 205, 206, 380

Case study (studies) 3, 31, 107, 129, 130, 136, 137, 157, 162, 234, 263, 264, 391
  atypical/exceptional case(s) 4, 15, 39, 77, 80, 81, 92, 95–97, 123, 127, 136, 148, 153, 188, 198, 208, 213, 316, 402
  self-study 3, 19, 92, 95–97, 203, 204, 340, 402
China/Chinese
  Confucian precepts/view 276
  Confucianism 15–17, 39, 44, 111, 172, 173, 175, 176, 289, 311, 322, 326, 338
  demographics 293, 298
  folk values 227, 292
  Great Cultural Revolution 19, 83, 248–250, 292
  ideal values 226, 227, 292
  little emperors 292
  Mao Zedong Thought 249, 250
  one-child policy 8, 292, 294–297
  open-door policy 275, 291, 294, 298
  population policy (policies) 295, 296
  social organization 260, 284–286
  socialist values 291, 292
  traditional Chinese medicine 247, 251
  traditional Chinese values 226
Cognitive superefficiency 139, 211, 212
Collectivism 82, 199, 257, 260, 262, 277–279, 281287
  collectivist(s) 33, 260, 261, 286
Colonialism 18, 31
Compassion 10, 27, 85, 144, 157, 187, 215, 237, 297, 326, 338, 357, 358, 359
Conformity 7, 75, 126, 171, 184, 221, 226, 256, 257, 285, 288, 311

Contradictions 31, 197, 199, 261, 397
Coping 29, 97, 113, 120, 130, 155, 242, 339, 361, 362, 364
  see also forbearance, forgiveness, hope, meaning reconstruction
Creativity 16, 45, 52, 56, 58, 62, 68, 69, 74, 87–89, 91, 93–95, 97, 99, 101, 104, 111, 119, 134, 139, 140, 144, 155, 161, 162, 178, 203–207, 210–213, 216, 249, 260, 271, 300, 321, 322, 330, 342, 387, 389, 394, 405, 407
  creative activity 339
  creative brain 405
  creative energy 161, 164, 194, 202–204, 213, 320, 323, 401
  creative forces of madness 87, 91, 92, 161, 320
  creative ideas 88, 89, 210, 406
Culture 4, 5, 15, 19, 20, 25, 29, 30, 31, 38–40, 44, 112, 194, 197, 209, 221–227, 231, 248, 257, 258, 260, 269, 275, 285, 286, 291, 292, 298, 299, 304, 305, 308–310, 335, 399
  bilingual/bicultural competence 3, 5, 95, 167, 275
  Confucian-heritage cultures 226
  cross-cultural studies 284
  cultural norms 221–224
  cultural parents 30, 275
  cultural relativism 219, 220, 221, 223–225, 317
  cultural universals 222
  culture shock 30, 31
  culture specific 222, 223
  deviance 221, 223, 226
  high culture 292
  mass culture 258, 292
  multiculturalism 194
  pathogenic aspects/demands of culture 276, 309, 310
  pathogenic culture/subculture 223
  transcultural applicability 325–329, 340

universalism 224, 225, 317, 319
  see also universality/ecumenicity
Curative measures 219, 244, 254, 260

Democracy 21, 25, 237, 247, 260, 268, 269, 273, 274, 281, 288
Denial 97, 101, 116, 117, 232, 233, 264, 271, 281, 331, 335, 336, 343, 351–353
Depression 33, 47, 59, 69, 76, 91, 95, 99–101, 113, 137, 155, 207–210, 233, 305, 316, 334, 349, 361, 382, 401–405
  coping with depression 113, 155
Despair 27, 52, 53, 79, 113, 117, 118, 133, 143, 145, 146, 183, 234, 242, 245, 254, 259, 319, 361, 370–375, 386, 387, 397, 398
Dialectics 159, 186, 198, 199, 250, 260, 262, 328, 375
  dialectical synthesis 199, 225, 283
  dialectical thinking 15, 197–199, 229, 247, 250, 251
  inner dialectics 199
  Maoist dialectics 260, 262
  outer dialectics 199
  between the particular and the universal 219, 222
Dialogic Action Therapy (DAT) 81, 105, 114
Dogmatism 232, 331, 343, 344, 346, 347
Dynamic Relaxation and Meditation (DRM) 76, 105, 108, 393, 396
  see also Body-Mind-Spirit (BMS) interconnectedness

Egocentricity 331, 332, 343–347
Egoism 107, 147, 174, 175, 177, 178, 189, 193, 337, 338, 357, 358, 359
Embitterment 32, 51, 156, 328, 333, 334, 349, 350, 386

Emptiness 22, 54, 56, 70, 71, 84, 93, 113, 122, 136, 140–145, 154, 175, 194, 197, 207, 313, 321, 325–330, 333, 334, 339–341, 343, 344, 347–349, 357, 358, 360, 388
  empty mind 71, 96, 159, 175, 321
  mindless mind 71
Encounter movement 257
Enlightenment 29, 34, 45, 48, 56, 66, 70, 88, 92, 118, 127, 139, 142, 144, 148, 155–160, 163, 176–179, 187, 190–192, 194, 209, 233, 237, 389
  see also nirvana
Entrenchment 119, 361, 375–377
Equifinality 150, 225
Eros versus Thanatos 321
Ethical relativism 223–225
Ethical-legal orientation 288
Evil 16, 23, 32, 97, 142, 159, 192, 202, 224, 231–233, 235, 236, 238, 241, 244, 265, 267, 313, 315, 316, 322, 323, 328
Existential quest 141, 328, 331, 336, 337, 339, 344, 355–358
Expressive dance to music 108, 381, 384, 385, 395, 396
  see also Dynamic Relaxation and Meditation (DRM)
Extraordinary experiences 66, 92, 93, 97, 155, 160, 163, 169, 315, 316, 321, 333, 348
  mystical-transcendental state (of enlightenment) 48, 144
  see also religious experience(s)

Filial piety 4, 11, 15, 222, 276, 292, 301, 303–311
Filicide 276, 297, 299–301, 303, 305, 311, 312
  see also patricide
Forbearance 113–115, 118, 241, 242, 329, 335, 351, 361–365, 375

Forgiveness 28, 29, 42, 113, 115–117, 336, 361, 365–370
Free association 38, 48, 60–63, 160, 204, 379, 380, 389, 392–394

Golden Rule 37, 169, 171, 173, 174
Grandparenthood 11, 15
Guanyin 110, 135
Guilt 7, 35, 43, 115, 116, 139, 162, 169, 232, 305, 334, 349, 363, 366–369
  guilt induction 6, 7

Hallucination 48, 54, 56, 93, 97, 106, 144, 156, 207, 216, 232, 233, 379, 388
  willful hallucination 48, 54, 97, 156, 216, 388
Hedonism 337, 355, 357
Holistic health 60, 72, 73, 103, 108, 342, 380, 393, 395, 396
Homicide(s) 239
Hope 11, 20, 27, 58, 106, 113, 117–119, 132, 146, 158, 169, 194, 243, 251, 280, 294, 315, 335, 340, 353, 361, 370–375, 392, 397, 399
Human dignity 5, 223–226, 237, 238, 262, 315–319, 322
  dignity-in-madness 313, 317, 320, 322
  madness-in-dignity 313, 320, 322
Human nature 32, 142, 162, 228, 249, 289, 326, 374
Humility 36, 37, 52, 118, 119, 132, 133, 194, 195, 206, 215, 232, 331, 336, 339, 344, 353, 354, 358, 386, 387, 396

Idiographic methods 198
  see also nomothetic methods
Ideology 82, 236, 249, 255, 275, 291, 292, 294, 298, 370
Independence 14, 77, 288, 308, 359, 384

Individualism 33, 82, 147, 171, 172, 184, 199, 249, 255–258, 260, 262, 277–280, 283–287, 294, 296, 300, 337, 357
  individualists 21, 275, 277, 278, 284, 287
  individuals-in-isolation (versus individuals-in-community) 262
  self-contained individualism 33, 147, 257, 258, 260, 280, 283, 337, 357
Infanticide 306
Infantilization 5, 6, 14, 17
  see also mother worship
Interdependence 199, 257, 281, 285, 288
Investigative research 269, 293, 294

Karma 37, 44, 110, 147, 149, 171, 175, 179, 191, 193, 195
Kinship 8, 276, 290, 295, 298

Laozi 15, 164, 176, 177, 178
Life cycle 289
Locus of responsibility 288
Loneliness 56, 66, 67, 118, 127, 145, 146, 148, 169, 258–260, 382

Mad genius 234, 238, 405
Marginality 30, 38, 39
Materialism 337, 355, 357
Meaning reconstruction 113, 118, 119, 242, 261, 375–378
Mental disorder(s) 47, 50, 91, 92, 95, 96, 100, 101, 127, 129, 136, 140, 141, 192, 199, 201, 202, 208–210, 219, 220, 223, 240, 247, 264, 316, 317, 402–404
Mental health 85, 97, 105, 134, 136, 161, 203, 240–251, 253–256, 259, 261, 262, 264, 321
  collective mental health 242
  mental health crisis 242, 245, 251
  mental health services 246
  societal mental health 242, 250

Metacognition 139, 216, 235, 331, 332, 341, 344–347
  degrees of complexity 332
  reflective metacognition 331, 332, 341, 344, 346, 347
Misanthropy 338, 339, 358, 359
Modesty 41, 336, 353
Mood disorder(s) 87, 95, 136, 137, 203, 208–210, 213, 316, 403, 404
  bipolar disorder(s) 95, 208–210, 401–407
  elevated mood disorder 203
  hypomania 39, 47, 50, 63, 64, 66–76, 84, 86–89, 92, 93, 95, 98–100, 102–104, 107, 108, 121, 129, 135, 137, 147, 151, 161, 163, 182, 188, 209, 213, 379–385
  mania 38, 47–50, 52, 55–61, 64, 66, 69, 87, 88, 92, 95, 96, 98, 100, 104, 106, 108, 117, 118, 132, 139, 144, 145, 156, 160, 161, 166, 176, 179, 183, 205, 206, 208–210, 212, 213, 379, 380, 382, 385, 387, 389, 394, 401–407
  unipolar disorder/mood elevation 48, 76, 95, 203, 208, 213, 214, 316, 321, 381, 385
Mother worship 5
  see also infantilization
Multidimensional Evaluations of Spirituality (MES) 326, 343
Music 37, 50, 53, 54, 63, 64, 69–71, 75, 80, 81, 86, 88, 89, 91, 94, 101, 107–109, 149, 156, 168, 182, 189, 210, 214, 216, 217, 329, 356, 379, 381, 383–385, 387, 388, 393, 395–398, 401

Nirvana 178, 179, 209, 210
  see also enlightenment
Nomothetic methods 198
  see also idiographic methods
Normality 4, 24, 45, 49, 55, 60, 94–96, 98, 105, 121, 141, 163, 177, 197, 199, 201, 203, 221, 231, 321, 382, 389

Oedipal myth 276, 299–301, 303, 308, 312
Opioid addiction 239

Patricide 276, 299–301, 303, 311, 312
  see also filicide
Poetry 22, 38, 39, 64, 66, 70, 89, 104, 108, 156, 167–169, 210
Politics 266
  political orientation 288
  of societal pathology 266
  theocracy 273, 274
  see also religion(s)
Prevention 69, 248, 250, 256, 259, 260, 382
  communitarian programs 260
  primary prevention 256
Pseudodichotomy (pseudodichotomies) 198, 201
Psychiatry 24, 53, 95, 127, 140, 141, 154, 192, 209, 219, 221, 231, 247, 248, 251, 402
Psychiatric diagnosis 140, 141, 201, 202, 219–222, 229
  diagnostic issues 203, 208
  Diagnostic and Statistical Manual of Mental Disorders (DSM) 201
  Self-diagnosis 129, 204
Psychic numbing/turmoil 54, 145, 331–334, 343, 347–351
Psychoanalysis 61, 87, 179, 209, 322, 393
  impulse control 13, 49, 50, 57, 92, 96, 111, 159, 162, 169, 175, 198, 214, 221, 226, 227, 229, 292, 321, 322, 334, 351, 385, 406
  repression 36, 55, 56, 69, 71, 74, 96, 108, 139, 140, 144, 159, 162, 169, 204, 205, 211, 321, 322, 389, 406
  thought control 16, 322
  unconscious 48, 49, 54, 55, 61–63, 69, 87, 96, 134, 140, 144, 159, 162, 204, 206, 211, 321, 322, 335, 352, 389, 393, 406

Psychohistory 5, 13, 17, 19, 43, 44, 84
Psychology 4, 6, 7, 22, 24, 25, 28, 30, 35, 37, 38, 44, 53, 57, 66, 78, 82, 88, 96, 105, 106, 108, 112, 122, 126, 129, 133, 159, 162, 166, 172, 182, 199, 202, 204, 244, 247, 249–251, 253, 254, 257, 260, 262, 267–269, 277, 278, 280, 283, 287, 294, 296, 297, 321, 326, 341, 387, 395
   abnormal psychology 166
   clinical psychology 25, 35, 38, 53, 96, 129, 162, 202, 204, 244, 250, 251, 257, 387, 395
   cross-cultural psychology 287
   dialectical psychology 199
   environmental and population psychology 250
   health psychology 112
   of madness 16, 33, 37, 40, 45, 60, 76, 81, 87, 89, 91, 92, 96, 97, 100, 102, 103, 106–108, 115, 126, 129, 134, 140, 143, 144, 152, 154, 155, 157, 158, 160–164, 169, 175, 192, 201, 203, 204, 208, 210, 231, 232, 238, 313, 317, 320–323, 340, 407
   psychological decentering 172, 173, 178, 179, 331, 332, 341, 344–347
   psychological illiteracy 11, 13, 30
   psychologism 244, 254, 262
   of religion 180, 232, 254, 325
Psychopath 25, 57, 62, 85, 91, 97, 120, 127, 199, 201, 202, 210, 221, 233, 239, 255, 263–265, 280, 309, 310, 316, 321, 322, 338, 339, 358, 390
Psychopathology 25, 97, 120, 127, 199, 201, 202, 210, 221, 233, 239, 255, 265, 309, 310, 338
   childhood psychopathology 309, 310
   family pathology 276

Quakerism 185–187, 201, 234, 236, 237
   George Fox 158, 201, 233–235, 236

Religious Society of Friends 185, 201, 234, 236
Quakers 185, 187, 188, 236–238

Religion(s) 110, 114, 115, 120, 142, 149, 150, 154, 180, 182, 185, 188, 232, 235, 237, 254, 266, 269, 273, 325, 327
   Buddhism 96, 110, 116, 132, 139, 149, 150, 172, 174, 178, 179, 187, 215, 237, 289, 321, 325, 326, 329, 338, 339, 357
   Christian nationalism 274
   Christianity 115, 150, 180, 183, 186, 236, 241, 269, 325, 329, 335, 338, 339
   Daoism 96, 116, 149, 172, 174–176, 178, 179, 289, 321, 326, 338
   Evangelicalism 266, 268, 270, 271
   Evangelicals 267–273
   Fundamentalism 256, 271, 273
   Judeo-Christian heritage 274
   religiosity 115, 143, 155, 160, 183, 201, 232, 233, 235, 236, 238, 326, 328, 329
   religious experience(s) 55, 89, 104, 188, 190, 232, 235, 388
      see also extraordinary experiences
   religious luminaries 158, 201, 202, 231, 339
   religious movement 233, 234

Self-actualization 221, 253, 254, 279, 330, 331, 339, 344, 358, 360
Self-deprecation 306
Self-encapsulation 147
Self-enchantment 101, 138, 209, 210
Self-mastery 41, 42, 156, 193, 313, 342
Self-observations 137, 202, 213
Self-rejection 41–43, 156, 210, 334, 335, 349, 351
Selflessness 37, 71, 96, 114, 172, 174–176, 178, 193, 220, 221, 260, 293, 321, 323, 332, 338, 346, 358, 359
   selfless self 48, 69–71, 93, 96, 97, 156, 159, 160, 175, 193, 321, 379

Shame 15, 16, 21, 43, 57, 67, 111, 115, 116, 124, 144, 156, 169
Shared psychotic disorder (Folie à deux) 240
Socialization 11, 124, 226, 291, 292
  parenting 6, 15, 291–294, 298, 303
Societal disorders 199
  societal pathology (pathologies) 266
Sociology 250
  of mental disorders 50, 95, 199, 201, 209, 210, 219, 240, 247, 317, 402–404
  sociopathology 239
Spirituality 18, 22, 43–45, 53, 60, 63, 84, 88, 97, 101, 105, 108, 109, 110, 113, 115, 129, 132, 139, 141–145, 147, 148, 150, 153–164, 169, 171, 176, 179, 180, 182–186, 188, 190, 192–194, 197, 232, 233, 237, 258, 313, 320, 321, 325–348, 351, 356, 357, 359, 387, 397
  assessment of spirituality 180, 313
  dialectics of spirituality and madness 159–161
  relational/ecumenical spirituality 36, 105, 109, 147, 148, 150, 172, 176, 184, 288, 318, 337, 357, 359
  spiritual adventure 21
  spiritual development 130, 169, 179, 194, 198, 313, 325, 330, 342
  spiritual emptiness 22, 84, 113, 122, 136, 140–143, 154, 194, 197, 313, 321, 325–328, 330, 331, 333, 334, 339–441, 343, 344, 347–349, 357
  spiritual journey 44, 68, 93, 104, 108, 118, 121, 141, 142, 144, 148, 149, 153, 158, 162, 169, 171, 174, 179, 183, 185, 190–193, 195, 326, 344, 385

spirituality-in-communion 45, 127, 171, 179, 184, 188, 193, 194, 258
spirituality-in-isolation 148, 169, 184, 258
St. Vitus's dance 239
  dancing manias 239
Suicides of despair 239, 259
Temporal orientation 289
  child-centeredness 15, 290
  elder-centeredness 15, 290

Thought liberation 15, 177
Transcendence 22, 147, 178, 313, 331, 337, 339, 344, 357–359
Trump 27, 240, 261, 263–274, 280
  Trump phenomenon 240, 261, 263, 265, 266, 267, 269, 271, 273, 274

Unitarian Universalists 185, 187, 188
Universality/ecumenicity 149, 150, 186, 194, 222, 223, 225, 237, 318, 319, 322, 326, 327, 338, 358

Values 11, 30, 60, 84, 91, 119, 127, 141, 145, 188, 199, 221–227, 240, 255–258, 260, 267, 274, 278, 279, 284–286, 288, 291, 292, 294, 298, 308, 311, 318, 325, 327, 329, 336, 337, 340, 355–357, 360, 378
Violence 19, 28, 57, 97, 114, 228, 231, 232, 234, 238, 245, 246, 260, 267, 274, 295, 299–301, 306, 308, 311–313, 315–317, 319, 320, 322

World citizenship 38, 39, 40, 169

Zhuangzi 15, 77, 134, 135, 175–178, 334, 338

Made in the USA
Monee, IL
28 April 2026

49137067R00246